Arteriogenesis

Dedicated to
Dr. Paul A. J. Janssen
in memoriam

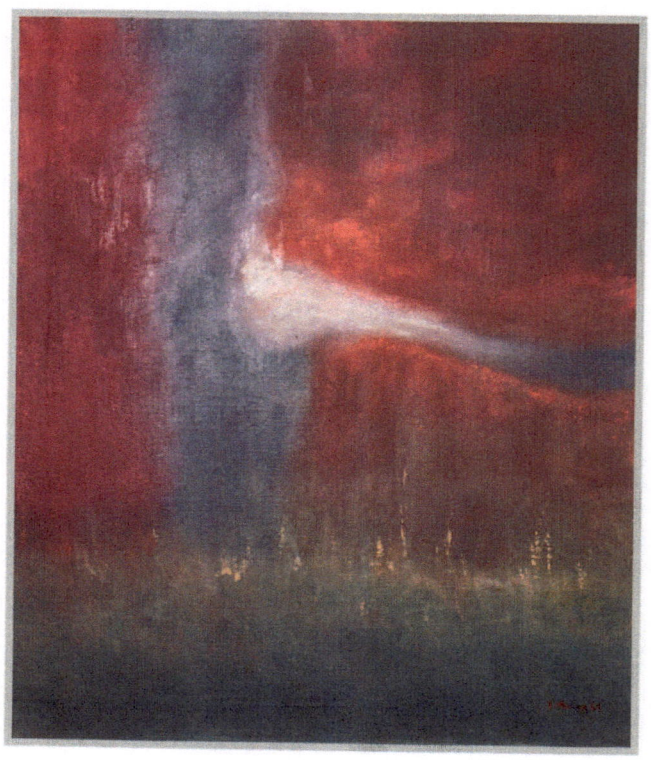

"Arteriogenesis"
Painting by Thomas Maciag

Kind gift to Wolfgang Schaper
at the occasion of Dr. Maciag's
visit in Bad Nauheim.

Arteriogenesis

edited by
Wolfgang Schaper & Jutta Schaper

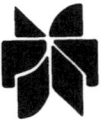 Springer Science+Business Media, LLC

Library of Congress Cataloging-in-Publication Data

A C.I.P. Catalogue record for this book is available
from the Library of Congress.

Arteriogenesis edited by Wolfgang Schaper and Jutta Schaper
ISBN 978-1-4757-8888-4   ISBN 978-1-4020-8126-2 (eBook)
DOI 10.1007/978-1-4020-8126-2

Design by Schaper Kommunikation, Bad Nauheim

Table of Contents

List of Contributors

MIROSLAV BARANCIK*
Institute for Heart Research, Slovak Academy of Sciences, Bratislava, Slovakia

STEFANIE BOEHM
Max-Planck-Institute for Physiological and Clinical Research, Dept. of Experimental Cardiology, Bad Nauheim, Germany

KERSTIN BOENGLER
Max-Planck-Institute for Physiological and Clinical Research, Dept. of Experimental Cardiology, Bad Nauheim, Germany

KERSTIN BROICH
Max-Planck-Institute for Physiological and Clinical Research, Dept. of Experimental Cardiology, Bad Nauheim, Germany

ALEXANDRA BUEHLER
University Maastricht, Cardiovascular Research Institute Maastricht (CARIM), Dept. of Cardiology, Maastricht, The Netherlands

HANS-JOERG BUSCH
University Freiburg, Research Group, 'Experimental and Clinical Arteriogenesis', Freiburg im Breisgau, Germany

IVO R. BUSCHMANN
University Freiburg, Research Group, 'Experimental and Clinical Arteriogenesis', Freiburg im Breisgau, Germany

WEI-JUN CAI*
Central South University, Xiangya School of Medicine, Dept. of Anatomy & Neurobiology, Changsha, Hunan, PR China

ELISABETH DEINDL*
University München Grosshadern, Medical Clinic, München, Germany

INKA EITENMUELLER
Max-Planck-Institute for Physiological and Clinical Research, Dept. of Experimental Cardiology, Bad Nauheim, Germany

BORJA FERNÁNDEZ
Max-Planck-Institute for Physiological and Clinical Research, Dept. of Experimental Cardiology, Bad Nauheim, Germany

WILLIAM F.M. FULTON
Professor emeritus, Braemar, Grampian, Scotland

MATTHIAS HEIL
Max-Planck-Institute for Physiological and Clinical Research, Dept. of Experimental Cardiology, Bad Nauheim, Germany

ARMIN HELISCH*
Dartmouth-Hitchcock Medical Center, Dept. of Cardiology, Lebanon, New Hampshire, USA

KONSTANTIN-ALEXANDER HOSSMANN
Max-Planck-Institute for Neurological Research, Dept. of Experimental Neurology, Köln, Germany

ANDREAS KAMPMANN
Max-Planck-Institute for Physiological and Clinical Research, Dept. of Experimental Cardiology, Bad Nauheim, Germany

ALEXANDER KLUGE
Kerckhoff-Clinic, Dept. of Radiology, Bad Nauheim, Germany

SAWA KOSTIN
Max-Planck-Institute for Physiological and Clinical Research, Dept. of Experimental Cardiology, Bad Nauheim, Germany

THOMAS KUBIN
Kerckhoff-Clinic, Res. Group 'Vascular Genomics', Bad Nauheim, Germany

ALESSANDRA MARTIRE
Max-Planck-Institute for Physiological and Clinical Research, Dept. of Experimental Cardiology, Bad Nauheim, Germany

FREDERIC PIPP
Max-Planck-Institute for Physiological and Clinical Research, Dept. of Experimental Cardiology, Bad Nauheim, Germany

RALF RITTER
University of Frankfurt, Faculty of Medicine, Vascular- and Endovascular Surgery, Frankfurt/Main, Germany

JUTTA SCHAPER
Max-Planck-Institute for Physiological and Clinical Research, Dept. of Experimental Cardiology, Bad Nauheim, Germany

WOLFGANG SCHAPER
Max-Planck-Institute for Physiological and Clinical Research, Dept. of Experimental Cardiology, Bad Nauheim, Germany

THOMAS SCHMITZ-RIXEN
University of Frankfurt, Faculty of Medicine, Vascular- and Endovascular Surgery, Frankfurt/Main, Germany

EDDA SCHNEELOCH
University Freiburg, Research Group, 'Experimental and Clinical Arterio-genesis', Freiburg im Breisgau, Germany

CHRISTIAN SEILER
University of Bern, Dept. of Cardiology, Bern, Switzerland

DIMITRI SCHOLZ
Max-Planck-Institute for Physiological and Clinical Research, Dept. of Experimental Cardiology, Bad Nauheim, Germany

CLAUDIA STROHM
Max-Planck-Institute for Physiological and Clinical Research, Dept. of Experimental Cardiology, Bad Nauheim, Germany

NIELS VAN ROYEN
University Freiburg, Research Group, 'Experimental and Clinical Arterio-genesis', Freiburg im Breisgau, Germany

SABINA VOGEL
Kerckhoff-Clinic, Research Group 'Vascular Genomics', Bad Nauheim, Germany

DIETMAR VON DER AHE
Kerckhoff-Clinic, Research Group 'Vascular Genomics', Bad Nauheim, Germany

SHAWN WAGNER
Max-Planck-Institute for Physiological and Clinical Research, Dept. of Experimental Cardiology, Bad Nauheim, Germany

SWEN WOLFRAM*
DSM Nutritional Products, Human Nutrition and Health, Basel, Switzerland

TIBOR ZIEGELHOEFFER
Max-Planck-Institute for Physiological and Clinical Research, Dept. of Experimental Cardiology, Bad Nauheim, Germany

RENÉ ZIMMERMANN
Kerckhoff-Clinic, Research Group 'Vascular Genomics', Bad Nauheim, Germany

*Work carried out during tenure at the Max-Planck-Institute, Bad Nauheim, Germany

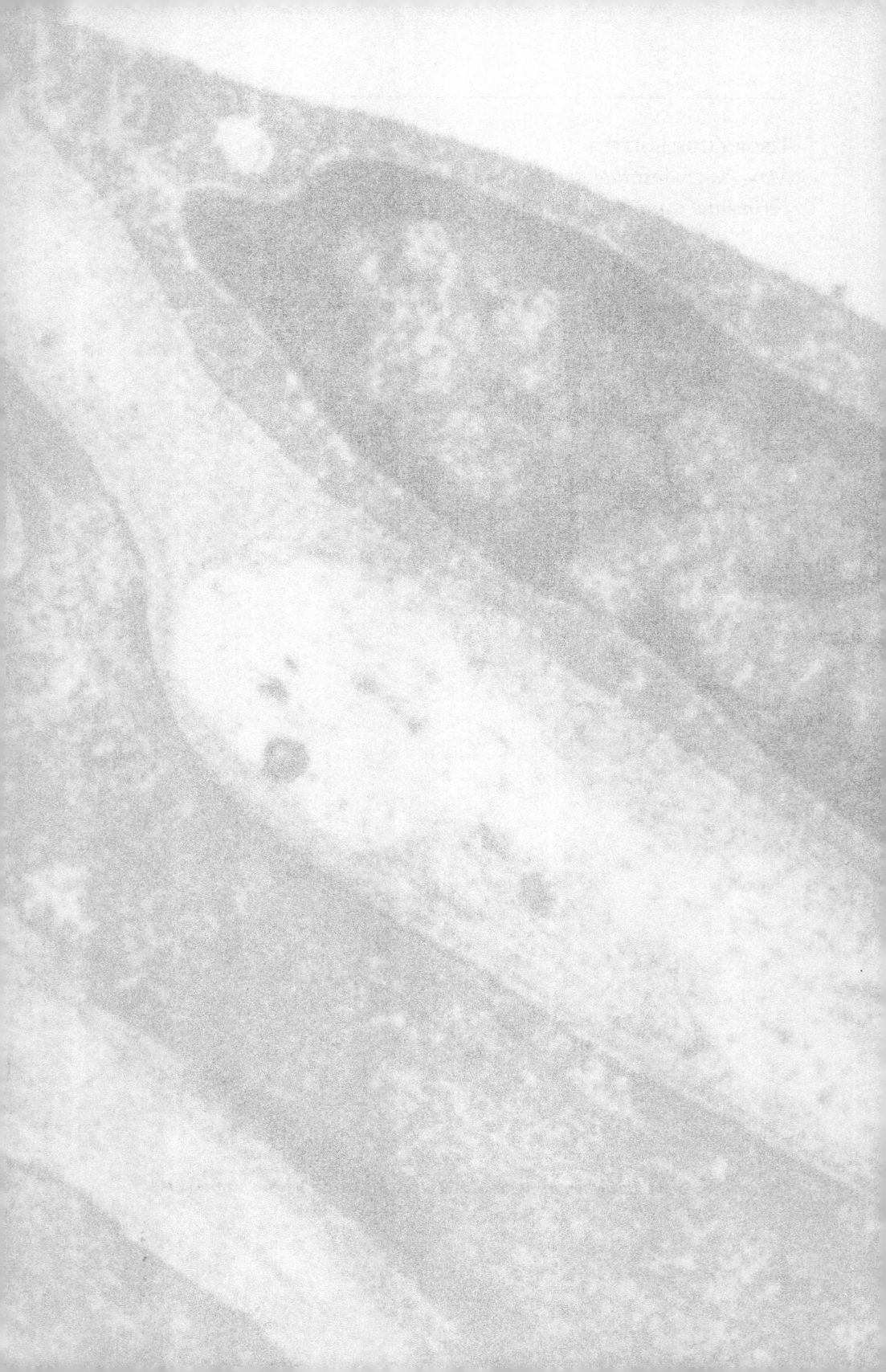

Chapter 1

Introduction

Wolfgang Schaper

This monograph describes primarily the activities of the Nauheim group of investigators, previous and present, in the field of collateral artery growth and is the result of many years of involvement with this topic. In our first book (1971) we had concentrated on the collateral circulation in the canine heart after chronic coronary artery occlusion, its hemodynamics, histology, histochemistry and electron microscopy[1]. It contained our first forays into endothelial and smooth muscle cell proliferation and DNA-replication and we are still in the possession of old slides showing, in histological sections of collateral arteries, radioactive RNA, first in the nuclei of vascular cells and later in the cytoplasm, after perfusion of a dog heart with chronic occlusions of 2 of the 3 coronary arteries (but no infarction) with tritiated uridine. Since, at that time, gene cloning had still a long way to go, we did not know which transcripts we had detected with our autoradiographic studies and stopped doing those experiment for a good number of years. However, our interest was rekindled by the cloning of angiogenic growth factors around 1986.

Our first book was twice updated with outside contributions in 1981 and in 1991 concentrating on our discovery that monocytes play an important role in arteriogenesis and we made extensive use of the new tool of immunofluorescence creating a "molecular histology" of collateral artery growth[2,3].

The present volume tries to integrate the older findings with modern molecular approaches, i.e., gene expression profiling, subtractive cloning, transgene approaches and phenotyping of targeted gene disruptions in mice. We developed or perfected new tools for the measurement of physiological parameters like blood flow using Laser-Doppler Imaging and magnetic resonance imaging in mice and rabbits and CT-scans in rabbits or surrogates of flow like infrared thermography. Even gene expression in the living transgenic mouse is now visible in real time when gene promoters were coupled to reporter genes like luciferase and the animals are placed in a dark chamber where the light flashes from the luciferase-luminol reaction are detected by a CCD camera. In the morphological section extensive use was made of confocal microscopy and for the characterization of blood cells FACS cell sorting was employed. These modern techniques were used to better address remaining problems that had been with us for a long time but resisted to be solved.

Why Arteriogenesis?

The differences between arteriogenesis, the growth and remodeling of preexisting arterioles into mature arteries, and angiogenesis - the sprouting or splitting of preexisting capillaries- are now much clearer, compared to our last, the "blue book", where we struggled with terminology and finally came up with "recapitulated vasculogenesis". However those active in the field of embryonic vascular development were unhappy with this. Recently the term vasculogenesis was again introduced to describe the still hypothetical development of blood vessels from bone marrow-derived stem cells.

Ever since "angiogenesis" was accepted as the most fitting name for capillary sprouting and vasculogenesis for the embryonic development of vessels from angioblasts, the postnatal development of collateral arteries from arteriolar networks, useful adaptations in cases of arterial occlusions, was left linguistically undefined. Since the growth of collateral vessels is the most important adaptive process in the vascular system, the only one of patho-physiological significance to compensate for the loss of an artery, we felt that **this important mechanism deserves a fitting name.** In many clinical studies where angiogenic growth factors were tried and where, besides capillary density, also larger arterial vessels were observed (whether or not caused by the agent in question) these were subsumed also under "angiogenesis". We found this not applicable because we had shown earlier that the mechanisms of angiogenesis and the development of a collateral circulation differ, in parts fundamentally.

Ramon Munoz-Chapuli, a developmental biologist from the University of Malaga/Spain, proposed "Arteriogenesis" during a seminar discussion here in Bad Nauheim and Werner Risau and I found that a fitting name and we proposed that in a chapter of Michel Simons and Anthony Wares book[4] and later in several reviews and original papers. The most fundamental differences between angiogenesis and arteriogenesis are that tissue hypoxia/ischemia are not required for arteriogenesis which relies on physical factors notably on fluid shear stress and on the help of circulating cells, notably monocytes, that adhere to the shear stress-activated endothelium. Arteriogenesis is the more complex process in the same way that an artery is different from a capillary: it is a much more complex tissue that has to cope with strong physical forces and the signal originating in the endothelium has to overcome the barrier of the internal elastic lamina and several layers of smooth muscle cells which do not normally exhibit tight junctions among themselves nor with the endothelium. That this primitive information system changes during arteriogenesis will be described in the following chapters.

Arteriogenesis is not restricted to pathophysiological situations like arterial occlusions but plays also an important role under physiological conditions: the increased demand for blood flow in the growing uterus during pregnancy is met by marked growth of the uterine artery which increases its diameter several fold but shrinks again after completion of pregnancy (Moll). The morphological changes are very similar to the changes described for the growth of collateral arteries. Other conditions, like the arterialization of veins[5] and the outward remodeling of arteries proximal to arterio-venous shunts follow basically the same mechanisms as in arteriogenesis except that the difference between starting and final dimensions are very much smaller.

This book discusses several problems that have not hitherto been solved or had remained controversial. One of these problems is:

■ **The importance of preexisting arteriolar connections**
Dr. Fulton delves into the history of the debate about coronary collateral vessels and he shows that the concept of their preexistence was embattled from the beginning and that it was always a matter of technique: those in the possession of the method with a high resolution were able to show

them, the others denied their existence. This battle continues into our time where the question of "neo-arteriogenesis" was brought up because of the believe that newly formed capillaries from the angiogenic process are able to recruit smooth muscle and transform into arterioles, thereby repeating in the adult organism an important embryonal developmental stage. Although this is an interesting concept it does not apply to the type of arteriogenesis that we describe here: interconnecting arterioles must be present as a substrate; when they are not (as in the hearts of pigs, rabbits and rats), no arterial collaterals can form. Greatly enlarged and numerous capillaries can assume part of the role of collateral arteries in the pig heart but are inferior because of their subendocardial position and because of the low driving pressure at their source vessels. This makes them prone to the "subendocardial crunch" when the diastolic intraventricular pressure rises.

Dr. Ritter describes typical pathways of collateral vessels in human pathology. This is important within the context of our discussion about the preexistence of an arteriolar network of collateral vessels. Not only are preexisting arterioles needed, they form and follow, in the human body, avenues along which typical rescue pathways develop. Dr. Ritter illustrates cases of astounding feats of adaptation, i.e., where the circulation of both legs is supplied via collaterals formed from enlarged preexisting vessels surrounding the ureter after occlusion of both iliacal arteries. He also shows the formation of secondary networks when the feeder arteries of the primary collaterals became occluded. He raises the question why in some cases the adaptation proceeds so well so that the patient was able to lead a normal life without symptoms whereas in others the adaptation by collaterals remained incomplete and stopped before a satisfying result was obtained. In other chapters the question is discussed, **whether**

■ collateral formation **follows always the same basic mechanisms** be it in the heart, brain or the peripheral circulation. The answer is yes, the same mechanisms apply. They are only modified by the metabolic needs of the organ supplied and, perhaps, by the size of the animal: mouse collaterals do not need much remodeling because just one cell division satisfies the need.

■ **The genetic background does play a quantitative role** with regard to the density of the preexistent arteriolar network, which is poorly developed in the white laboratory mouse (Balb/C) in comparison with the black C57BL/6 strain which exhibits a denser network and a surprisingly fast ability to adapt to femoral occlusion by collateral growth. It would be highly interesting to identify the genes that are responsible for these differences.

■ Another controversial topic under discussion is that of the **role of the intima, which becomes the most active cell layer in the wall of the transforming collaterals.** Mitosis and apoptosis occur here suggesting a high turnover of the cell population. The dedifferentiated SMCs exhibit a pattern of embryonal gene expression with a downregulation of desmin, upregulation of fibronectin etc. These observations suggest that the intima may be the incubator for the new and larger vessel, the supplier of new cells, which may leave the incubator for maturation in the new media. This view is somewhat at odds with the conventional opinion that the intima is a symptom of degeneration, the bed for atherosclerosis or, in our context, the mechanism of pruning. However, new experiments show that even an excessive intima formation in mouse collateral vessels (after restoration of blood flow) is an asset at re-occlusion: intimal cells rearrange much faster into a large lumen than would have been possible from cell proliferation.

■ **The influence of tissue ischemia on arteriogenesis** was taken for granted since many decades in spite of Fulton's pioneering studies 40 years ago showing that in the diseased human heart collaterals often develop far away from areas of ischemia. We have gathered several new arguments against a role of ischemia in arteriogenesis and we hope that the discussion can now be closed.

■ A grave problem is **which of the known (or yet to be discovered) vascular growth factors is essential for arteriogenesis.**
We recently carried out some experiments that illustrate the complexity of the role of growth factors in arteriogenesis. In spite of a substantial

body of literature no clear favorite is apparent. In our own experiments the two most favored factors bFGF and VEGF-A do not change expression in growing collaterals nor in the adjacent tissue. Other factors like PDGF and HGF are also absent from expression profiles of collateral artery tissue. Targeted disruption of the FGF-1 and-2 genes and injection of soluble receptors for VEGF and FGF do not interfere with arteriogenesis. Transgenic mice expressing the VEGF promoter coupled to a reporter gene fail to express the reporter in growing collaterals after femoral occlusion. The only hint that the mentioned growth factors do play a role is their activity when the proteins are administered locally (VEGF, PlGF, MCP-1). However they accelerate growth rather than changing the final level of adaptation, which is reached without treatment but after a longer time of observation and which remains well below the physiological level of conductance of the artery before occlusion. However, these factors may not act directly on vascular cells but rather via attraction of monocytes that adhere and invade and produce a cocktail of factors that are essential for collateral artery growth. On the other hand we recently found that the FGF receptor 1 in FGF-2 knockout mice, upregulated during a brief time window after femoral occlusion, is phosphorylated in collateral tissue. This strongly argues for the deputy role of one of the now 25 known FGF ligands.

■ It is of note that **the arteriogenic process may be primarily controlled via the availability of the receptors** (ligands are present anyway in the ECM), which may explain the often observed inefficiency of infused ligands into normal tissue. Most receptors may have only a brief time window of activity early after arterial occlusion, which explains why growth factors infused some time after occlusion appear to be inactive. Furthermore infusion of PAS interferes with the ligand receptor complex of the FGF system and strongly inhibits collateral artery growth. The intracellular signaling in collateral vessels proceeds via the Ras/ERK pathway, which is a strong indication for the involvement of the FGF system but does not exclude PDGF, which employs the same signal pathway.

However, smooth muscle cells in culture react only to PDGF-AB but not to FGF-2 with an increase in PKB/Akt phosphorylation. On the other hand shear stress activated collateral vessels do not show an upregulation of PKB/Akt, which argues for an involvement of FGF- but not of PDGF ligands. Desmin and destrin are downregulated in FGF-2- (but not in PDGF AB-) exposed SMCs in culture and show a downregulation just as in growing collateral vessels, which argues for a key role of FGF ligands. Transgenic overexpression of FGF-2, mainly in skeletal muscle, greatly stimulates blood flow recovery in femoral occluded mice, but mainly in combination with exercise.

Another argument against an involvement of PDGF is that Gleevec®, an anticancer drug that inhibits PDGF receptor signaling, had no effect on arteriogenesis in our rabbit model when locally infused over 7 days by Alzet minipump into the proximal stump of the occluded femoral artery. Mice with deletion of the PDGF retention motif do not show a grossly abnormal course of blood flow recovery after femoral ligation (preliminary unpublished experiments).

■ **Is it imaginable that arteriogenesis can occur without growth factors?**
We have shown that arteriogenesis can proceed without changes in the local concentration of the classical ligands. This can be explained away by the brief appearance of the receptor. But is it imaginable that integrin activation by fluid shear stress leading to phosphorylation of kinases (Rho-pathway) finally activates the cell cycle without interference of extracellular mitogens? Can it be imagined that SMCs enter the cell cycle when the transcription of elastin is downregulated? A recent report showed massive proliferation of SMCs in an elastin knockout model[6]. On the other hand: downregulation of elastin in SMCs in culture occurs only in the presence of FGF (Kubin, unpublished). It is known that arterial SMCs are heterogeneous and that isolated subpopulations can proliferate in culture without serum support. Are these cells (arterial smooth muscle stem cells?) the ones that migrate into the intima or proliferate *in situ*? However, bone marrow stem cells do not incorporate into the wall of collateral arteries.

■ **The role of monocytes**
We were the first to observe the invasion of monocytes into growing collaterals in the canine coronary collateral circulation more than 35 years ago[7]. Since then the importance of this cell type was supported by several

other findings: the discovery that the monocyte-attractant chemokine MCP-1, when infused into the proximal stump of the occluded artery stimulated arteriogenesis, the finding that interfering with monocyte adhesion to the adhesion molecule ICAM-1 inhibited arteriogenesis, that targeted disruption of the MCP-1 receptor CCR2 also inhibited arteriogenesis, that increasing the life span of monocytes with GMCSF stimulated arteriogenesis and that transient elimination of monocytes from the peripheral blood by liposome-packaged bisphosphonates stopped arteriogenesis. Likewise chemical elimination of monocytes by 5-fluorouracil inhibited (and recovery from chemotherapy with an overshoot of the monocyte count stimulated) arteriogenesis. Monocytes are particularly important during the early phases after arterial occlusion. Their role in later stages, especially in situations with chronically increased shear stress, is presently under study and preliminary results suggest an even greater invasion with very high shear stress. Most certainly matrix-lysing enzymes play an important role probably by inactivating TIMP, their tissue inhibitor, by releasing stored growth factors and by digesting elastin, which leads to de-inhibition of SMC mobility and proliferative quiescence.

■ **Physical forces**

Our studies and those of others have shown that fluid shear stress, a weak force in physical terms compared to the circumferential wall stress, is a surprisingly strong morphogen that is able to remodel arterioles into arteries and these into even larger structures. Fluid shear stress is difficult to manipulate over a longer period of time. With our new model of distal stump anastomosis of the occluded femoral artery in pigs and rabbits side-to-side with the accompanying vein we have created a relatively stable situation of chronically increased shear stress. Our hemodynamic studies with this new model showed that **the restoration of the physiological maximal conductance after arterial occlusion by collateral blood vessels is a realistic goal!** These AV-shunt experiments also enabled us to employ new methods of expression profiling and of proteomics to search for the factors responsible for the drastic remodeling as it occurs in arteriogenesis. **To unravel the morphogenic power of blood flow, to understand the transmission of the mechanical force into the genome that changes expression to enable existing vessels to grow, is the central problem in arteriogenesis.**

Our gene profiling and proteomic studies in rabbits, pigs and mice have provided a wealth of information which is difficult to analyze because of the sheer number of sequences to be tested for functional significance. Hybridizing rabbit RNA obtained from shear stress stimulated collateral vessels (in comparison with collaterals of the same stage of development from the same animal) to micro-arrays we obtained 713 sequences that were identified (and are shear stress-related) of which 136 were, at first analysis, relevant because they contained many transcription factors, cell cycle related genes, genes coding for signaling molecules and matrix proteins. It will take time to extract the most significant information from these studies. We will update our web site with new genetic information soon after the appearance of this book (www.kerckhoff.mpg.de)

References

1. SCHAPER W. The Collateral Circulation of the Heart. *Amsterdam London: Elsevier North Holland Publishing Company;*1971.
2. SCHAPER W. The Pathophysiology of Myocardial Perfusion. *Amsterdam, New York, Oxford: Elsevier/North-Holland Biomedical Press;*1979.
3. SCHAPER W, SCHAPER J. Collateral Circulation - Heart, Brain, Kidney, Limbs. *Boston, Dordrecht, London: Kluwer Academic Publishers;*1993.
4. SCHAPER W, PIEK JJ, MUNOZ-CHAPULI R, WOLF C, ITO W. Collateral circulation of the heart, in Ware JA ,Simons M (eds.): Angiogenesis and Cardiovascular Disease. *New York, NY, Oxford: Oxford University Press;* 1999:159-198.
5. KWEI, S, STAVRAKIS, G, TAHAKAS, M, TAYLOR, G, FOLKMAN, MJ, GIMBRONE, M, GARCIA-GARDENA, G. Early adaptive responses of the vascular wall during venous arterialization in mice. *Am J Pathol.* 2004;164:81-89
6. LI DY, BROOKE B, DAVIS EC, MECHAM RP, SORENSEN LK, BOAK BB, EICHWALD E, KEATING MT. Elastin is an essential determinant of arterial morphogenesis. *Nature.* 1998;393:276-280.
7. SCHAPER J, KOENIG R, FRANZ D, SCHAPER W. The endothelial surface of growing coronary collateral arteries. Intimal margination and diapedesis of monocytes. A combined SEM and TEM study. *Virchows Arch A (Pathol Anat).* 1976;370:193-205.

Embryonic Development of Collateral Arteries

Borja Fernández

In the embryo, the early vascular system derives from mesoderm precursor cells called angioblasts, which colonize different embryonic structures and coalesce *in situ*, to form a network of endothelial channels devoid of mural cells. This morphogenetic mechanism receives the name of vasculogenesis, and the resulting vascular network is called primary plexus. During early embryonic stages the plexus grows and expands by sprouting and intussusception, similar to the angiogenic type of growth of adult capillary networks, and supplies the primitive organ primordia with oxygen. As development proceeds however, the plexus is inefficient to perfuse the more compact tissues, and differentiation into an arterio-venous system is required. The primordia of arteries and veins appear when the endothelial channels of the primary plexus become invested with un-differentiated mural cells. Putative chemoattractant signals recruit perivascular mesenchymal cells, which are then committed in situ to the musculo-vascular phenotype. Both, recruitment and differentiation seem to be induced by the endothelium. The whole process has received the name of arterialization [1-6].

During the last decade, the molecular signals governing the process of arterialization began to be elucidated [4-12]. Angiopoietins secreted by perivascular mesenchymal cells bind to Tie receptors on the surface of endothelial cells, stabilizing the vessel wall and promoting vessel maturation. Both, stabilization and maturation rely on perivascular cell recruitment and contact to the endothelial cells. Upon contact, mesenchymal cells differentiate into pericytes and smooth muscle cells through the

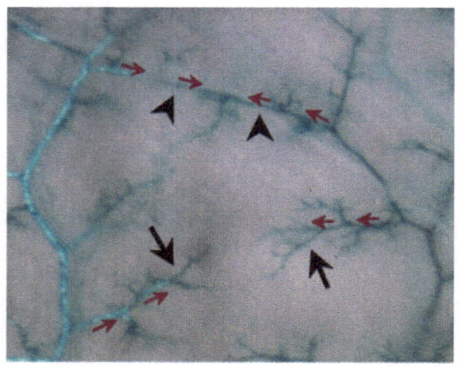

Fig. 1

Micrograph of a portion of the epigastric vascula-ture of a pLac-Z transgenic mouse stained with the β-galactosidase. pLac-Z transgenic mice show Lac-Z expression (blue) in vascular smooth mus-cle cells and pericytes[30]. Black arrows point to conventional "ending" arteries of two independ-ent arterial trees. Black arrowheads point to a collateral artery connecting the two independent arterial trees. Red arrows show the direction of blood flow.

action of differentiation growth fac-tors such as PDFG and TGF. Al-though several transcription factors are known to be involved in the dif-ferentiation of mesenchymal cells into smooth muscle cells, there is no single pathway that can initiate the whole musculo-vascular differentia-tion program.

The anatomy of the arterial sys-tem follows a basic tree-branching pattern, where big arteries branch into smaller arteries, and these into arterioles, which connect with the capillary network. Thus, conven-tional arteries show a proximal-to-distal axis, where the blood flows in one direction from the proximal ex-treme of the vessel (connected to a larger artery) to the distal extreme of the vessel (connected to a smaller artery or capillary). Collateral arteries do not show a proximal-to-distal axis with respect to the blood flow. In collateral arteries, the blood flows from the two opposite extremes of the vessel to the branches localized along the collateral length (Fig. 1). Thus, it is the anatomy of the vessel that distinguishes a preexisting quiescent collateral from a conventional artery, and both types of vessels are indis-tinguishable from their histology and ultrastructure in normal physio-logical conditions.

During embryonic development, the differentiation of the arterial system follows also a proximal-to-distal direction with respect to the blood flow. Big conducting arteries develop first, and the differentiation wave extends distally through smaller arteries and arterioles. A good example of this type of differentiation pattern can be found in the mor-phogenesis of the coronary arteries (coronariogenesis)[13-17]. The primordi-um of the coronary system consists of a plexus of endothelial channels, called coronary plexus, which grows into the cardiac matrix and sub-epi-cardial space covering the whole heart. This coronary plexus expands by angiogenesis, until it makes contact with the aortic root at the base of the heart, initiating the differentiation of the capillary plexus into coronary arteries. The sudden increase of blood flow at the proximal portion of the plexus seems to be a crucial trigger for arterialization. Epicardium-derived mesenchymal cells close to the aortic root are then recruited, differentiating into smooth muscle cells. Recruitment and differentiation propagate in a proximal-to-distal direction, starting at the coronary ostia (forming the main trunk of the coronary arteries) towards the apex of the heart (forming the small precapillary arterioles). Thus, the proximal-to-distal anatomical axis of arterial segments is developed as a consequence of an ordered and directional propagation of the musculo-vascular differentiation wave. Then, how do collateral arteries develop?

Very few studies describe the formation of collateral arteries. Price and collaborators showed that collateral arteries of the rat gracilis muscle develop during the postnatal period by arterialization of two opposing arteriole endings, proceeding along capillary pathways[18]. Smooth muscle cells of the collateral vessel wall derive from recruitment of perivascular mesenchymal cells and/or from proliferation and migration of smooth muscle cells at the terminal end of the opposing arterioles to finally form a continuous arteriolar vessel. The formation of collateral arteries can then be considered a continuation of the arterialization process along capillary domains of opposing arterioles. What is then restricting or inducing arterialization in terminal arterioles to finally form a collateral *versus* a conventional "ending" artery?

Analyzing how arterialization stops at the distal end of arterioles might be a good hint. In mammals, the right and left coronary arteries branch throughout the right and left ventricles respectively, and do not usually surpass the interventricular limit. During coronariogenesis, when terminal branches of the two developing coronary arteries meet at the interventricular borders, arterialization stops. In some cases, a defect in the connection of the coronary plexus to the aortic root gives rise to a single coronary artery, the arterialization of which starts in one coronary ostium, continues through its respective ventricle, surpass the interventricular limit, and continue branching throughout the other ventricle, compensating for the missing coronary artery[19,20]. Thus, the irrigation domain of one particular artery is limited by adjacent arteries that irrigate

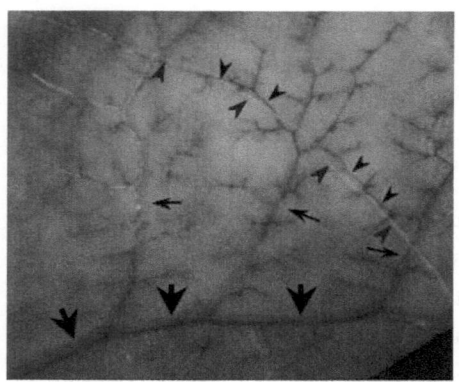

Fig. 2

Micrograph of the epigastric vasculature of a pLac-Z transgenic mouse stained with the β-galactosidase. The main epigastric artery (big black arrows) branches into smaller arteries (small black arrows), which are inter-connected by collateral arteries (black arrowheads). The pathway of the main epigastric nerves (red arrowheads) coincides with the anatomical localization of collateral arteries.

the surrounding tissue. Inhibitory signals from arterialized tissue seem to limit differentiation of the adjacent vasculature. Development of collateral arteries might rely on suppression of the inhibitory signals that limit arterialization of one particular segment of the plexus.

One recent relevant finding adding complexity to the process of arterialization was reported by Mikouyama and collaborators[21]. They found that mutations in genes relevant for axon guidance alter the nerve branching pattern, as well as the arterial branching pattern. The concept that arterial differentiation relies on putative inductive signals from the nerve system is not new, however. One decade ago, researches on coronariogenesis already showed that differentiation of the coronary arteries is in close anatomic association with neural crest-derived cardiac ganglia[16]. Moreover, cardiac defects associated with experimental ablation of the cardiac neural crest include anomalies in the origin and course of the main coronary arteries[17]. How this morphogenetic dependency between the nervous and the arterial systems can affect the development of collateral *versus* conventional arteries is unknown. However, the fact that in some vascular systems the anatomical localization of collateral arteries coincides with the pathway of the main nerve trunks is suggestive in this regard (Fig. 2).

Shear stress from the blood flow, inhibitory stimuli from the surrounding arterialized tissue, and inductive cues from the nerve system seem to be important factors regulating the differentiation of conventional *versus* collateral arteries. How are these physiological stimuli translated into molecular signals?

Two molecular pathways recently found to regulate vascular differentiation might be crucial for collateral artery development. The Ephrin/Eph and the Jagged/Notch signaling systems are both composed of membrane bound ligands (Ephrin and Jagged) and membrane bound receptors (Eph and Notch). Thus, signaling through these molecular pathways relies on cell-to-cell contacts. Interestingly, both signaling pathways are also required for proper development of the nervous system [22,23].

In the embryonic capillary plexus, future arterial endothelial cells express Ephrin-B2 ligand, whereas the corresponding receptor Eph-B4 is expressed

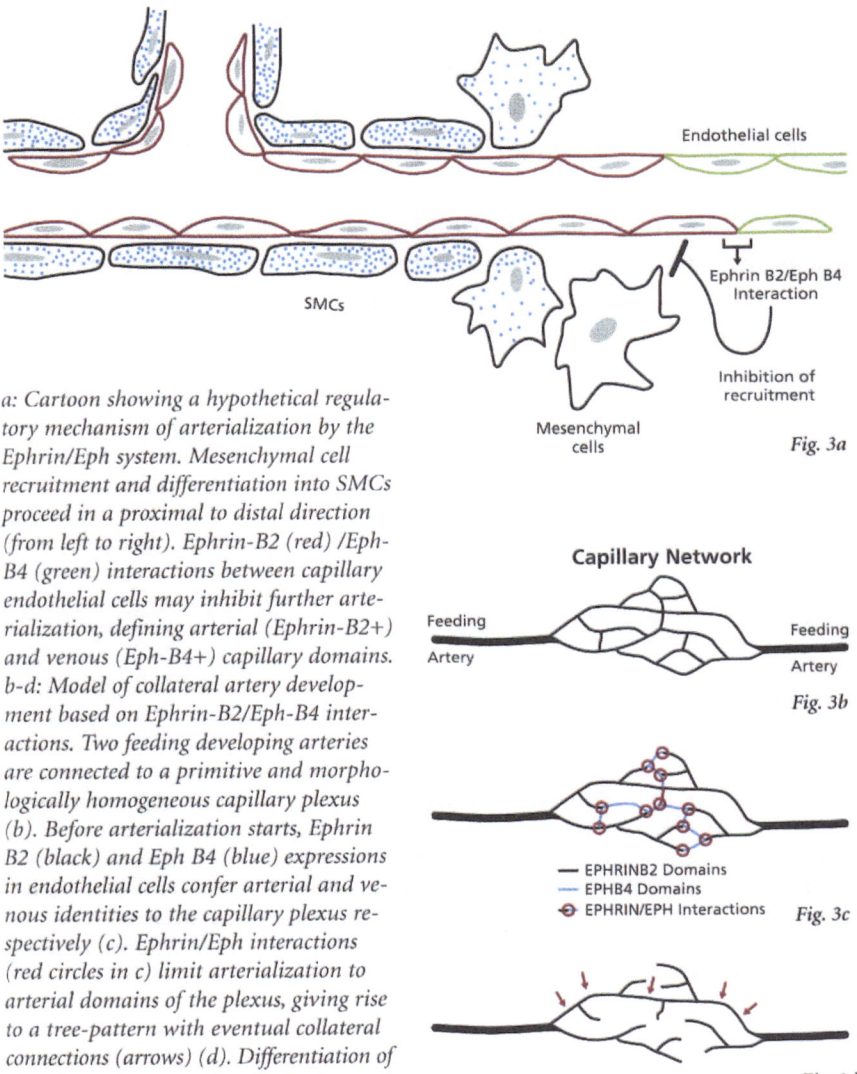

Endothelial cells

SMCs

Ephrin B2/Eph B4 Interaction

Inhibition of recruitment

Mesenchymal cells

a: Cartoon showing a hypothetical regulatory mechanism of arterialization by the Ephrin/Eph system. Mesenchymal cell recruitment and differentiation into SMCs proceed in a proximal to distal direction (from left to right). Ephrin-B2 (red) /Eph-B4 (green) interactions between capillary endothelial cells may inhibit further arterialization, defining arterial (Ephrin-B2+) and venous (Eph-B4+) capillary domains. b-d: Model of collateral artery development based on Ephrin-B2/Eph-B4 interactions. Two feeding developing arteries are connected to a primitive and morphologically homogeneous capillary plexus (b). Before arterialization starts, Ephrin B2 (black) and Eph B4 (blue) expressions in endothelial cells confer arterial and venous identities to the capillary plexus respectively (c). Ephrin/Eph interactions (red circles in c) limit arterialization to arterial domains of the plexus, giving rise to a tree-pattern with eventual collateral connections (arrows) (d). Differentiation of the vein system occurs later in development.

Fig. 3a

Capillary Network

Feeding Artery

Feeding Artery

Fig. 3b

—— EPHRINB2 Domains
—— EPHB4 Domains
⊖ EPHRIN/EPH Interactions

Fig. 3c

Fig. 3d

by future venous endothelial cells[24]. Ligand-receptor interactions may confer identity to the endothelial cells, restrict cell intermingling, and create a boundary that represents the arterio-venous transition[25,26] (Fig. 3a). The Ephrin/Eph system may then serve to avoid abnormal connections between arteries and veins and to regulate inter-arterial connections (Fig. 3b-d).

Mutations in the genes coding for Jagged (ligand) and Notch (receptor) cause disorders of the human cardiovascular system[27,28]. Some morphogenetic functions of this evolutionary conserved signaling system were discovered in studies with the zebra fish embryo. In this experimental model angioblasts that express Notch will form the aorta, whereas angioblasts not expressing Notch will form the cardinal vein[29]. Thus, Notch is able to confer vascular identity to precursor cells before they differentiate into a particular cell type (Fig. 4). The Jagged/Notch signaling system may have special relevance in the embryonic development of collateral arteries, as we have found consistent, time-dependent, and cell-type restricted regulation of Jagged and Notch protein expression during the growth of collateral arteries after arterial stenosis in the adult (see chapter 9).

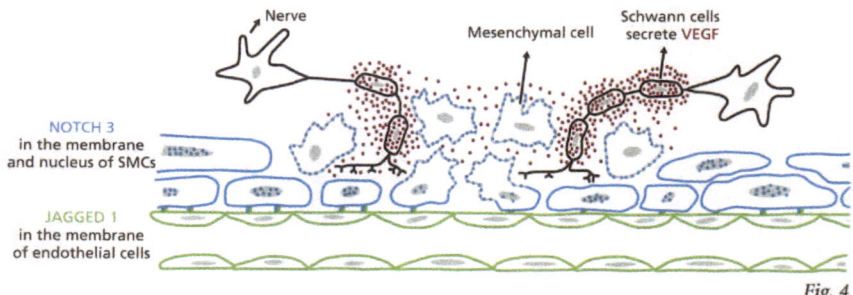

Fig. 4

Cartoon showing the possible involvement of the Jagged/Notch system in collateral artery development. Schwann cells secrete VEGF (red), inducing Notch expression (blue) in perivascular mesenchymal cells, which become then committed to the SMC linage[31]. Upon contact with Jagged-expressing endothelial cells (green), Notch is activated and translocated to the nucleus of presumptive SMCs, regulating the transcription of differentiation genes. In this model, development of collateral vs. terminal arterioles relies on the anatomical pathway of the developing sensory nerve system.

During the last decades, the discovery of the morphogenetic and the molecular bases of vasculogenesis and angiogenesis allowed the development of new therapeutical strategies to fight against ischemia. In the future, the discovery of the basic mechanisms of arterialization and collateral artery formation may allow us to induce experimentally the development and growth of conducting and collateral arteries, to completely restore the maximal physiological conductance of the occluded artery.

References

1. OWENS GK. Regulation of differentiation of vascular smooth muscle cells. *Physiol Rev.* 1995;75:487-517
2. THAYER JM, MEYERS K, GIACHELLI CM, SCHWARTZ SM. Formation of the arterieal media during vascular development. *Cell Molec Biol Res.* 1995;41(4):251-262
3. KATOH Y, PERIASAMY M. Growth and differentiation of smooth muscle cells during vascular development. *Trends Cardiovasc Med.* 1996;6:100-106
4. FOLKMAN J, D'AMORE PA. Blood vessel formation: what is its molecular basis? *Cell* 1996; 87:1153-1155
5. CONWAY EM, COLLEN D, CARMELIET P. Molecular mechanisms of blood vessel growth *Cardiovasc Res.* 2001;49:507–521
6. CARMELIET P. Mechanisms of angiogenesis and arteriogenesis. *Nature Med.* 2000;6(3):389-395
7. OETTGEN P. Transcriptional regulation of vascular development. *Circ Res.* 2001;89:380-388
8. GORSKI DH, WALSH K. The role of homeobox genes in vascular remodeling and angiogenesis. *Circ Res.* 2000;87:865-872
9. SURI C, JONES PF, PATAN S, BARTUNKOVA S, MAISIONPIERRE PC, DAVIS S, SATO TN, YANKOPOULOS GD. Requisite role of angiopoietin-1, a ligand for the TIE2 receptor, during embryonic angiogenesis. *Cell* 1996;87(7):1171-1180
10. VIKKULA M, BOON LM, CARRAWAY III KL, CALVERT JT, DIAMONTI AJ, GOUMNEROV B, OASYK KA, MARCHUK DA, WARMAN ML, CANTLEY LC, MULLIKEN J.B, OSEN BR. Vascular dysmorphogenesis caused by an activating mutation in the receptor tyrosine kinase TIE2. *Cell* 1996; 87(7):1181-1190
11. SORIANO P. Abnormal kidney development and hematological disorders in PDGF beta-receptor mutant mice. *Genes Dev.* 1994 ;8:1888-1896
12. DICKSON MC, MARTIN JS, COUSINS FM, KULKARNI AB, KARLSSON S, AKHURST RJ. Defective haematopoiesis and vasculogenesis in transforming growth factor-beta 1 knockout mice. *Development.* 1995;121:1845-1854
13. BOGERS AJJC, GITTENBERGER-DE GROOT AC, POELMANN RE, PÉAULT BM, HUYSMANS HA. Development of the origin of the coronary arteries, a matter of ingrowth or outgrowth? *Anat Embryol.* 1989;180:437-441
14. VRANCKEN PEETERS M-PFM, GITTENBERGER-DE GROOT AC, MENTINK MMT, HUNGERFORD JE, LITTLE CD, POELMANN RE. The development of the coronary vessels and their differentiation into arteries and veins in the embryonic quail heart. *Dev Dyn.* 1997;208:338-34815. BERNANKE DH, VELKEY JM. Development of the coronary blood supply: changing concepts and current ideas. *Anat Rec.* 2002;269:198-208
16. WALDO KL, KUMISKI DH, KIRBY ML. Association of the cardiac neural crest with the development of the coronary arteries in the chick embryo. *Anat Rec.*1994;239:315-331
17. HOOD LC, ROSENQUIST TH. Coronary artery development in the chick: Origin and deployment of smooth muscle cells, and the effects of neural crest ablation. *Anat Rec.* 1992; 234:291–300
18. PRICE RJ, OWENS GK, SKALAK TC. Immunohistochemical identification of arteriolar development using markers of smooth muscle differentiation. Evidence that capillary arterialization proceeds from terminal arterioles. *Circ Res.* 1994;75:520-527

19. SANS-COMA V, ARQUÉ JM, DURÁN AC, CARDO M, FERNÁNDEZ B. Coronary artery anomalies and bicuspid aortic valves in the Syrian hamster. *Basic Res Cardiol.* 1991;86:148-153

20. DURÁN AC, ARQUÉ JM, SANS-COMA V, FERNÁNDEZ B, DE VEGA NG. Severe congenital stenosis of the left coronary artery ostium and its possible pathogenesis according to the coronary artery ingrowth theory. *Cardiovasc Pathol.* 1998;7:261-266

21. MUKOUYAMA YS, SHIN D, BRITSCH S, TANIGUCHI M, ANDERSON DJ. Sensory nerves determine the pattern of the arterial differentiation and blood vessel branching in the skin. *Cell* 2002;109(6):693-705

22. TEPASS U, GODT D, WINKLBAUER R. Cell sorting in animal development: signaling and adhesive mechanisms in the formation of tissue boundaries. *Curr Opin Genet Develop.* 2002;12:572–582

23. ARTAVANIS-TSAKONAS S, RAND MD, LAKE RJ. Notch signaling: cell fate control and signal integration in development. *Science* 1999;284:770–776

24. WANG HU, CHEN Z-F, ANDERSON DJ. Molecular distinction and angiogenic interaction between embryonic arteries and veins revealed by ephrin-B2 and its receptor Eph-B4. *Cell* 1998;93:741-753

25. ADAMS RH, KLEIN R. Eph Receptors and Ephrin Ligands: Essential Mediators of Vascular Development. *Trends Cardiovasc Med.* 2000;10:183-188

26. CHEN N, BRANTLEY DM, CHEN J. The ephrins and Eph receptors in angiogenesis. *Cytokine Growth Factor Rev.* 2002;13:75-8

27. LI L, KRANTZ ID, DENG Y, GENIN A, BANTA AB, COLLINS CC, QI M, TRASK BJ, KUO WL, COCHRAN J, COSTA T, PIERPONT ME, RAND EB, PICCOLI DA, HOOD L, SPINNER NB. Alagille syndrome is caused by mutations in human Jagged1, which encodes a ligand for Notch1. *Nat Genet* 1997; 16:243-251

28. JOUTEL A, CORPECHOT C, DUCROS A, VAHEDI K, CHABRIAT H, MOUTON P, ALAMOWITCH S, DOMENGA V, CECILLION M, MARECHAL E, MACIAZEK J, VAYSSIERE C, CRUAUD C, CABANIS EA, RUCHOUX MM, WEISSENBACH J, BACH JF, BOUSSER MG, TOURNIER-LASSERVE E. Notch3 mutations in CADASIL, an hereditary adult onset condition causing stroke and dementia. *Nature* 1996; 383:707–710

29. ZHONG TP, CHILDS S, LEU JP, FISHMAN MC. Gridlock signaling pathway fashions the first embryonic artery. *Nature* 2001;414:216-220

30. TIDHAR A, REISHENSTEIN M, COHEN D, FAERMAN A, COPELAND NG, GILBERT DJ, JENKINS NA, SHANTI M. A Novel Transgenic Marker for Migrating Limb Muscle Precursors and for Vascular Smooth Muscle Cells. *Devel Dyn.* 2001;220:60–73

31. CARMELIET P. Blood vessels and nerves: common signals, pathways and diseases. *Nat. Rev. Genet.* 2003;4:710–720

Structural Remodeling during Growth of Collateral Vessels

Wei-jun Cai, Dimitri Scholz, Tibor Ziegelhoeffer and
Jutta Schaper

I. Coronary collateral vessels in the dog heart

This chapter focusses mainly on collateral vessel development of the coronary circulation in the dog heart and it presents the general structural characteristics of vessel growth applicable also for collaterals of the peripheral circulation and in other species. In the second part, morphological features typical of and specific for arteriogenesis in the peripheral circulation will be discussed.

During collateral vessel development, a significant remodeling of all layers of the vascular wall takes place. This occurs in response to increased shear stress acting on endothelial cells as well as to elevated tangential wall stress that exerts its force on media and adventitia. The most characteristic feature of growing coronary collateral blood vessels is the appearance of a neointima consisting of smooth muscle cells, occasionally infiltrating mononuclear cells and extracellular matrix material. In contrast to normal arterioles or small arteries, that are characterized by the regular arrangement of circular smooth muscle cells, a growing collateral vessel consists of an intimal layer with irregularly arranged SMCs and the more or less regular original media, plus the widened adventitia. Growth of a collateral vessel thus occurs by addition of the neointima to the vessel wall structure but not by thickening of the medial layer. At late stages of development, the growth process is arrested, and the enlarged collateral vessel performs as a blood conductor saving tissue jeopardized by ischemia from destruction.

Classification of vessels

The classification of normal versus growing collateral vessels used in the present work is based on macroscopic appearance, on typical histological characteristics and on the presence or absence of proliferating cells in the vascular wall. Vessels with integrity of the internal elastic lamina and without smooth muscle cells in the intima were considered as quiescent or normal vessels. These were characterized by negative Ki-67 (proliferation marker) staining. Growing vessels showed a segmented internal elastic lamina and an enlarged neointima in the presence of Ki-67 positive cells. Mature vessels were characterized by an irregular internal elastic lamina, a moderate – extensive neointima and absence of Ki-67 immunostaining.

This classification rather than the dependence on time will be used throughout this chapter.

Endothelial cells

The endothelium is a single-cell lining covering the internal surface of blood vessels, which possesses multiple functions such as protection from thrombogenicity, regulation of selected blood cell adherence and of vascular dilatation and contraction. In normal small arterial vessels, endothelial cells oriented in the direction of flow are flat containing a central nucleus and a cytoplasm surrounded by a smooth cell membrane (Fig. 1a and b). In growing collateral vessels, the endothelium shows some disorientation, it is more prominent and blood cells may adhere to the ruffled membrane surface (Fig. 1c and d). While normal vessels show quiescent endothelial cells (fig. 2a), those in growing collateral vessels may be in mitosis (Fig. 2b), many are more prominent with numerous cellular organelles (Fig. 2c) and some are in apoptosis (Fig. 2d).

The endothelium modulates vascular tone by synthesis and release of nitric oxide (NO)[1,2], which was initially recognized as endothelium-derived relaxing factor [3] and now has been widely accepted as an important endogenous compound controlling blood pressure. In the vasculature, endothelial constitutive NO synthase (eNOS) is the main producer of NO, although other isoforms of NO synthase, inducible (iNOS) and neuronal (nNOS), exist. Increasing evidence established a plethora of diverse regulatory functions for NO, including vascular dilation, protection of endothelium from platelet aggregation and leukocyte adherence,

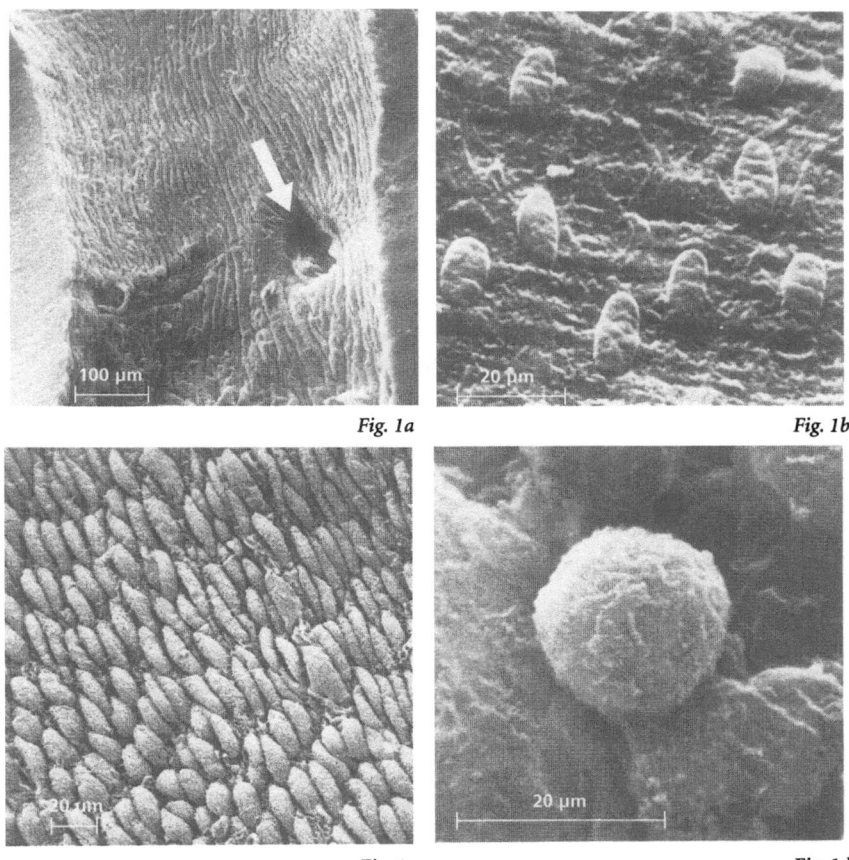

Fig. 1a *Fig. 1b*

Fig. 1c *Fig. 1d*

Appearance of normal and collateral vessel in the scanning electron microscope. 1a) The endothelial layer is continuous and oriented in the direction of flow. Note the orientation of the endothelial cells in the direction of the subbranch (arrow). 1b) Larger magnification showing the regular orientation of endothelial nuclei. 1c) The endothelium in growing collateral vessels is more prominent but still regularly arranged. 1d) Adhesion of a monocyte to an endothelial cell.

and inhibition of smooth muscle cell proliferation[4]. Confocal microscopy showed that in normal arterioles expression of eNOS is very low, but that in growing collateral vessels there is a 6-fold-increase (Fig. 3) that returned to normal levels in mature vessels. These findings and the role of NOS in collateral growth will be discussed more extensively in chapter 5.

Recently, the possibility has been discussed that endothelial cells may originate from bone marrow-derived progenitor cells circulating in blood (reviewed in[5]). Whether or not this is the case for endothelial cells in

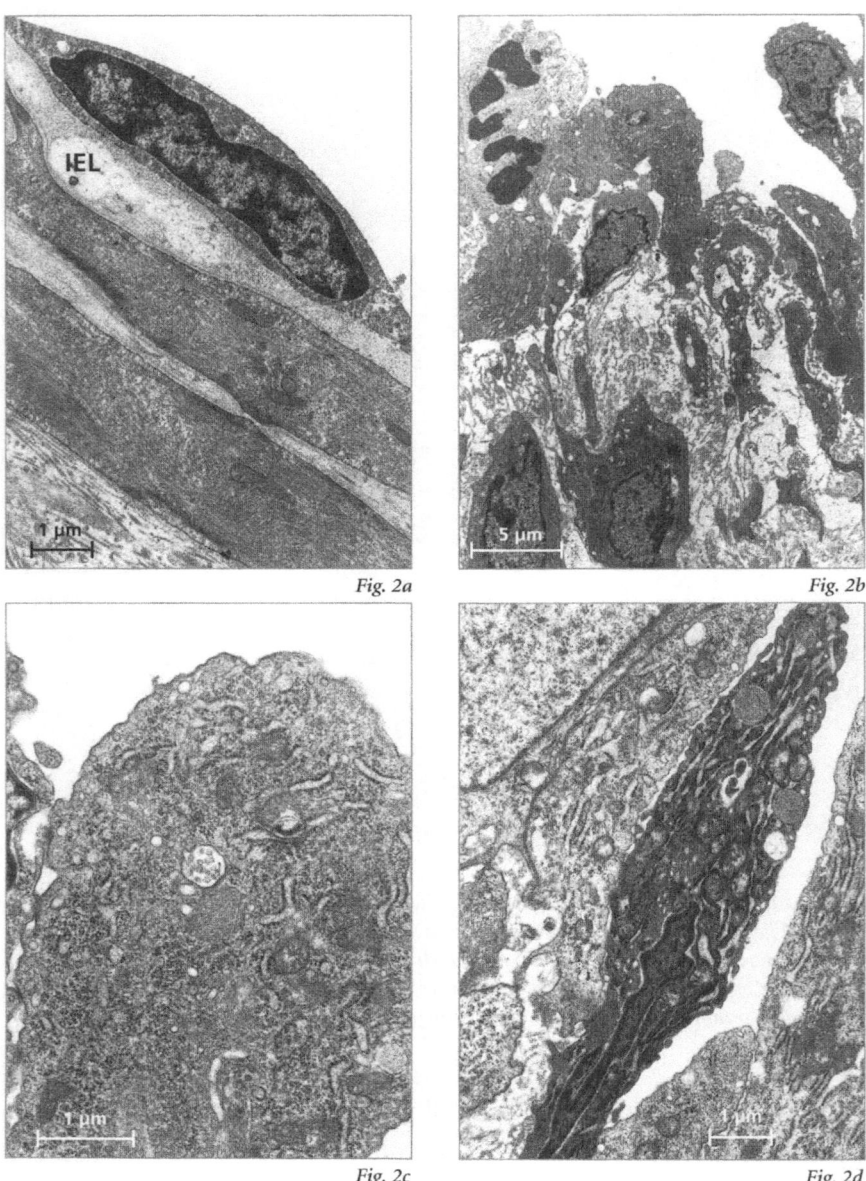

Fig. 2a

Fig. 2b

Fig. 2c

Fig. 2d

Ultrastructural appearance of endothelial cells in growing collateral vessels. 2a) Normal pre-existing collateral vessel with a quiescent endothelial cell, the internal elastic lamina (IEL) and 2 layers of SMCs. 2b) Prominent endothelial cells in a collateral vessel. Left upper corner: Mitosis of endothelial cell. 2c) An "activated" endothelial cell with increased cellular organelles. 2d) Apoptotic endothelial cell with a condensed nucleus and dark cytoplasm.

growing collateral vessels remains uncertain but is unlikely[5a]. The concept has been brought forward by several groups that endothelial progenitor cells can be recruited and mobilized by VEGF[6] and possibly other growth factors such as GM-CSF[7] or inhibition of metalloproteinases[8], and that homing and differentiation of progenitor cells into the endothelial layer are induced by the same factors. Induction of vascular networks in adult organs by VEGF has also been reported in experimental studies with transgenic „off and on" switching of the VEGF gene[9]. However, the majority of studies describing „neovascularization" or „angiogenesis"

report an increase in the number of capillaries but not of arterial blood conductors[5]. Obviously, an increase in the microvasculature without true arteriogenesis is ineffective in replacing a large occluded artery and in preventing ischemic injury, and its beneficial effect is questionable. Furthermore, rapid development of collateral vessels following abrupt LAD occlusion after bone marrow cell injection in swine heart as recently described[10] is unusual because pigs are known to possess a poor, almost non-existent preexisting collateral network. Collateral vessel formation requires not only endothelial cells but also smooth muscle cells, a fact not considered in this study.

At the present time, more experimental studies are needed to determine the arteriogenic properties of endothelial progenitor cells, which finally will determine whether or not this procedure has therapeutic potential.

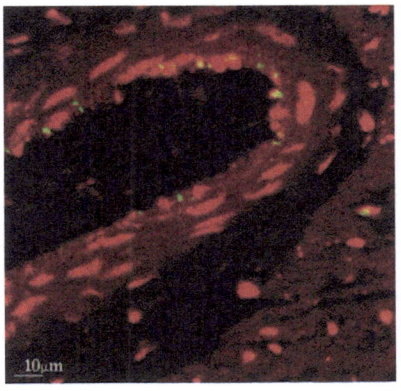

Fig. 3a

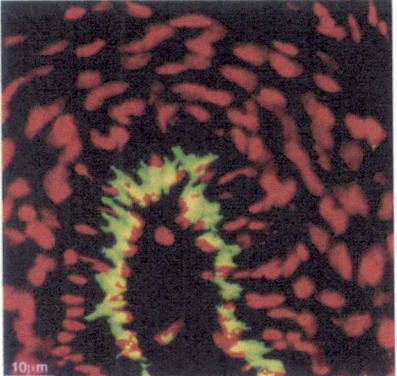

Fig. 3b

Localization of eNOS in blood vessels. Immunoconfocal microscopy. Specific fluorescence green, nuclei are red. 3a) In normal vessels, eNOS is present in the endothelial layer. 3b) The amount of eNOS is increased in a growing collateral.

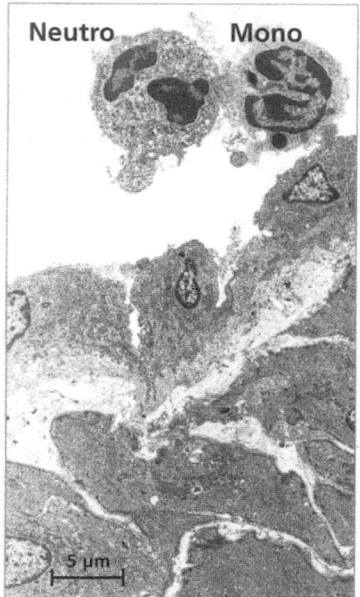
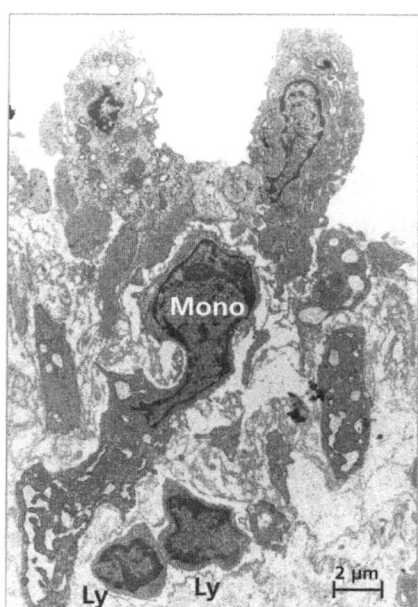

Fig. 4a   *Fig. 4b*

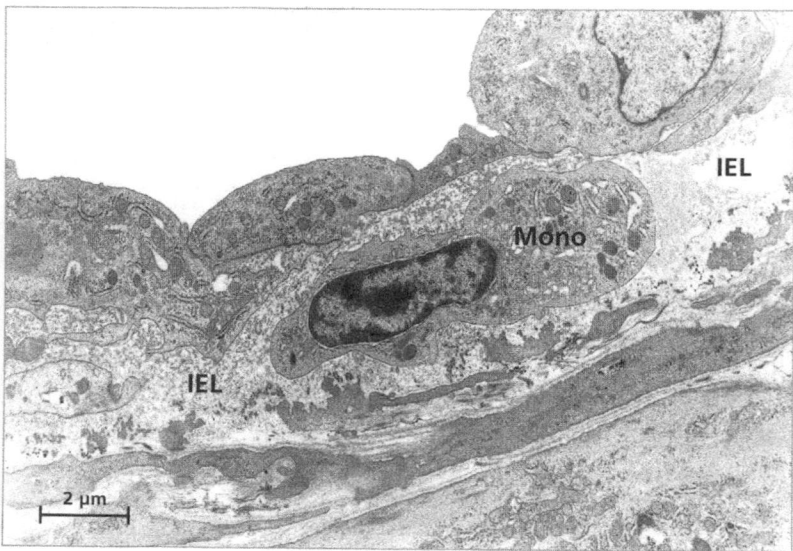

Fig. 4c

Adhesion and infiltration of mononuclear cells. 4a) Top: Adhesion of a monocyte (Mono) to an endothelial cell of a collateral vessel. A neutrophil (Neutro) is adhering to the monocyte. 4b) Prominent endothelial cells, damaged SMCs without basement membrane and two smaller lymphocytes (Ly) are present in a disorganized intimal layer of a growing collateral vessel. 4c) Infiltration of a monocyte into the intima between prominent endothelial cells and the fragmented IEL.

Adhesion and immigration of mononuclear cells

Mononuclear cells are seen to adhere to the endothelium in growing collateral vessels. Different stages may be defined: 1. Adhesion to the endothelium; 2. Penetration of the endothelial layer; 3. Infiltration of the neointima and media. In the first stage, mononuclear cells can be clearly identified as blood borne monocytes (Fig. 4a) but while they are immigrating the vessel wall they seem to alter their phenotype. They enlarge and the nucleus becomes more oval than horseshoe shaped but they still contain their dense granules and subcellular organelles are sparse, which identifies these cells to be monocytes (Fig. 4b). Occasionally, the immigrated non-muscle cells contain only a small cytoplasmic body, and the nucleus shows a chromatin distribution characteristic of lymphocytes (Fig. 4c). Monocytes typically exhibit small pseudopods along the cell membrane but the basement membrane is absent, which is a diagnostic criterion for the non-SMC nature of these cells (Fig. 5). The functional properties of monocytes and their role in vascular growth will be discussed in chapter 7. Here, it should only be emphasized that monocytes are important players in adaptive arteriogenesis because they provide numerous proangiogenic and proarteriogenic growth factors such as VEGF, the FGFs and others, they interact with the endothelium via specific adhesion molecules and MCP-1, and they represent the carriers of substances into the vascular wall.

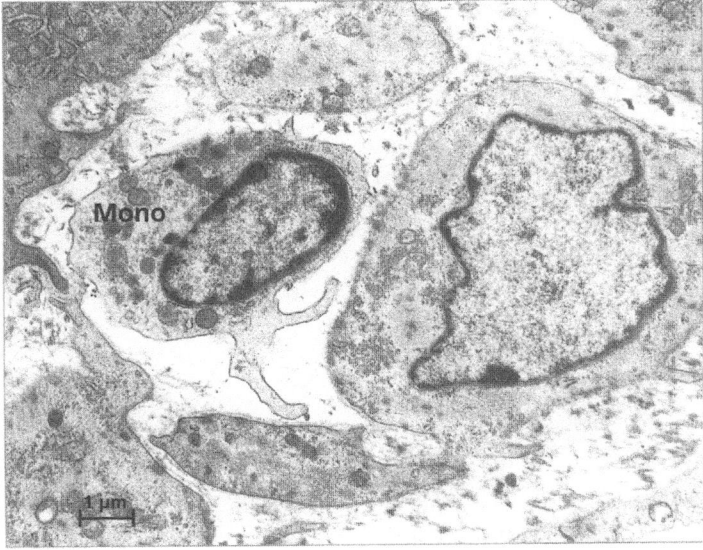

A monocyte (Mono) with several pseudopods is situated between the SMCs of a disorganized tunica media.

Fig. 5

Smooth muscle cells

In normal coronary arterioles and small arteries, SMCs in the media are arranged in a circular and very regular fashion. In growing collateral vessels, the media appears disorganized and the number of smooth muscle cell layers is reduced because migration of SMCs into the subendothelial space through the internal elastic membrane takes place (Fig. 6). This, however, is only possible when the basement membranes of the SMCs are dissolved so that the cells can move. This is obvious in numerous SMCs in the tunica media and intima. The basement membrane reappears in redifferentiated SMCs of mature collateral vessels. These observations

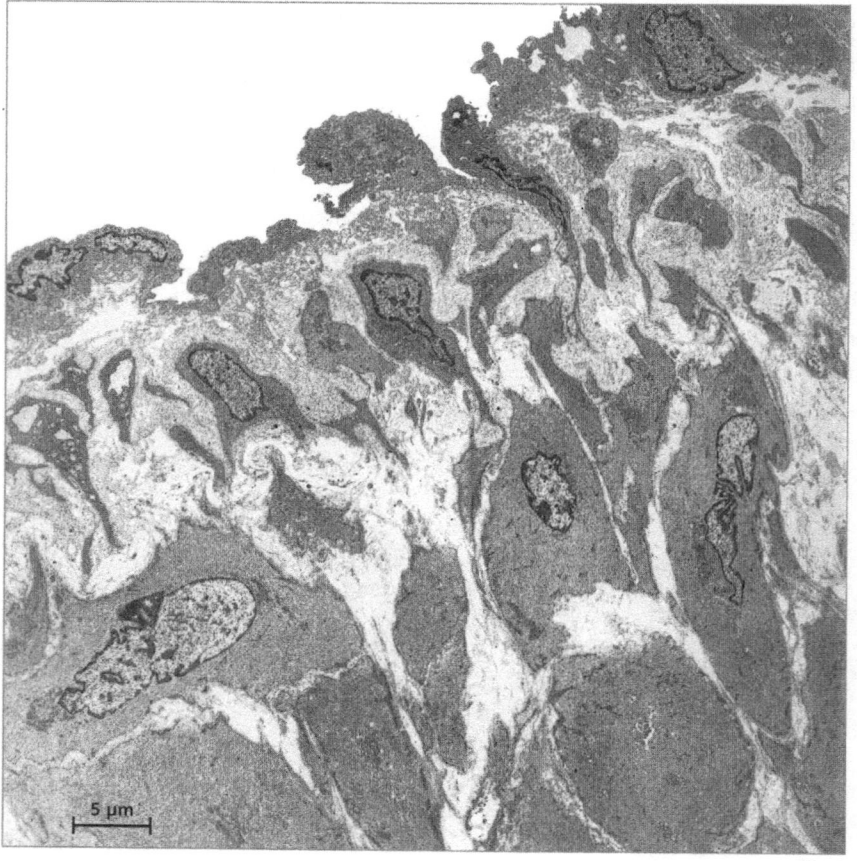

Fig. 6

Collateral vessel, actively growing. The IEL is absent, numerous smaller and larger SMCs are migrating towards the lumen. Note the large amount of ECM but absence of collagen fibrils between the migrating SMCs

strengthen the notion that laminin and other basement membrane components promote the differentiation of vascular SMCs[11,12], which may occur via receptor-mediated interaction and generation of signals that affect cell behavior. It is also possible that the network structure of the basement membrane prevents molecules with a dedifferentiating effect from contacting the cells. The disruption of the basement membrane would abolish such a function and allow for a direct interaction between SMCs and a number of growth factors produced by macrophages or the SMCs themselves, leading to the phenotypic modification of SMCs and subsequent migration and proliferation.

In addition to the modification of phenotypes, the disruption of the basal membrane may be of further importance functionally: Together with the degradation of internal and external elastic material, it paves the way for the expansion and outward growth of collateral vessels.

The basement membrane consists of laminin, collagen IV, fibronectin and other extracellular matrix proteins. It completely surrounds the SMCs and is connected with the intracellular milieu by binding to integrins, the dystrophin complex and the ankyrin-spectrin link-

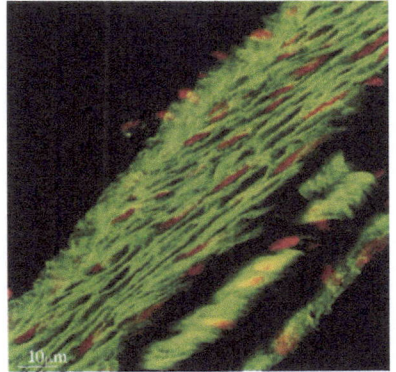

Fig. 7a

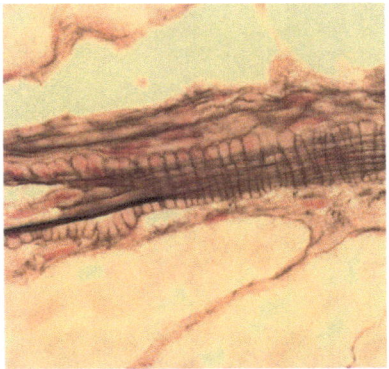

Fig. 7b

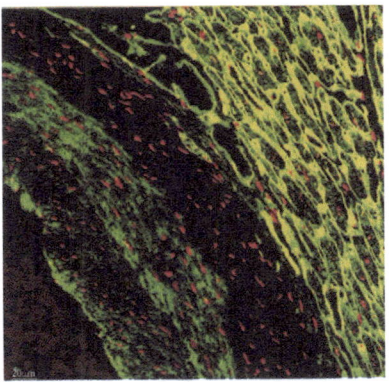

Fig. 7c

Localization of laminin by immunoconfocal microscopy. Specific fluorescence green, nuclei are red. 7a) In a normal vessel, laminin is situated between the SMCs. 7b) PUCHTLER-SWEAT staining for basement membranes (BM)in a small normal vessel (longitudinal section). BM: black, nuclei: pink. Elastic fibers are also black (longitudinal). Note: SMC are surrounded by BM. 7c) In a growing vessel, less laminin is present around the SMCs of the neointima and of the media.

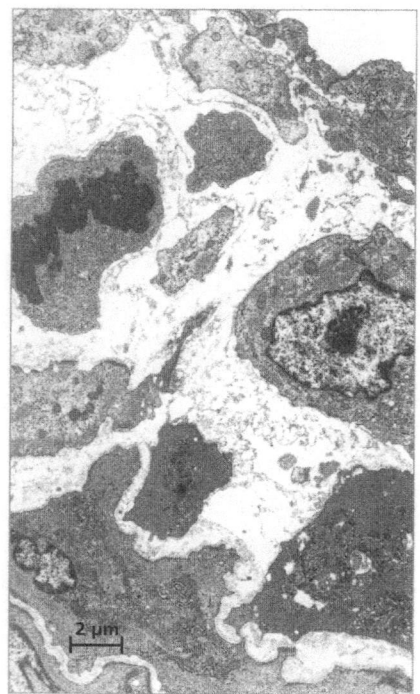

Fig. 8a

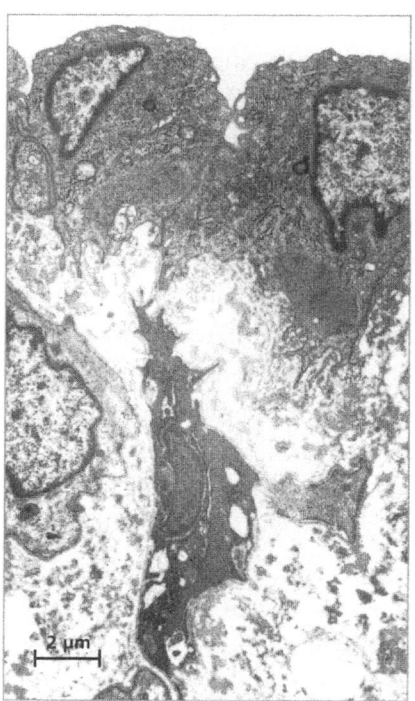

Fig. 8c

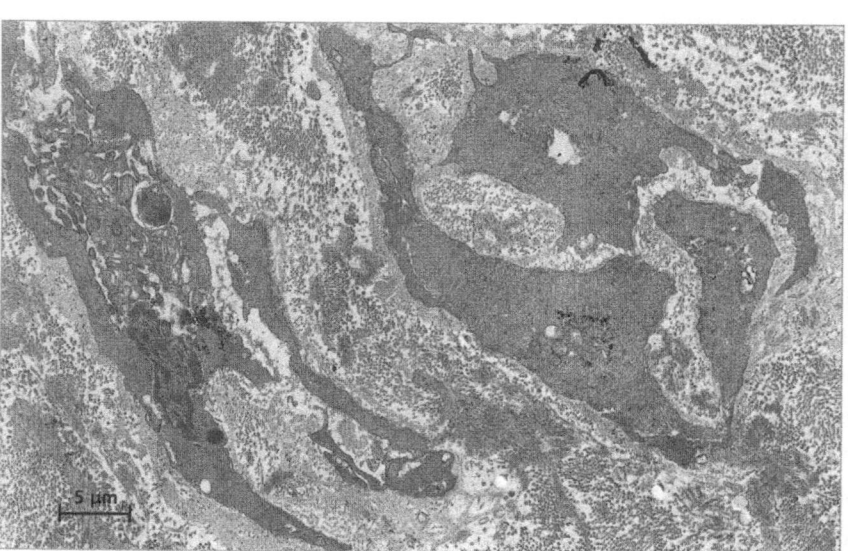

Fig. 8b

Smooth muscle cells in actively growing collateral vessels. 8a) A mitotic SMC (left) in a disorganized neointima. 8b) Irregularly shaped SMCs in abundant ECM in the media. Left: degenerating SMC. 8c) Apoptotic small SMC beneath the endothelial layer.

ing system (for review see[13]). Many integrins are capable of binding ECM proteins through a conserved arginine-glycine-aspartic acid (RGD) motif[14], and a tight connection between the ECM and the actin cytoskeleton seems to be essential for signal transduction[15] and cell migration[16] of SMCs. The role of integrins will be discussed in detail in chapter 9. Confocal microscopy shows that SMCs migrating or already situated in the neointima contain much less laminin or other matrix components of the basement membrane, which confirms ultrastructural findings (Fig. 7).

SMCs in the neointima frequently divide during the stage of active growth[17], but they also show signs of degeneration as indicated by the occurrence of cellular debris in the intercellular space and by the still persisting basement membrane delineating the original SMC size (Fig. 8a-c). Autophagic cell death is feasible and apoptosis can be observed[17]. Apoptosis may be caused by increased stretch of SMCs and is mediated by the beta1–integrin-rac-p38-p53 pathway[18]. The balance between the number of cells undergoing mitosis and the rate of cells dying will decide the final outcome of the vascular growth process[17]. Usually, the balance is in favor of cell division, which results in the formation of a multilayered neointima where the SMCs are arranged either circumferentially or in the direction of the longitudinal axis of the vessel. Proliferation of SMCs can be promoted by stretch[19], lack of elastin[20] as discussed below and by the direct action of growth factors (discussed in chapter 10). Many SMCs in the neointima transform from the

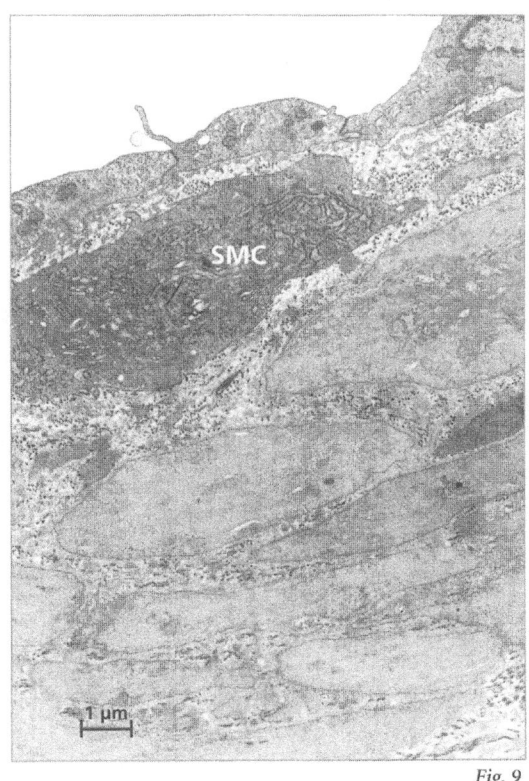

Fig. 9

Vascular wall of a growing collateral vessel characterized by almost complete absence of the IEL and presence of a large SMC of the synthetic phenotype below the endothelial layer.

contractile phenotype characterized by a high content of contractile filaments and scarcity of cellular organelles into the synthetic
phenotype with prominent rough
endoplasmic reticulum and Golgi
apparatus and numerous mitochondria while the contractile material is reduced (Fig. 9). Confocal
microscopy permits the identification of various proteins in the vascular wall by using specific monoclonal or polyclonal antibodies.
Employing this technique it became clear that in growing collateral vessels the majority of neoin-

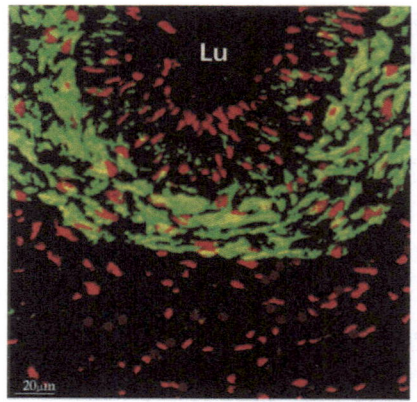

Fig. 10

Localization of α-smooth muscle actin by immunoconfocal microscopy. Specific fluorescence green, nuclei are red. The medial SMCs show intense α-smooth muscle actin staining but many neointimal cells are only weakly labeled. Lu-lumen

timal SMCs change not only their phenotype but exhibit an embryonal
expression pattern of their specific proteins[17]. While in normal non-
growing SMCs α-smooth muscle actin is the major protein, this is
reduced in growing collateral vessels (Fig. 10). Furthermore, the cytoskeletal protein desmin and the Ca-regulated calponin are decreased, whereas vimentin was strongly expressed (Figs. 11-13). This appearance corre-

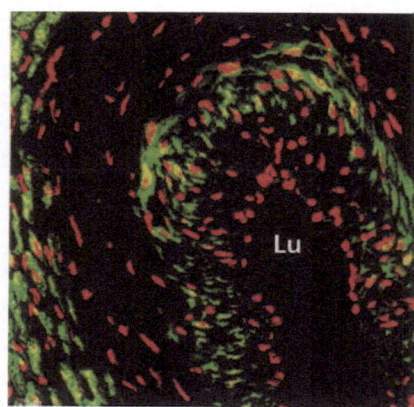

Fig. 11

Desmin (green, nuclei red) is present in SMCs of the media but absent from intimal SMCs. Lu-lumen

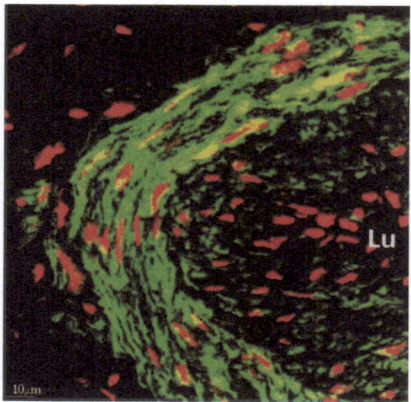

Fig. 12

Calponin (green-yellowish, nuclei red) is present in the media but significantly reduced in the neointima. Lu-lumen

sponds to the synthetic phenotype of SMCs as observed in the
electron microscope (Fig. 9). The
expression of vimentin instead
of desmin and the lack of α-
smooth muscle actin are typical
of embryonic SMCs[21], i.e., a reca-
pitulation of ontogeny occurs in
the cells of growing collateral vessels as previously described for
the ductus arteriosus in rabbits[22].

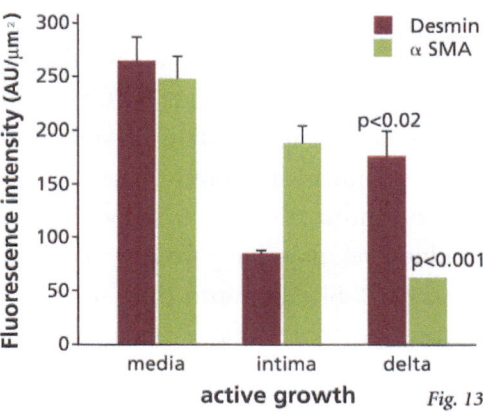

Fig. 13

Quantitative determination of fluorescence intensity of α-smooth muscle actin and desmin in the media and intima of actively growing vessels. The difference in intensity beween media and intima is statistically significant.

reprinted with permission from[17]

Desmin is one of the principal
intermediate filament proteins in
vascular smooth muscle. In SMCs
of smaller arteries and arterioles
the intermediate filaments contain
predominantly desmin. However, there is a relative paucity of information
regarding wether desmin expression is developmentally regulated in vascular smooth muscle. There exists one report that in the mammalian
embryo, from 9dpc onward desmin can be detected in vascular muscles[23].
Likewise, which role desmin plays in the regulation of SMCs functions remains unclear. However, the information from studies of desmin in skeletal
muscle indicates that desmin is essential to maintain tissue integrity, for
the tensile strength and integrity of myofibrils, and for terminal muscle
regeneration and maturation of muscle fibers. In desmin knockout mice,
the skeletal myofibers were disorganized, distended, and nonaligned. These
mice were weaker and fatigued easily[24,25]. Based on the findings from
skeletal muscle studies, it is concluded that the reduction of desmin in the
tunica media plays an important role in the development of collateral
vessels leading to a decrease in wall tension and facilitating the outward
expansion of the wall. Furthermore, the lack of desmin in SMCs of the
neointima and the reduction of α-smooth muscle actin indicate that these
cells will not significantly contribute to vasoconstriction or vasodilation.

Calponin, which is an actin-binding protein involved in the regulation
of smooth muscle shortening velocity, is a smooth muscle differentiation-
specific protein. It induces polymerization and inhibits depolymerization

of the thin filament actin[26], it shows a strong molecular resemblance with troponin T[27] and it possibly regulates crossbridge cycling during contraction[28]. Calponin inhibits SMCs growth, proliferation and migration, i.e., it maintains differentiation, and its reduction as observed in neointimal cells confirms the notion that SMCs may be susceptible to the action of pro-mitotic stimuli[29]. In calponin knockout mice a structural fragility of blood vessels accompanied by bleeding into the perivascular space was observed[30]. Bleeding into the neointima was not seen in collateral vessels, most probably because the intact endothelium and the media (still containing contractile SMCs with calponin) will prevent any direct contact with blood cells. The lack of calponin in the neointimal SMCs of growing vessels is taken to indicate SMC dedifferentiation into the synthetic phenotype.

Vinculin, a cytoskeleton-associated protein, is operative in establishing links between the extracellular matrix and the intracellular milieu via integrins[31]. It is reduced in SMCs of the neointima during the phase of active growth suggesting that the link with integrins might be weakened therefore allowing for cellular migration.

A new aspect of regulation of SMC proliferation might be disruption of N-cadherin cell-cell contacts mediated by MMP activity and involving ß-catenin release, which possibly induces ß-catenin-mediated cell signaling[32]. This, however, is data from cell culture experiments, which has to be confirmed *in vivo*, especially in view of the fact that SMCs in blood vessels lack any direct cell-cell contacts.

It is worth noting that some SMCs in the tunica media were still of the contractile phenotype indicated by high levels of calponin and α-SM actin although the basement membrane was fragmented. Apparently, there are more regulatory mechanisms involved in phenotype determination of SMCs. Many transcription factors as well as tissue-restricted proteins seem to be necessary to maintain or modulate the SMC phenotype (recently reviewed in [33]). Our own data indicate that matrix metalloproteinases (MMP, described below in detail) may be involved. The expression of MMP-2 and MMP-9 was very high in the early stage of collateral vessel growth, but reduced and low in the tunica media during active growth indicating that MMP activity is another important mediator controlling phenotype of SMCs. This view is supported by a recent study showing that the synthetic metalloproteinase inhibitor batimastat suppresses injury-induced phosphorylation of MAP kinase ERK1/ERK2 and phenotypic modification of arterial smooth muscle cells *in vitro*[34].

Degradation of the basement membrane facilitates SMC migration and expansion of the vascular wall, but if SMC migration were not controlled or limited, the integrity of the wall would be destroyed. MMPs promote SMC migration but tissue inhibitor of metalloproteinases (TIMP, discussed below) inhibits SMC migration. The low expression of MMPs and high amount of TIMP-1 and PAI-1 in the tunica media lead to the hypothesis that inhibition of MMPs most likely is an important contributor to limit the active movement of SMCs. This is in accordance with the findings that migration of SMCs in rabbit, rat and baboon explant cultures was inhibited using synthetic MMP inhibitors[36,37] or by overexpression of TIMP-1 in organ culture of human saphenous vein (HSV)[38].

Since a few years the possibility that SMCs can be derived from hematopoeitic progenitor cells is under investigation (reviewed in[39]). *In vitro*, bone marrow cells can differentiate into SMCs[40]. *In vivo*, SMCs in human atherosclerosis[41] or in neointimal lesions in rat aortic allografts[42] were shown to originate from injected bone marrow cells. Differentiation of Flk1 positive embryonic stem cells can be induced by adding VEGF for endothelial cells and PDGF-BB for mural (pericytes, SMCs) cells[43] indicating a higher degree of plasticity of a particular cell lineage than previously thought possible[44]. In a later study, it was confirmed that the fate of undifferentiated mesenchymal cells to develop into either endothelial cells or SMCs can be determined by exposure to growth factors or their receptors such as VEGF and PDGF-BB[45]. Since this is not the major topic of this chapter, only few examples regarding endothelial cells as well as SMCs have been cited here from the literature in order to show the beginning of an interesting field of research that may have implications later on for the therapeutic promotion of vascular growth. At the present time, it is too early to speculate on the role of bone marrow progenitor cells as contributing factors to collateral vessel growth because the role of circulating progenitors or of undifferentiated mesenchymal precursor cells is not yet satisfactorily established. One of the major uncertainties apparent in several studies is the fact that these undifferentiated cells are unsatisfactorily characterized before usage in animal experiments[46]. Methods, results and opinions vary widely regarding the possible potential of this new therapeutic principle as shown recently for cardiomyocytes[47]. Many more critical experimental studies have to be carried out before this question will be settled and a reliable concept established (see chapter 8).

The elastic membrane

The elastic membrane in normal vessels is a continuous sheath with multiple pores consisting of amorphous elastic material and surrounding microfibrils. In growing vessels, it is interrupted and may finally completely disappear (Figs. 6, 8, 9). New elastic material including the amorphous mass and its precursor tropoelastin and microfibrils can only sparsely be observed. These changes may have distinct functional consequences: loss of medial elasticity increases the possibility of endothelial damage and predisposition to atherosclerosis[48]. Furthermore, elastin has been shown to be essential for arterial morphogenesis and to regulate SMC proliferation, even in the absence of growth factors[20]. Lack of elastin results in vascular occlusion because of uninhibited SMC mitosis[20], which may play a role in collateral artery growth where elastic material is not fully replenished and its absence may be the cause of excessive neointima formation finally leading to vessel occlusion. In addition, the lack of a continuous elastic membrane may allow for passive outward movement of the vessel wall in response to elevated blood pressure. This process may be enhanced by disappearance of the SMC basement membranes and the elastic material of the adventitial layer (see below).

Interestingly, an ineffective elastogenesis seems to be ongoing in human atherosclerotic plaques and in abdominal aortic aneurysms, which would confirm the notion that dysregulated elastin synthesis accompanied by SMC proliferation causes vascular abnormalities[49].

Elastin and laminin can adhere to cells by a distinct transmembrane protein, the elastin-laminin receptor (ELR), which is different from the integrin family[50] and functions as a mechanotransducer sensitive for stretch in SMCs[19]. Moreover, a signaling pathway via the elastin receptor resulting in SMCs proliferation has recently been identified[51]. While lack of elastin results in SMCs proliferation, high dosages of elastin produce apoptotic and nonapoptotic cell death as shown in lymphocytes[52]. Further studies are needed to elucidate this possible effect in growing collateral vessels.

The extracellular matrix and matrix metalloproteinases

The extracellular matrix is situated between cells, either SMCs or fibroblasts in the media and in the adventitial layers. It consists of fibronectin and the proteoglycans, the different proteins of the basement membrane such as collagen IV and laminin and of the different types of fibrillar collagen, mostly collagen I but also collagen III and VI as well as fibronectin (Fig. 14). The amount of ECM differs, it is low in normal arterial vessels and it increases in growing collateral arteries, predominantly in the neointima (Fig. 15). It is collagen VI and fibronectin in particular that increase, whereas the fibrillar collagen I is rarely seen

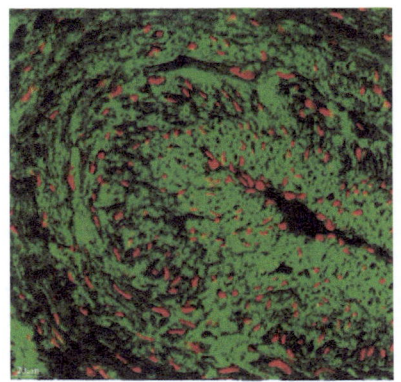

Fig. 14

Fibronectin (green, nuclei are red) in an actively growing vessel. Fibronectin is accumulated in the neointima and in the adventitia but the media only contains moderate amounts of this ECM protein.

reprinted with permission from[70]

in the neointima of vessels undergoing active growth. In mature vessels, collagen I is again detectable. Recently, it has been reported that polymerized collagen I suppresses SMC proliferation[53] as well as fibronectin, thrombospondin and tenascin-C expression and the migratory response of SMCs to fibronectin[54]. In view of these data, downregulation of collagen I can be interpreted as part of the shift of balance of protein expression (discussed below) to enable the vessel to enlarge. The overexpression of

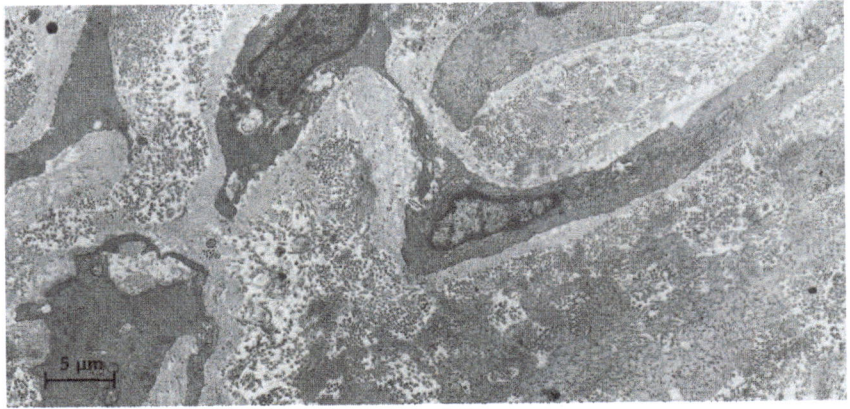

Fig. 15

Ultrastructural appearance of SMCs and the ECM in the neointima of a growing vessel. Large amounts of ECM separate the SMCs.

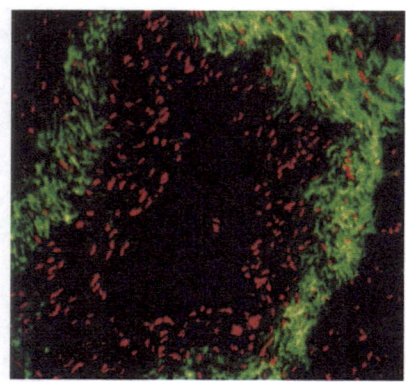

Fig. 16

Tenascin (green, nuclei red) is present in large amounts in the media but absent from the intima.

collagen VI provides further evidence that an embryonal protein pattern is recapitulated in growing collateral vessels[55]. Furthermore, an interaction between collagen VI and glycoproteins is particularly relevant in matrix assembly[56].

In the neointima, remnants of basement membrane material are abundant including laminin and collagen IV and glycoproteins are strongly increased[17]. The latter finding is especially interesting because several of the glycoproteins are capable of regulating synthesis of other structural components. Tenascin-C, which was significantly decreased in the intima (Fig. 16), is effective in preventing fibronectin induced cellular adhesion[57,58] and this effect can be neutralized by chondroitin sulfate[59]. The reduction of tenascin-C in combination with an increase in chondroitin sulfate and fibronectin in growing collateral vessels will then be responsible for cellular migration and adhesion (Fig. 16). In addition, tenascin has been described to possess proangiogenic properties, enhancing the sprouting, migratory, and survival effects of angiogenic growth factors, and it has distinct proliferative, migratory, and protective effects on endothelial cells in culture [60,61]. The data suggests that tenascin may act as a proangiogenic mediator in pathologic conditions involving neovascularization but that in arteriogenesis the inhibitory effect may be more prominent requiring downregulation or counteraction by other proteins. In general, the balance between the different matrix proteins seems to be decisive for the continuation or termination of the growth process.

The same consideration applies to the action of the proteolytic enzymes metalloproteinases (MMP) and their inhibitors, the tissue inhibitors of MMP (TIMP). Our own data show that in growing collateral vessels, MMP-2 and MMP-9 are upregulated in the intima and activated, compared to the media of the same vessel (Fig. 17). The opposite is true for TIMP-1, which is increased, however, in the intima of mature vessels (Fig. 17, 18). This led to the conclusion that vascular remodeling by protein

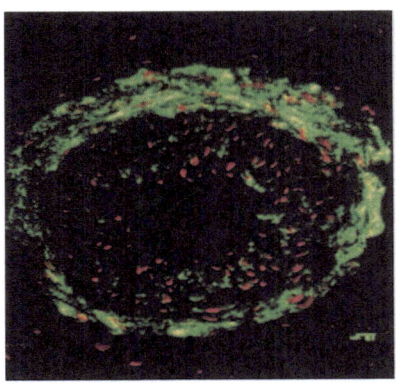
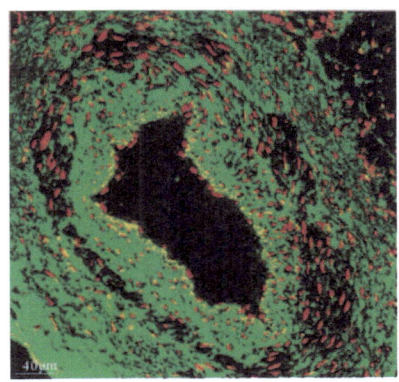

Fig. 17 a   Fig. 17 b

*Localization of MMP-2 and TIMP-1 (green, nuclei are red) in an actively growing vessel.
17a) The concentration of MMP is high in the neointima and low in the media. 17b) TIMP-1
is low in the intima and high in the media indicating a counterbalance between proteolysis
and its inhibition.*

degradation and lack of inhibition by TIMP was facilitated by the action
of MMP. Similar results were obtained by Tyagi on the mRNA level[62].

The intima of growing vessels contained more PAI-1 than the media, but
the media of both, growing and mature vessels showed an increase compared to control vessels (Fig. 18 and 19). It was suggested that PAI-1 plays
an important role in protecting the intima from excess proteolysis during
cell migration, proliferation and tissue remodeling[63,64]. In other studies it
was shown that PAI-1 inhibits cellular migration and neointima formation[65,66]. This confirms our previously postulated concept that proteolysis
and antiproteolysis need to be in balance in order to permit for effective
vascular remodeling[67]. The increased expression of PAI-1 in the presence
of downregulated TIMP-1 suggests a selfregulatory mechanism in collateral formation. A coordinated upregulation of bFGF and PDGF with that
of MMP-1 and MMP-9 was observed in growing vessels (Fig. 20) indicating
regulation of MMP expression by growth factors as described by others[68].

Regulation of MMPs by mechanical stress via the endothelin A receptor
has been reported[69] and this might be operative in growing collaterals,
where wall stress is increased as well. A contrasting observation is the fact
that selective MMP inhibition apparently elicited an angiogenic response
after myocardial infarction in rabbit hearts, and that it even doubled the
number of arterioles during ventricular remodeling[8], which shows that
much more evidence provided by careful experimental studies is needed
to clarify this issue.

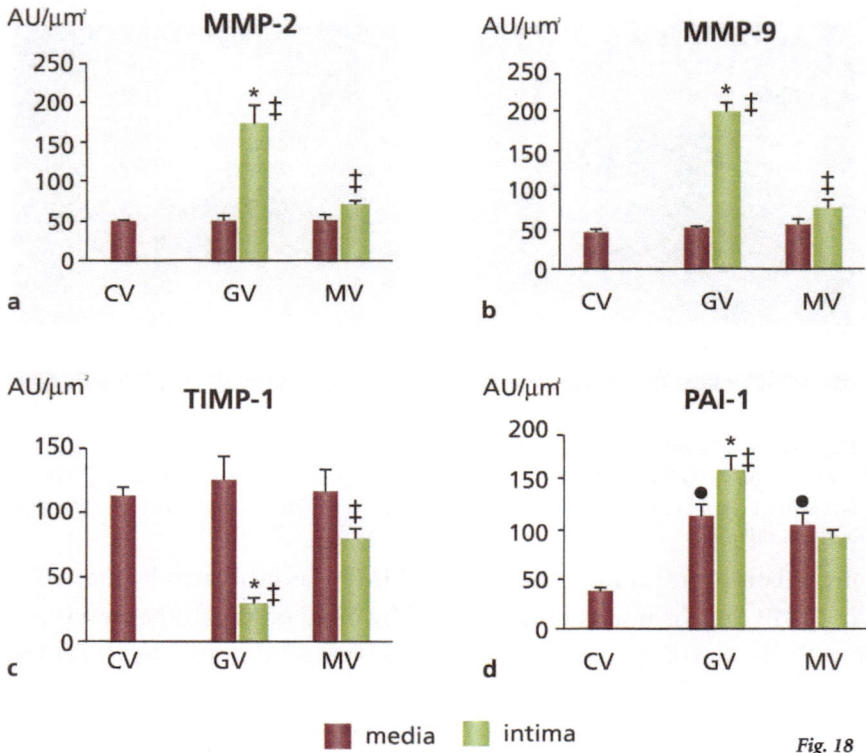

■ media ■ intima

Fig. 18

Measurements of fluorescence intensity of MMP-2 and MMP-9, TIMP-1, and PAI-1 in the media and intima of control (CV), growing (GV) and mature (MV) vessels. *p<0.001, intima of GV vs neointima of MV; ‡p<0.001 intima vs media in same vessels; •p <0.001, media of GV or MV vs media of CV. AU = arbitrary units

reprinted with permission from [67]

There is no doubt, however, that controlled proteolysis plays an important role in collateral vessel growth. The temporal and spatial expression pattern of MMPs and their inhibitors TIMP and PAI-1 is associated with migration, proliferation and rearrangement of SMCs. The balance between these factors, proteolysis, antiproteolysis and proliferation of SMCs will decide the outcome of the growth process.

The adventitia

In normal arteriolar vessels or small arteries, the adventitia is a small rim of connective tissue surrounding the medial layer and it consists mostly of ECM and few fibroblasts. In growing collateral vessels, the adventitia is widened and proliferation of fibroblasts is evident. The number of fibroblasts was 5-fold elevated in growing vessels[70]. There was no evidence for the presence of myofibroblasts, neither in the adventitia nor in other layers of the vessel. This is in accordance with a report by Maeng that adventitial fibroblasts do not play a role in neointima formation[71], but it is in contradiction to another report describing migration of adventitial fibroblasts into the neointima[72], both in cases of vascular injury. Apparently, this problem is not solved yet. However, in collateral arteries adventitial myofibroblasts do not seem to be involved in the growth process.

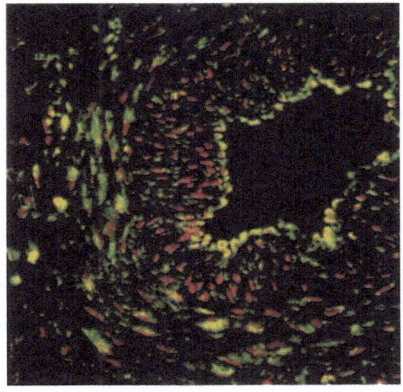

Fig. 19

Localization of PAI-1 (green, nuclei red) in a growing collateral vessel. PAI-1 is highest in the subendothelial part of the neointima.

Fibroblasts in the adventitia show signs of activation such as increased number of cellular organelles. They proliferate but some of them undergo apoptosis. In mature vessels, these changes disappear. In accordance with a recent report[73], it may be postulated that the cause of activation lies in the elevation of mechanical tension, represented by increased blood pressure and increased shear stress.

Interestingly, the elastic fiber content in normal vessels was 25-fold higher than in

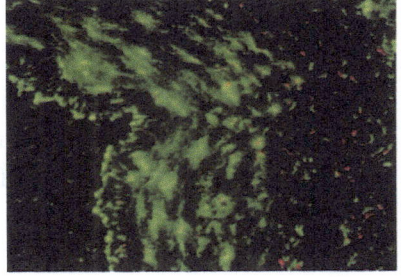

Fig. 20

Localization of bFGF (green, nuclei are red) in an actively growing vessel corresponding to that of Fig. 19. bFGF is abundant in the neointima.

collaterals, a phenomenon, which may support proliferation of medial SMCs and adventitial fibroblasts[70]. Mast cells were more numerous in the adventitia of collaterals than in normal vessels[17].

Adventitial MMP-2, MMP-9 and fibronectin as well as bFGF and PAI-1 were strongly upregulated as compared to normal vessels (Fig. 21). Perivascular myocyte damage and induction of eNOS in capillaries between the adventitia and the myocardium indicate expansion of growing vessels. It is concluded that adventitial activation is associated with the development of collateral vessels through cell proliferation, production of growth factors, and induction of extracellular proteolysis thereby contributing to remodeling during adaptive arteriogenesis[70].

Early markers of vascular growth

In search of early structural markers of arteriogenesis, we studied the expression of gap junction proteins. Gap junctions are specialized regions of the sarcolemma containing intercellular channels, which provide a pathway for ions, metabolites, fluid and messenger proteins. Connexins (Cx) of various isoforms are the gap junction proteins. In normal vessels, Cx37 and Cx40 were found bridging the endothelial cells. Cx43 was absent. SMCs were not connected by connexins. In growing vessels, Cx 37, but not the other isoforms of Cx was expressed in the SMC layer (Fig. 22). This may have been caused by an altered hemodynamic situation, i.e., by increased tangential wall stress[74]. From this study it was concluded that induced Cx37 is an early signal of adaptive arteriogenesis.

Furthermore, calponin, α-SM actin, desmin and vinculin that are evenly expressed in SMCs in normal vessels, are suitable as early markers because they are reduced in the neointimal SMCs of growing vessels. Of these proteins, desmin was the most sensitive showing a 3-fold reduction in the stage of early growth where the other proteins were still within the normal range. In actively growing vessels, α-SM actin, calponin and vinculin were 3-, 3.3- and 2.9-fold lower, respectively, in the neointima compared to the media. In comparison, Cx37 was 3 times higher in the media than in the neointima. Desmin was almost absent in the neointima and 5-fold reduced in the media. Our findings indicate that induction of Cx37 and reduction of desmin precede the phenotypic changes of SMCs, which are characterized by downregulation of α-SM actin, calponin and vinculin, and the formation of a neointima. An altered expression of Cx37 and desmin, therefore, is recommended as early markers for arteriogenesis[75].

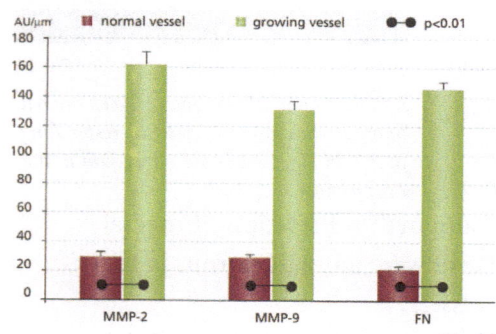

Fig. 21

Measurements of fluorescence intensity of MMP-2, MMP-9 and fibronectin (FN) in the adventitia of normal and growing collateral vessels. A significant increase in the concentration of the proteolytic enzymes as well as of the ECM protein fibronectin can be observed. AU = arbitrary units

reprinted with permission from[70]

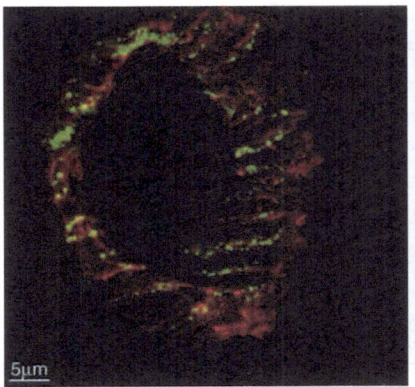 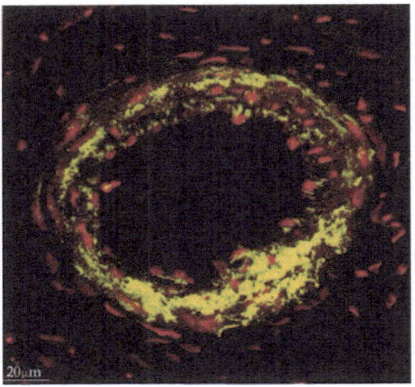

Fig. 22 a   *Fig. 22 b*

Connexin 40 and 37 show similar localization (green, nuclei are red). 22a) In normal vessels Cx40 is localized exclusively in the endothelial layer. 22b) In growing vessels, Cx37 is present in the SMC layer (yellow).

II. Collateral vessels in the peripheral circulation of rabbit and mouse

The model employed in both animal species consists of acute occlusion of one femoral artery while the contralateral side is used as control. Since the model uses acute occlusion, the time course is different from that in canine cardiac collaterals where a phase of stenosis precedes that of occlusion. Another difference is the extension of the neointima, which is much smaller in rabbit collaterals as compared to dog coronary collateral vessels, and which is almost nonexistent in mouse collateral vessels. The growth of rabbit collateral vessels finally results in a well-organized vessel wall where a neointimal layer cannot be discerned anymore at later stages.

Proliferation and phenotype changes

In rabbit collateral arteries, the nuclear proliferation marker Ki-67 detected the first mitotic activity after 24 hours. It achieved its maximum between days 3-7 and faded slowly thereafter, distinguishable still at day 21 (Fig. 23). Mitosis was observed in all layers of the vessel, in endothelial cells and medial SMCs as well as in the fibroblasts of the adventitia. By electron microscopy, endothelial cells and a large number of the SMCs contained many free ribosomes and rough endoplasmic reticulum sug-

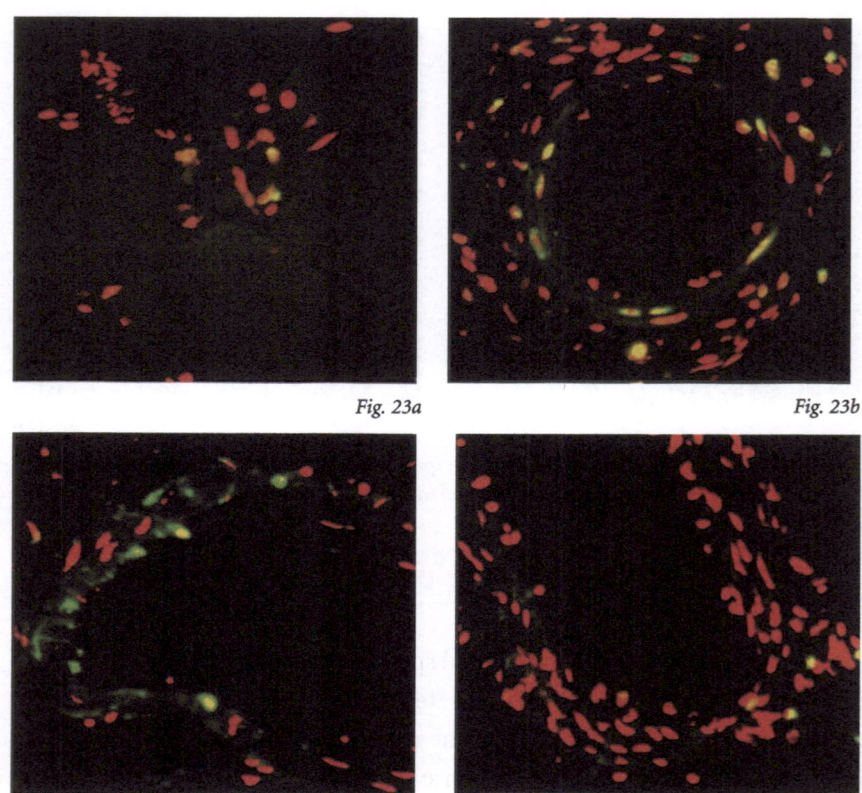

Fig. 23a

Fig. 23b

Fig. 23c

Fig. 23d

Cellular proliferation in growing collateral arteries. 23a) 2 days, 23b) 3 days, 23c) 7 days, 23d) 21 days after occlusion of the femoral artery. All proliferative cells are labeled yellow in contrast to Ki 67, nuclei are red.

gesting that these cells were transforming from the contractile into the proliferative-synthetic phenotype. Five to seven days after occlusion a very prominent rough endoplasmic reticulum indicated strong synthetic activity in all layers of the arterial wall.

Lamina elastica interna and neointima formation, extracellular matrix

Ten to fourteen days after femoral occlusion in rabbit a neointima becomes evident. While SMCs in the lamina media are circularly arranged, the intimal SMCs are directed helically, and are smaller than the medial cells.

Fragments of the original internal elastic lamina were still present in growing vessels, but newly synthesized elastic material including the amorphous mass and microfibrils was also found. In contrast with cardiac collateral vessels, the fragmentation of the original internal elastica was only partial. Asymmetry of neointima formation was obvious. It appeared half-moon-like with foci of subendothelial growth under which ·the lamina elastica interna was disrupted and the media disorganized. These regions probably represent the sites of immigration of the medial SMCs into the neointima.

The process of neointima formation and lysis of the internal elastic membrane is thus spatially restricted and involves matrix metalloproteinases[67]. Electron microscopic and immunohistochemical data suggests that all cells in the arteriogenic neointima are SMCs[76,77] as described originally in the intimal injury model in rabbits[78].

Besides the role of matrix metalloproteinases in neointima formation, these enzymes have also been shown to play an important role in monocyte transmigration[79]. In numerous studies using different *in vitro* as well as *in vivo* models the monocytes/macrophages were found to have the capacity to produce various MMPs, including MMP-1, MMP-3, MMP-7, MMP-9, MMP-12 and MT1-MMP (for review see[80]). MMP-9 expression by monocytes has been shown to be induced by exposure to lipopolysaccharide[81] or by direct contact with T-lymphocytes[82] and endothelial cells [83]. Endothelial cells alone may also secrete stimulators for MMP-9 secretion in monocytes[83]. The central role of monocytes in the early phases of collateral artery growth was functionally proven by the modulation of the arteriogenic response which depended on the monocyte concentration in peripheral blood[84]. Moreover, stimulation of monocyte activation and chemotaxis with monocyte chemoattractant protein-1 (MCP-1) promoted arteriogenesis[85]. Recently, we found that stimulation of collateral artery growth by MCP-1 in rabbits was accompanied by a local increase in protein content and/or activity of MMP-1, MMP-2, MMP-3 and MMP-9[86] (Fig. 24). We also demonstrated the presence of MMPs in the intima of growing rabbit hind limb collateral arteries and in the perivascular space. In order to inhibit MMP activity we used the synthetic MMP inhibitor BB-94. BB-94 treatment resulted in reduction of protein content

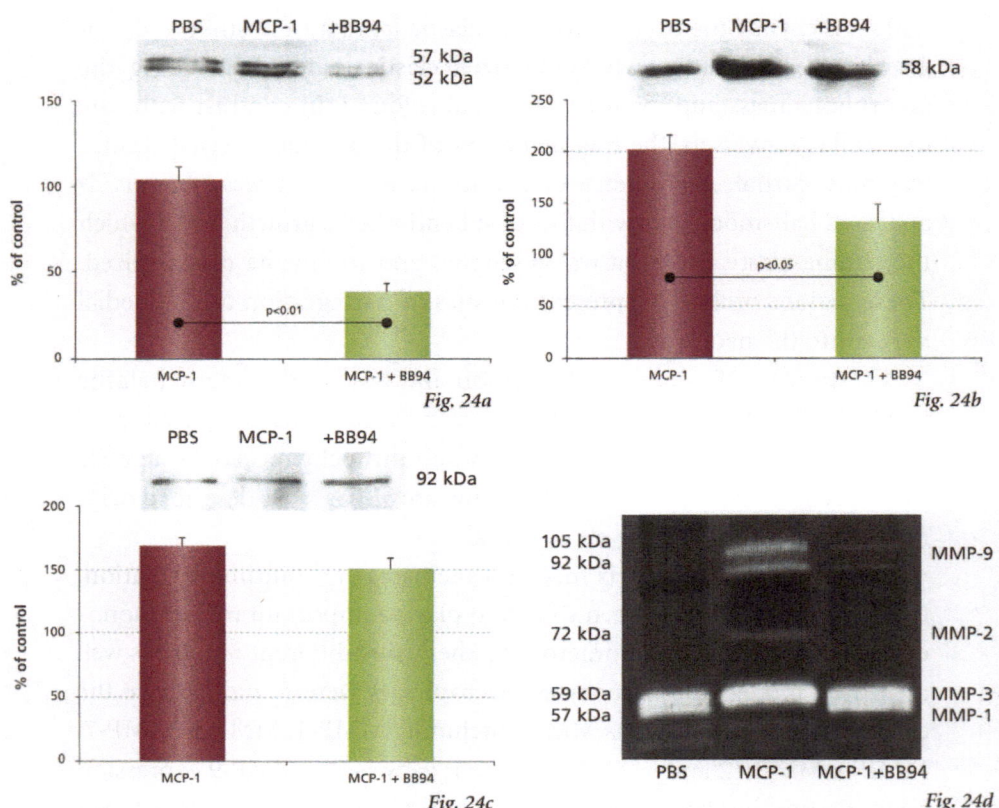

MMP-1 (a), MMP-3 (b) and MMP-9 (c) protein content (Western blot analysis) and activity (d, gelatin zymography) in growing collateral arteries 1 week after femoral artery occlusion in rabbits receiving either PBS, MCP-1 or MCP-1 + BB94.

and/or activity of MMP-1, MMP-2, MMP-3 and MMP-9 (Fig. 24). In addition, this treatment strongly attenuated the positive effect of MCP-1 stimulation on collateral artery growth as shown by the decrease in collateral conductance and angiographic score[86] (Fig. 25). Thus, these data accentuated the physiological importance of matrix metalloproteinases in collateral artery growth and particularly in monocyte transmigration and neointima formation.

At twenty-one days after occlusion the neointima contained maximally 3-4 and at 42 days maximally 6-7 layers of SMCs with new elastic material between the new layers.

Six to eight months after arterial occlusion the ultrastructure of collateral vessels was similar to that after 21-42 days. All SMCs exhibited the contractile phenotype. Endothelial cells were quiescent.

Differences of morphological aspects in arteriogenesis of the peripheral circulation between rabbits and mice are minimal with regard to time course. The formation of a neointima is less pronounced in mice than in rabbits. Preexistent collateral arterioles contain usually only one layer of SMCs in mice and 1-2 layers in rabbits. Proliferative activity of SMCs results in additional layers of SMCs in rabbits but not in mice. There, the circular layer is widened by addition of more SMCs; the cells are hypertrophied with large nuclei resulting in

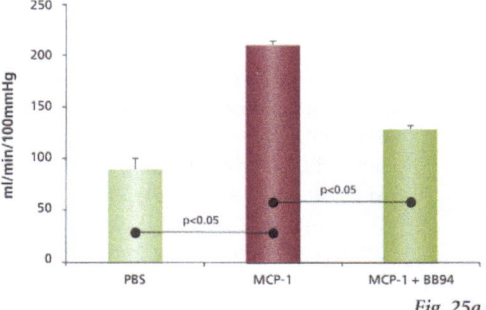

Fig. 25a

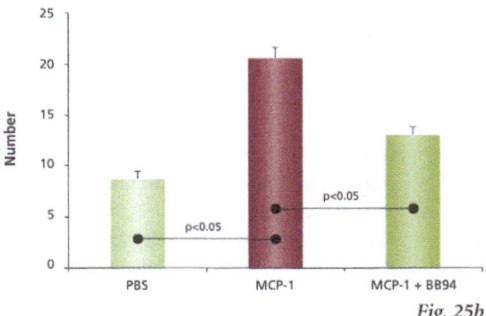

Fig. 25b

Collateral conductance (a) and number of visible collateral arteries (b) of the hind limb 1 week after femoral artery occlusion in rabbits receiving either PBS, MCP-1 or MCP-1 + BB94.

thickening of the vessel wall. Vessel wall thickening, therefore, occurs by enlargement of the media and less by neointima formation. Migration of SMCs seems to play a minor role in collateral vessel growth of smaller animals.

References

1. PALMER RM, FERRIGE AG, MONCADA S. Nitric oxide release accounts for the biological activity of endothelium-derived relaxing factor. *Nature.* 1987;327:524-6.
2. MYERS PR, MINOR RLJ, GUERRA RJ, BATES JN, HARRISON DG. Vasorelaxant properties of the endothelium-derived relaxing factor more closely resemble S-nitrosocysteine than nitric oxide. *Nature.* 1990;345:161-3.
3. FURCHGOTT RF, ZAWADZKI JV. The obligatory role of endothelial cells in the relaxation of arterial smooth muscle by acetylcholine. *Nature.* 1980;288:373-6.
4. SCHMIDT HH, WALTER U. NO at work. *Cell.* 1994;23:919-25.
5. SZMITKO PE, FEDAK PW, WEISEL RD, STEWART DJ, KUTRYK MJ, VERMA S. Endothelial progenitor cells: new hope for a broken heart. *Circulation.* 2003;107:3093-100
5a. ZIEGELHOEFFER T, FERNÁNDEZ, B, KOSTIN S, HEIL M, VOSWINCKEL R, HELISCH A, SCHAPER W. Bone Marrow-Derived Cells Do Not Incorporate Into the Adult Growing Vasculature. *Circ Res.* Dec 2003; online
6. KALKA C, MASUDA H, TAKAHASHI T, GORDON R, TEPPER O, GRAVEREAUX E, PIECZEK A, IWAGURO H, HAYASHI SI, ISNER JM, ASAHARA T. Vascular endothelial growth factor(165) gene transfer augments circulating endothelial progenitor cells in human subjects. *Circ Res.* 2000;86:1198-202.
7. KOCHER AA, SCHUSTER MD, SZABOLCS MJ, TAKUMA S, BURKHOFF D, WANG J, HOMMA S, EDWARDS NM, ITESCU S. Neovascularization of ischemic myocardium by human bone-marrow-derived angioblasts prevents cardiomyocyte apoptosis, reduces remodeling and improves cardiac function. *Nat Med.* 2001;7:430-6.
8. LINDSEY ML, GANNON J, AIKAWA M, SCHOEN FJ, RABKIN E, LOPRESTI-MORROW L, CRAWFORD J, BLACK S, LIBBY P, MITCHELL PG, LEE RT. Selective matrix metalloproteinase inhibition reduces left ventricular remodeling but does not inhibit angiogenesis after myocardial infarction. *Circulation.* 2002;105:753-8.
9. DOR Y, DJONOV V, KESHET E. Induction of vascular networks in adult organs: implications to proangiogenic therapy. *Ann N Y Acad Sci.* 2003;95:208-16.
10. KAMIHATA H, MATSUBARA H, NISHIUE T, FUJIYAMA S, TSUTSUMI Y, OZONO R, MASAKI H, MORI Y, IBA O, TATEISHI E, KOSAKI A, SHINTANI S, MUROHARA T, IMAIZUMI T, IWASAKA T. Implantation of bone marrow mononuclear cells into ischemic myocardium enhances collateral perfusion and regional function via side supply of angioblasts, angiogenic ligands, and cytokines. *Circulation.* 2001;104:1046-52.
11. HEDIN U, BOTTGER BA, LUTHMAN J, JOHANSSON S, THYBERG J. A substrate of the cell-attachment sequence of fibronectin (Arg-Gly-Asp-Ser) is sufficient to promote transition of arterial smooth muscle cells from a contractile to a synthetic phenotype. *Dev Biol.* 1989;133:489-501.
12. THYBERG J. Phenotypic modulation of smooth muscle cells during formation of neointimal thickenings following vascular injury. *Histol Histopathol.* 1998;13:871-91.
13. MOISEEVA EP. Adhesion receptors of vascular smooth muscle cells and their functions. *Cardiovasc Res.* 2001;52:372-86.
14. RUOSLAHTI E. INTEGRINS. *J Clin Invest.* 1991;87:1-5.
15. LAFRENIE RM, YAMADA KM. Integrin-dependent signal transduction. *J Cell Biochem.* 1996;61:543-553.

16. PALECEK SP, LOFTUS JC, GINSBERG MH, LAUFFENBURGER DA, HORWITZ AF. integrin-ligand binding properties govern cell migration speed through cell-substratum adhesiveness. *Nature.* 1997;385:537-40.

17. WOLF C, CAI W-J, VOSSCHULTE R, KOLTAI S, MOUSAVIPOUR D, SCHOLZ D, AFSAH-HEDJRI A, SCHAPER W, SCHAPER J. Vascular remodeling and altered protein expression during growth of coronary collateral arteries. *J Mol Cell Cardiol.* 1998;30:2291-305.

18. WERNIG F, MAYR M, XU Q. Mechanical stretch-induced apoptosis in smooth muscle cells is mediated by beta1-integrin signaling pathways. *Hypertension.* 2003;41:903-11.

19. SPOFFORD CM, CHILIAN WM. The elastin-laminin receptor functions as a mechanotransducer in vascular smooth muscle. *Am J Physiol Heart Circ Physiol.* 2001;280:H1354-60.

20. LI DY, BROOKE B, DAVIS EC, MECHAM RP, SORENSEN LK, BOAK BB, EICHWALD E, KEATING MT. Elastin is an essential determinant of arterial morphogenesis. *Nature.* 1998;393:276-80.

21. GABBIANI G, SCHMID E, WINTER S, CHAPONNIER C, DE CHASTONAY C, VANDEKERCKHOVE J, WEBER K, FRANKE WW. Vascular smooth muscle cells differ from other smooth muscle cells: predominance of vimentin filaments and a specific alpha-type actin. *Proc Natl Acad Sci USA.* 1981;78:298-301.

22. GIURIATO L. Rabbit ductus arteriosus during development: anatomical structure and smooth muscle cell composition. *Anat Rec.* 1993;235:95-110.

23. LI Z, MARCHAND P, HUMBERT J, BABINET C, PAULIN D. Desmin sequence elements regulating skeletal muscle-specific expression in transgenic mice. *Development.* 1993;117:947-59.

24. LI Z, MERICSKAY M, AGBULUT O, BUTLER-BROWNE G, CARLSSON L, THORNELL L-E, BABINET C, PAULIN D. Desmin is essential for the tensile strength and integrity of myofibrils but not for myogenic commitment, differentiation, and fusion of skeletal muscle. *J Cell Biol.* 1997;139:129-144.

25. AGBULUT O, LI Z, PERIE S, LUDOSKY MA, PAULIN D, CARTAUD J, BUTLER-BROWNE G. Lack of desmin results in abortive muscle regeneration and modifications in synaptic structure. *Cell Motil Cytoskeleton.* 2001;49:51-66.

26. KAKE T, KIMURA S, TAKAHASHI K, MARUYAMA K. Calponin induces actin polymerization at low ionic strength and inhibits depolymerization of actin filaments. *Biochem J.* 1995;-312:587-92.

27. SMALL J, FUERST D, THORNELL L. Review: The cytoskeletal lattice of muscle cells. *Eur J Biochem.* 1992;208:559-572.

28. MATTHEW JD, KHROMOV AS, MCDUFFIE MJ, SOMLYO AP, TANIGUCHI S, TAKAHASHI K. Contractile properties and proteins of smooth muscles of a calponin knockout mouse. *J Physiol.* 2000;529:811-24

29. TAKAHASHI K, TAKAGI M, OGHAMI K, NAKAI M, KOJIMA A, NADALL-GINARD B, SHIBATA N. Inhibition of smooth muscle cell migration and proliferation caused by transfection of the human calponin gene is associated with enhanced cell matrix adhesion and reduced PDGF responsiveness. *Circulation.* 1993;88:1-174.

30. TANIGUCHI S, TAKEOKA M, EHARA T, HASHIMOTO S, SHIBUKI H, YOSHIMURA N, SHIGEMATSU H, TAKAHASHI K, KATSUKI M. Structural fragility of blood vessels and peritoneum in calponin h1-deficient mice, resulting in an increase in hematogenous metastasis and peritoneal dissemination of malignant tumor cells. *Cancer Res.* 2001;61:7627-34.

31. BURRIDGE K, FERAMISCO JR. Microinjection and localization of a 130 K protein in living fibroblasts: A relationship to actin and fibronectin. *Cell.* 1980;19:587-597.

32. UGLOW EB, SLATER S, SALA-NEWBY GB, AGUILERA-GARCIA CM, ANGELINI GD, NEWBY AC, GEORGE SJ. Dismantling of cadherin-mediated cell-cell contacts modulates smooth muscle cell proliferation. *Circ Res.* 2003;92:1314-21.

33. KUMAR MS, OWENS GK. Combinatorial control of smooth muscle-specific gene expression. *Arterioscler Thromb Vasc Biol.* 2003;23:737-47.

34. RONNOV-JESSEN L, PETERSEN OW. A function of filamentous α-smooth muscle actin: retardation of. 1996;

35. DENGER S, JAHN L, WENDE P, WATSON L, GERBER SH, KUBLER W, KREUZER J. Expression of monocyte chemoattractant protein-1 cDNA in vascular smooth muscle cells: induction of the synthetic phenotype: a possible clue to SMC differentiation in the process of atherogenesis. *Atherosclerosis.* 1999;144:15-23.

36. PAULY RR, PASSANITI A, BILATO C, MONTICONE R, CHENG L, PAPADOPOULOS N, GLUZBAND YA, SMITH L, WEINSTEIN C, E.G. L. Migration of cultured vascular smooth muscle cells through a basement membrane barrier requires type IV collagenase activity and is inhibited by cellular differentiation. *Circ Res.* 1994;75:41-54.

37. KENAGY RD, HART CE, STETLER-STEVENSON WG, CLOWES AW. Primate smooth muscle cell migration from aortic explants is mediated by endogenous platelet-derived gowth factor and basic fibroblast growth factor acting through matrix metalloproteinases 2 and 9. *Circulation.* 1997;96:3555-3560.

38. GEORGE SJ, JOHNSON JL, ANGELINI GD, NEWBY AC, BAKER AH. Adenovirus-mediated gene transfer of the human TIMP-1 gene inhibits smooth muscle cell migration and neointimal formation in human saphenous vein. *Hum Gene Ther.* 1998;10:867-77.

39. CHIU RC. Adult stem cell therapy for heart failure. *Expert Opin Biol Ther.* 2003;3:215-25.

40. KASHIWAKURA Y, KATOH Y, TAMAYOSE K, KONISHI H, TAKAYA N, YUHARA S, YAMADA M, SUGIMOTO K, DAIDA H. Isolation of bone marrow stromal cell-derived smooth muscle cells by a human SM22alpha promoter: *in vitro* differentiation of putative smooth muscle progenitor cells of bone marrow. *Circulation.* 2003;107:2078-81.

41. CAPLICE NM, BUNCH TJ, STALBOERGER PG, WANG S, SIMPER D, MILLER DV, RUSSELL SJ, LITZOW MR, EDWARDS WD. Smooth muscle cells in human coronary atherosclerosis can originate from cells administered at marrow transplantation. *Proc Natl Acad Sci USA.* 2003;100:4754-9.

42. RELIGA P, BOJAKOWSKI K, MAKSYMOWICZ M, BOJAKOWSKA M, SIRSJO A, GACIONG Z, OLSZEWSKI W, HEDIN U, THYBERG J. Smooth-muscle progenitor cells of bone marrow origin contribute to the development of neointimal thickenings in rat aortic allografts and injured rat carotid arteries. *Transplantation.* 2002;74:1310-5.

43. YAMASHITA J, ITOH H, HIRASHIMA M, OGAWA M, NISHIKAWA S, YURUGI T, NAITO M, NAKAO K, NISHIKAWA S. Flk1-positive cells derived from embryonic stem cells serve as vascular progenitors. *Nature.* 2000;408:92-6.

44. D'AMORE PA. Kissing cousins-evidence for a common vascular cell precursor. *Nat Med.* 2000;6:1323-4.

45. MUNOZ-CHAPULI R, GONZALEZ-IRIARTE M, CARMONA R, ATENCIA G, MACIAS D, PEREZ-POMARES JM. Cellular precursors of the coronary arteries. *Tex Heart Inst J.* 2002;29:243-9.

46. ORKIN SH. Stem cell alchemy. *Nature Medicine.* 2000;6:1212-1213.

47. LAFLAMME MA, MYERSON D, SAFFITZ JE, MURRY CE. Evidence for cardiomyocyte repopulation by extracardiac progenitors in transplanted human hearts. *Circ Res.* 2002;90:634-40.

48. Avolio A, Jones D, M. T-S. Quantification of alterations in structure and function of elastin in the arterial media. *Hypertension.* 1998;32:170-5.
49. Krettek A, Sukhova GK, Libby P, . Elastogenesis in human arterial disease: a role for macrophages in disordered elastin synthesis. *Arterioscler Thromb Vasc Biol.* 2003;23:582-7.
50. Hinek A. Biological roles of the non-integrin elastin/laminin receptor. *Biol Chem.* 1996;377(7-8):471-80.
51. Mochizuki S, Brassart B, Hinek A. Signaling pathways transduced through the elastin receptor facilitate proliferation of arterial smooth muscle cells. *J Biol Chem.* 2002;277: 44854-63.
52. Peterszegi G, Robert L. Cell death induced in lymphocytes expressing the elastin-laminin receptor by excess agonists: necrosis and apoptosis. *Biomed Pharmacother.* 1998;52: 369-77.
53. Koyama H, Raines EW, Bornfeldt KE, Roberts JM, Ross R. Fibrillar collagen inhibits arterial smooth muscle proliferation through regulation of Cdk2 inhibitors. *Cell.* 1996; 87: 1069-78.
54. Ichii T, Koyama H, Tanaka S, Kim S, Shioi A, Okuno Y, Raines EW, Iwao H, Otani S, Nishizawa Y. Fibrillar collagen specifically regulates human vascular smooth muscle cell genes involved in cellular responses and the pericellular matrix environment. *Circ Res.* 2001;88:460-7.
55. Burke RD, Wang D, Jones VM. Ontogeny of vessell wall components in the outflow tract of the chick. *Anat Embryol.* 1994;189:447-456.
56. Wiberg C, Klatt AR, Wagener R, Paulsson M, Bateman JF, Heinegard D, Morgelin M. Complexes of matrilin-1 and biglycan or decorin connect collagen VI microfibrils to both collagen II and aggrecan. *J Biol Chem.* 2003;ahead of print:
57. Chiquet-Ehrisman R, Kalla P, Pearson CA, Beck K, Chiquet M. Tenascin interferes with fibronectin action. *Cell.* 1988;53:383-390.
58. Mackie EJ, Scott-Burden T, Hahn AWA, Kern F, Bernhardt J, Regenass S, Weller A, Buehler FR. Expression of tenascin by vascular smooth muscle cells. *Am J Pathol.* 1992; 141:377-388.
59. Murphy-Ullrich JE, Lightner VA, Aukhil I, Yan YZ, Erickson HP, Hoeoek M. Focal adhesion integrity is downregulated by the alternatively spliced domain of human tenascin. *J Cell Biol.* 1991;115:1127-1136.
60. Castellon R, Caballero S, Hamdi HK, Atilano SR, Aoki AM, Tarnuzzer RW, Kenney MC, Grant MB, Ljubimov AV. Effects of tenascin-C on normal and diabetic retinal endothelial cells in culture. *Invest Ophthalmol Vis Sci.* 2002;43:2758-66.
61. Zagzag D, Shiff B, Jallo GI, Greco MA, Blanco C, Cohen H, Hukin J, Allen JC, Friedlander DR. Tenascin-C promotes microvascular cell migration and phosphorylation of focal adhesion kinase. *Cancer Res.* 2002;62:2660-8.62.
62. Tyagi SC, Kumar S, Cassatt S, Parker JL. Temporal expression of extracellular matrix metalloproteinases and tissue plasminogen activator in the development of collateral vessels in the canine model of coronary occlusion. *Can J Physiol Pharmacol.* 1996;74::983-95.
63. Reidy M, Irvin C, Lindner V. Migration of arterial wall cells: Expression of plasminogen activators and inhibitors in injured rat arteries. *Circ Res.* 1996;78:405-414.
64. Hasenstab D, Forough R, Clowes AW. Plasminogen activator inhibitor type 1 and tissue inhibitor of metallo proteinases-2 increase after arterial injury in rats. *Circulation Research.* 1997;80:490-496.

65. CARMELIET P, MOONS L, LIJNEN R, JANSSENS S, LUPU F, COLLEN D, GERARD RD. Inhibitory role of plasminogen activator inhibitor-1 in arterial wound healing and neointima formation: a gene targeting and gene transfer study in mice. *Circulation.* 1997;96:3180-91.

66. CARMELIET P, MOONS L, HERBERT JM, CRAWLEY J, LUPU F, LIJNEN R, COLLEN D. Urokinase but not tissue plasminogen activator mediates arterial neointima formation in mice. *Circ Res.* 1997;81:829-39.

67. CAI W-J, VOSSCHULTE R, AFSAH-HEDJRI A, KOLTAI S, KOCSIS E, SCHOLZ D, KOSTIN S, SCHAPER W, SCHAPER J. Altered balance between extracellular proteolysis and antiproteolysis is associated with adaptive coronary arteriogenesis. *J Mol Cell Cardiol.* 2000;32:997-1011.

68. RUTHERFORD C, MARTIN W, SALAME M, CARRIER M, ANGGARD E, FERNS G. Substantial inhibition of neo-intimal response to balloon injury in the rat carotid artery using a combination of antibodies to platelet-derived growth factor-BB and basic fibroblast growth factor. *Atherosclerosis.* 1997;130:45-51.

69. ERGUL A, PORTIK-DOBOS V, GIULUMIAN AD, MOLERO MM, FUCHS LC. Stress Upregulates Arterial Matrix Metalloproteinase Expression and Activity via Endothelin A Receptor Activation. Am J Physiol Heart Circ Physiol. 2003; online: 70. CAI W-J, KOLTAI S, KOCSIS E, SCHOLZ D, KOSTIN S, LUO X, SCHAPER W, SCHAPER J. Remodeling of the adventitia during coronary arteriogenesis. *Am J Physiol Heart Circ Physiol.* 2003;284:H31-40.

71. MAENG M, MERTZ H, NIELSEN S, VAN EYS GJ, RASMUSSEN K, ESPERSEN GT. Adventitial myofibroblasts play no major role in neointima formation after angioplasty. *Scand Cardiovasc J.* 2003;37:34-42.

72. SIOW RC, MALLAWAARACHCHI CM, WEISSBERG PL. Migration of adventitial myofibroblasts following vascular balloon injury: insights from *in vivo* gene transfer to rat carotid arteries. *Cardiovasc Res.* 2003;59:212-21.

73. HINZ B, MASTRANGELO D, ISELIN C, CHAPONNIER C, GABBIANI G. Mechanical tension controls granulation tissue contractile activity and myofibroblast differentiation. *Am J Pathol.* 2001;159:1009-1020.

74. CAI W-J, KOLTAI S, KOCSIS E, SCHOLZ D, SCHAPER W, SCHAPER J. Connexin37, not Cx40 and Cx43, is induced in vscular smooth muscle cells during coronary arteriogenesis. *J Mol Cell Cardiol.* 2001;33:957-967.

75. CAI W-J, KOCSIS E, SCHOLZ D, LUO X, SCHAPER W, SCHAPER J. Presence of Cx37 and lack of desmin in smooth muscle cells are early markers for arteriogenesis. *Submitted to Mol Biochem.* 2003;

76. SCHOLZ D, CAI W-J, SCHAPER W. Arteriogenesis, a new concept of vascular adaptation in occlusive disease. *Angiogenesis.* 2001;4:247-257.

77. SCHOLZ D, ITO W, FLEMING I, DEINDL E, SAUER A, WIESNET M, BUSSE R, SCHAPER J, SCHAPER W. Ultrastructure and molecular histology of rabbit hind limb collateral artery growth (arte riogenesis). *Virchows Arch.* 2000;436:257-270.

78. SPAET TH, STEMERMANN MB, VEITH FJ, LEIJNIEKS I. Intimal injury and regrowth in the rabbit aorta: medial smooth muscle cells as a source of neoinitma. *Circ Res.* 1975;36:58-70.

79 WU L, TANIMOTO A, MURATA Y, FAN J, SASAGURI Y, WATANABE T. Induction of human matrix metalloproteinase-12 gene transcriptional activity by GM-CSF requires the AP-1 binding site in human U937 monocytic cells. *Biochem Biophys Res Commun.* 2001;285:300-7.

80. SHAPIRO SD. Diverse roles of macrophage matrix metalloproteinases in tissue destruction and tumor growth. *Thromb Haemost.* 1999;82:846-9.

81. SUZUKI T, HASHIMOTO S, TOYODA N, NAGAI S, YAMAZAKI N, DONG HY, SAKAI J, YAMASHITA T, NUKIWA T, MATSUSHIMA K. Comprehensive gene expression profile of LPS-stimulated human monocytes by SAGE. *Blood.* 2000;96:2584-91.

82 LACRAZ S, ISLER P, VEY E, WELGUS HG, DAYER JM. Direct contact between T-lymphocytes and monocytes is a major pathway for induction of metalloproteinase expression. *J Biol Chem.* 1994;269:22027-33.

83 AMORINO GP, HOOVER RL. Interactions of monocytic cells with human endothelial cells stimulate monocytic metalloproteinase production. *Am J Pathol.* 1998;152:199-207.

84. HEIL M, ZIEGELHOEFFER T, PIPP F, KOSTIN S, MARTIN S, CLAUSS M, SCHAPER W. Blood monocyte concentration is critical for enhancement of collateral artery growth. *Am J Physiol Heart Circ Physiol.* 2002;283:H2411-H2419.

85. ITO WD, ARRAS M, WINKLER B, SCHOLZ D, SCHAPER J, SCHAPER W. Monocyte chemotactic protein-1 increases collateral and peripheral conductance after femoral artery occlusion. *Circ Res.* 1997;80:829-37.

86. ZIEGELHOEFFER T, HOEFER IE, VAN ROYEN N, BUSCHMANN IR. Effective reduction in collateral artery formation through matrix metalloproteinase inhibitors. *Circulation.* 1999;100:I-705.

Chapter 4

Magnetic Resonance Imaging

Shawn Wagner, Armin Helisch and Tibor Ziegelhoeffer

Introduction

Small animals are becoming a widely accepted medium for research due to the availability of transgenic mice and the need to minimize the quantities of the biological agents. However, many of the invasive techniques used to monitor recovery in larger animals can not be performed in mice. Currently, Laser-Doppler imaging has fulfilled the criteria by providing a surface weighted perfusion value for blood flow recovery in hind limb ischemia models allowing researchers to track limb reperfusion. While this technique may be far from an exact measurement since it cannot be calibrated and only provides arbitrary units as a measure, it is currently the only widely accepted method[1-8] which provides longitudinal study capability. Microsphere injections at the termination of a study have also been used in rats[9] and mice[10] and even proposed unilaterally and without validation as a "gold standard" by one group[11]. Besides lacking the day-to-day follow-up results, microspheres are a measure of tissue perfusion since the microspheres are trapped in the capillaries, and due to the small size of mouse capillaries, may embolize relatively large vessels which restricts repeatability. Additionally, this method is notorious for being unreliable as can be seen in[10] where 50% of the mice were excluded from the analysis due to failure of the procedure. We have thoroughly investigated this method and found it to be too unreliable to warrant use in mouse hind limb ischemia studies as a method for assessing collateral artery development.

Magnetic resonance imaging (MRI) techniques are currently the most suitable method to measure non-invasively inside tissue. The measurement of blood flow by MRI has long been established for the use in human and larger animals but no method has been presented for measuring hind limb larger vessel blood flow in mice. The difficulty in utilizing MRI in small animals to measure blood flow is that contrast injections into the tail vein are invasive and result in damage to the vessels precluding follow-up studies. Therefore, methods that utilized spin labeling are the most suitable for longitudinal studies since these methods require no injections of contrast agent and rely on manipulation of the spin states to achieve contrast.

Nuclear Magnetic Resonance

Unlike many other analysis techniques, magnetic resonance can be utilized to give an immense variety of information ranging for images of internal tissue to molecular motions of molecules. A simple review of where the signal come from in magnetic resonance can answer many questions as to the resolution limits of imaging.

A magnetic nucleus, e.g. a proton atom of water, in a magnetic field will have a defined frequency of precession around the axis of a magnetic field as a result of the angular momentum. The angular frequency, ω, of the precession was first calculated by Sir Joseph Larmor in 1900 and is known as the Larmor's theorem:

$$\omega = \gamma B \tag{1}$$

The *Larmor frequency*, $\omega/2\pi$, is then a function of the gyromagnetic ratio, γ, and the field strength of the magnetic field, B. For a proton, ^1H, which has a natural abundance of 99.98% of all hydrogen atoms the gyromagnetic ratio is 42.6 MHz/Tesla which is derived from the ratio of the magnetic moment, μ, to the angular momentum, $I\hbar$:

$$\gamma = \mu/I\hbar \tag{2}$$

The spin, I, of the 1/2 nuclei has two quantized values in a magnetic field having two possible eigenstates with a defined energy, E:

$$E = \pm \mu B \tag{3}$$

The difference between these two states is then 2μB, therefore, if this amount of energy is introduced via photons or quanta having an energy, *hv*, equal to the separation then a proton can be promote to the higher energy state or be stimulated to emitted a photon and enter the lower energy state. It is important to note that all spin transitions in NMR are stimulated and do not occur spontaneously, transitions between energy states are therefore only induced by the local environment. This principle has been utilized to obtain various information about local molecular motions and in a later section on spectroscopy uses this principal to determine chemical exchange rates between ATP and phosphocreatine in skeletal muscle tissue.

If we consider the bulk of all protons at or around room temperature the number of proton in each energy state is nearly equal. This ratio between states, N, can be determined by the Boltzmann factor, *k*:

$$N = \exp(2\mu B/kT) \tag{4}$$

The difference in the number of protons in each state will determine the overall signal obtained in experiments and since the temperature, T, can not be varied to any large degree for *in vivo* studies, the magnetic field strength will be the most important factor in determining the population difference. If this ratio is calculated at body temperature, 310 K, there is only approximately a 3 proton difference between energy states for every 1 million protons in a 1 Tesla magnetic field. A typical human imaging scanner is about 1.4 Tesla and small animal scanners are about 4.7 Tesla. This small difference has become one the most limiting factors in sensitivity and resolution in magnetic resonance imaging.

While an in depth analysis of magnetization and imaging can be obtained elsewhere [12], we will briefly describe how imaging is accomplish. Since the Larmor frequency is dependant on the magnetic field strength then localized changes in a fixed magnetic field can yield information on position. In a fixed magnetic field the resonance frequency for water produces a single line in a spectrum with a linewidth dependant on the homogeneity of the field and local changes in the homogeneity due to motions of charge bearing atoms and molecules. During imaging a magnetic field gradient is applied thus resulting in the water resonance frequency being dependant on the location in magnetic field. These gradients can and are applied in the x,y, and z axes or various combinations of axial planes. The location and concentration can then be mathematically determine by solving equations defining the frequency spectra associated with these various gradient fields.

The prior explanation defines how magnetic resonance imaging worked before advanced computers and Fourier transform calculations. What really occurs now is that the spectra are acquired in the time domain from a free induction decay of the net magnetization of the excited state as the surrounding magnetic noise relaxes the observed nuclei in a changing magnetic field. The free induction decays or echo, produced by refocusing of this decay is transformed from the time domain to the frequency domain and empirically solved for location and intensity (concentration). These solutions require that the number of variables at least equal the number of solutions. If we want to produce an image with the resolution of 4 x 4 x 4, defined in space by different magnetic field gradients, we must produce 4^3 equations and solutions. One can see that as the resolution requirements increase the number of different equations and solutions increases by a cubic power. The increasing time for acquisition and the limited signal-to-noise ratio due to the lower net number of nuclei observed have lead to limitations of resolution of around 100 μm *in vivo*.

Measuring Blood Flow with Magnetic Resonance Imaging (Time-of-Flight imaging)

One of the main objectives in a mouse vascular occlusion model is to quantitatively measure the return of blood flow past the occlusion as well as to understand the method of redistribution of the blood flow, the latter will be addressed in the following section. Quantitative measurements of distal hind limb flow by MRI in mice have not been reported, even though it would be a very important endpoint for assessing the development of a collateral circulation after arterial occlusion. Time-of-flight experiments are not novel and have been employed using FLASH[13], MSE[14] and EPI[15] to assess blood flow. Contrast boluses have also been utilized in a pig coronary occlusion model[16] and a mouse hind limb ischemia model[17], however, these methods require the administration of contrast agents and do not give exact measures of blood volume flow. In mice, tail and jugular vein injections are difficult and result in local damage of the veins precluding serial studies requiring non-invasive techniques to obtain mouse information for longitudinal studies.

Two-dimensional TOF imaging saturates a single image slice through the use of large flip angles and fast repetition times[18]. The large flip angles produce a sort of spin labeling where blood and tissue outside the image slice are in an equilibrium state and blood and tissue inside the acquisition slice are in an a saturation state where there is no net population difference between the two energy states. The acquired signal is then highly contrast weighted from motions of fluid, blood, entering the acquired slice in the interval between signal acquisition pulses. This method has been employed on a 7 Tesla magnet to obtain maps of the relative calf blood flow recovery (error bar is the standard error of the mean) in longitudinal studies for three different strains (Figure 1). Traditionally, we have imaged three slices from different heights of the calf muscle and obtained intensities from the different leg muscles by selecting a region of interest (ROI) containing the blood vessels and setting a threshold of two standard deviations to eliminate 95% of the noise from the ROI.

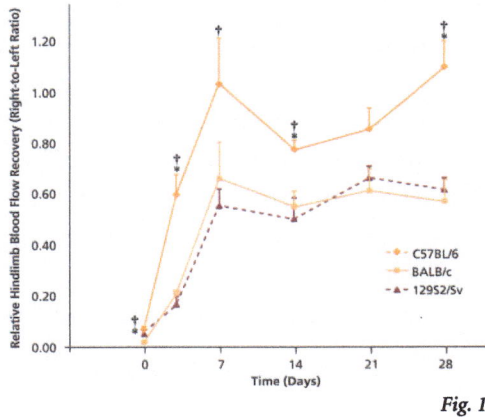

Fig. 1

The right-to-left ratio of the blood flow determined by time-of-flight magnetic resonance imaging for recovery after right femoral artery occlusion

We found that there was little differences in the Balb/C and 129S2/Sv strains with regard to relative blood recovery and significant differences between C57BL/6 and Balb/C (†, $p<0.05$) or 129S2/Sv (✱, $p<0.05$). The volume flows where also examined in a separate study with the mice sedated with 1.5% isofluorane in a mixture of air/oxygen (80/20). An external standardizing tube connected to an infusion pump placed on the mouse hind limb area was used to calibrate the flow measurements twenty-one days after surgical occlusion. (Table 1)

Volumetric calf blood flow in a mouse hind limb ischemia model for three mouse strains			
Mouse Strain	Blood Flow Left Hind limb (ml/min)	Blood Flow Right Hind limb (ml/min)	Right-to-Left[1] Ratio
C57BL/6	0.28 ± 0.04[2]	0.21 ± 0.02	0.88 ± 0.11
Balb/C	0.23 ± 0.05	0.12 ± 0.02	0.61 ± 0.10
129Sv	0.50 ± 0.07	0.31 ± 0.05	0.73 ± 0.04

[1] Calculated average ratio from the individual right-to-left blood flows for each mouse in the group.
[2] All values are the mean ± standard error of the mean

Table 1

The flow values from the table are mainly a combination of the venous and arterial flow from the great vessels in the calf muscle and do not represent tissue perfusion. However, we can approximate what the maximum perfusion could be at the testing conditions in healthy mice from the left hind limb assuming the values from Table 1 represent only arterial flow (Table 2), however, half this value is a more reasonable estimate of the potential blood available for tissue perfusion.

Approximate maximum blood perfusion in resting mice for three tested mouse strains		
Mouse Strain	Muscle Weight (mg)	Maximum Blood Perfusion[1] [ml/(min·100 g)]
C57BL/6	239.40 ± 12.58[2]	117 ± 18
Balb/C	224.00 ± 5.47	103 ± 22
129Sv	170.40 ± 3.90	393 ± 42

[1] Calculated maximum for the resting mouse using the combined venous and arterial flow measured and the muscle weight assuming all blood flows though the tissue.
[2] All values are the mean ± standard error mean

Table 2

To figure out if these are reasonable values they can be compared to previous studies. Terjung found for different rat tissues in resting animals using microspheres 5-6 ml/(min·100 g) in fast-twitch white (FTW) fiber sections; 10-12 ml/(min·100 g) fast-twitch red (FTR) and slow-twitch red (STR) muscle)[9] which compares nicely with the TOF MRI mouse data, since maximum blood perfusion in humans has been found to be about 10-30 times higher than resting tissue[19,20]. Perfusion imaging using spin labeling inversion recovery technique has measured muscle tissue perfusion at a much higher level of 96 ± 10 ml/(min·100 g)[21]. While this number is considerably higher it may not be unreasonable considering Terjung found a 12-15 times increase in perfusion in isometric twitch contractions, so the differences may be reconciled by the depth of narcosis and the ambient temperature affecting the perfusion.

Mast Cell Growth Factor analysis by Magnetic Resonance Blood Flow Measurements

Recently mast cells have been suggested to play a role in arterial vessel development since they were found to accumulate in the adventitia of growing collateral arteries. [22] Mast cells have been reported to be a significant source of FGF-2. [23] They are involved in the activation of metalloproteinases and tryptases [24] contributing to the lysis of the extracellular matrix. Additionally, mast cell have been reported to play a role in stimulation of angiogenesis. [25]

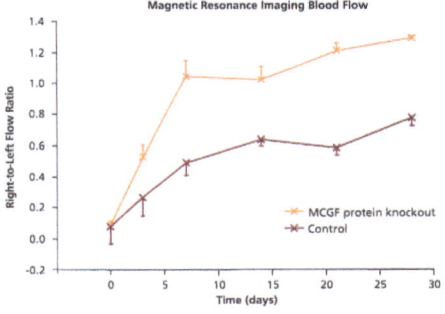

In order to further elucidate the role of mast cells in arteriogenesis we applied our hind limb ischemia model to two types of mast cell growth factor knockout mice. The WCB6F1/J Kitl^{Sl}/Kitl^{Sl-d} mice are knockout mice for the protein and WBB6F1/J-Kit^W/Kit^{W-v} are knockout mice for a receptor of mast cell growth factor (MCGF). The most profound effects were measured in the MCGF protein knockout mice. The deviation from the control mice was apparent in both the perfusion measurement by Laser-Doppler imaging analysis and the blood flow measurement by magnetic resonance imaging. While these stud-

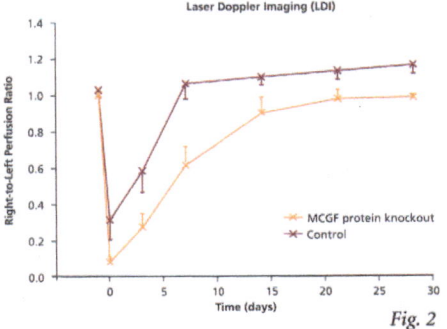

Fig. 2

Magnetic resonance inflow imaging and Laser-Doppler imaging recovery curves after right-sided femoral artery occlusion. Error bars show the standard error mean.

ies have not been completed, we will not elaborate on a possible role for mast cells but we will demonstrate the difference between the two measurements and demonstrate how by just using one measurement the data could be misinterpreted. Figure 2 shows the recovery by both methods.

The MRI data suggests a better recovery for mast cell protein knockout mice and the LDI data shows a decreased recovery. The question is how to reconcile the differences between these two data sets. MRI is measuring the average blood flow in the calf muscle with three slice planes selected along the length of the muscle. If we examine the individual slices, we see that there is a decrease of the blood flow along the length of the muscle as should be expected since blood supplying the tissue will be diverted through arterioles to the capillaries (Figure 3). In the case of the MCGF protein knockout mice the blood flow on the right (occluded side) is greater than the flow on the non-occluded side at the proximal end of the muscle and diminishes along the length of the muscle to less than the left side blood flow. The end result is an inversion of the relative right-to-left ratio by the end of the muscle. Since Laser-Doppler imaging is measuring a perfusion value in the foot, it should be expected that the LDI values would be higher for the control mice. This leads to an interesting question as to the reliability of just LDI results for predicting the growth of collateral vessels or MRI results estimating the potential for salvage of the tissue in the acral parts of the limb, which is a major concern in peripheral arterial disease. In cases were changes in blood perfusion in the muscle may occur than LDI may underestimate the recovery. This becomes a serious problem especially when vasodilating agents are tested or when genetically altered mice may have impaired or increased vasomotor responses.

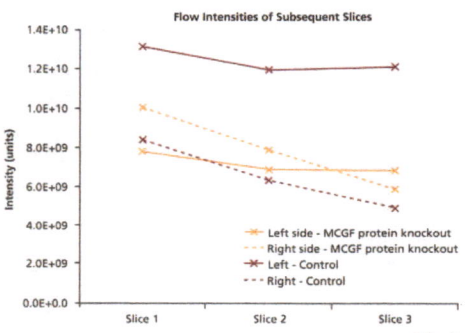

Plotted intensity values for the averaged slice which compose the magnetic resonance blood flow ratio for the right (occluded side) and left (non-occluded side) muscles seven days after occlusion.

Magnetic Resonance Angiography of Collateral Vessels

X-ray angiograms through the use of contrast agent injected post-mortem give a visualization of collateral vessels but only a static picture of the growth; a very difficult technique with limited ability to quantify the

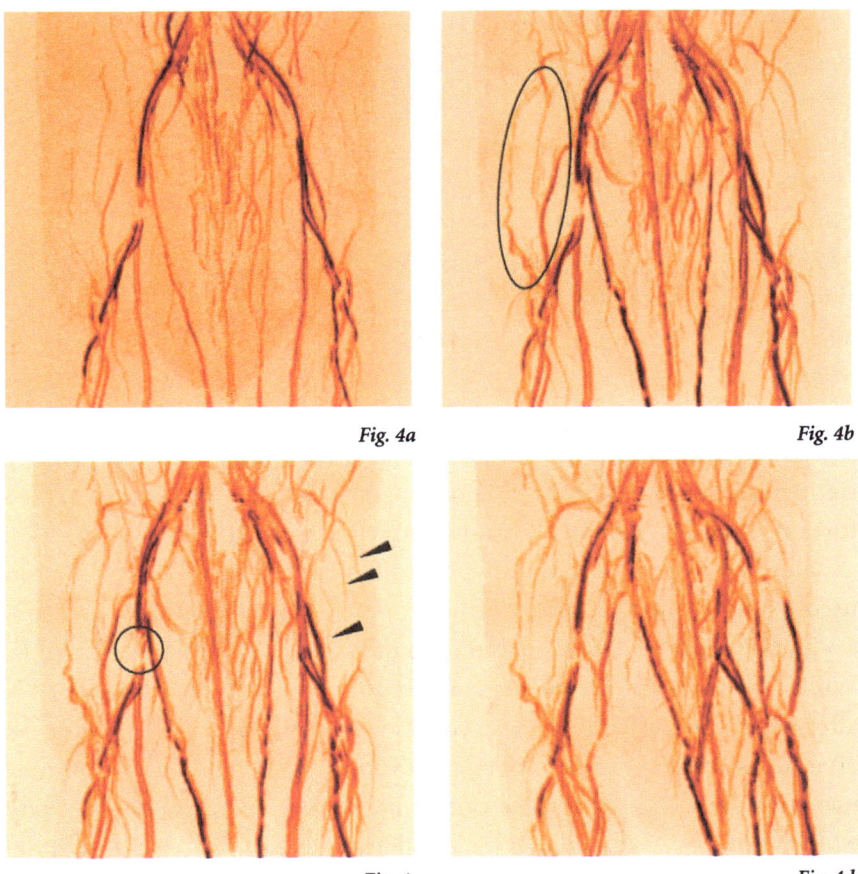

Fig. 4a

Fig. 4b

Fig. 4c

Fig. 4d

Three-dimensional angiography of a mouse three months after femoral artery ligation. Images with different times of acquisition a.) 11 minutes, b.) 22 minutes c.) 44 minutes d.) 44 minute acquisition rotated to better show the collateral vessels. The circle indicates the site of occlusion of the femoral artery and the oval the enlarged collateral arteries. Arrow heads indicate the preexisting vessels on the contra-lateral side.

obtained images for assessment of blood flow. *The more important questions are how do collateral vessels grow and where?* While direct measurement of blood available through collateral vessels is possible through the use of MRI, how this blood is re-distributed is still an open question. Magnetic resonance angiography has been performed in rat[26,27] and mouse brains[28] using time-of-flight techniques. This technique has been extrapolated to the mouse hind limbs with a good deal of success, however, extensive longitudinal studies still need to be perform to fully understand the growth and enlargement and possible regression of arterial vessels bridging the arterial occlusion. The feasibility of these types of experiments has already been shown [18]. Repetitive exams of different numbers of repetitions have shown that collateral vessels can be visualized in 11 minutes in high resolution scans of the lower hind limbs of a mouse, 100 μm isometric volume. Further repetitions added to the visual quality of the images (Figure 4). The collateral vessels (oval) from the quadriceps were clearly visible as contributing vessels to the peripheral hind limb blood flow distal to the surgical occlusion (circle). The utility of having a 3D image can be seen in the fourth image where an addition collateral vessel can be seen in a different rotation.

A complimentary experiment measured the number of collateral vessels in five C57BL/6 mice 6 weeks after femoral artery ligation and assigned them to one of three categories: quadriceps collaterals [1], adductor collaterals [2], and the deep adductor collateral [3] (Figure 5, Table 3).

The inability to image inductor collateral vessels which have been used to show collateral artery growth and explain the blood flow recovery by Scholz et. al. [5] must lead one to question the role of these vessels. While they may be significant contributors to blood flow immediately after occlusion, the role of these vessels is most likely minimal six weeks after occlusion. While the MRI angiograms are not quantitative measurements qualitative assumptions can be made based on size and intensity which indicates that the quadriceps collateral vessels are the most important for maintaining blood flow to the distal limb after occlusion.

Number of collateral vessels counted for 3D MRI angiograms obtained in 22 minutes			
Mouse	Quadriceps Vessel	Adductor[1] Vessel	Deep Adductor[2] Vessel
#1	1	0	0
#2	1	0	1
#3	2	0	0
#4	2	0	1
#5	4	0	1
Average ± SD	2.0 ± 1.2	0.0 ± 0.0	0.6 ± 0.5

[1] Surface collateral vessel as defined by Scholz et. al. [5]
[2] Collateral vessel connecting the end of the a. profunda to the a. superficialis   *Table 3*

31P Spectroscopy

The discussion of blood flow is not complete without information about the physiological impact of blood deficit on tissue and metabolism. Magnetic resonance spectroscopy could play a key role in understanding *in vivo* the effects of decreased oxygen supply and the reduction of the blood drainage which can carry away detrimental byproducts of anaerobic metabolism. Magnetic resonance spectroscopy has the unique characteristic that the concentrations of all the products and reactants of metabolism can be measured as well as reaction rate constants *in vivo*. A detailed review of this topic in humans has been published by A. Heerschap.[30] Phosphocreatine (PCr) is one of the high energy metabolic storage molecules used to rapidly produce

$$PCr + ADP + H^+ \overset{kf}{\underset{kr}{\rightleftharpoons}} ATP + Cr \tag{5}$$

adenosine triphosphate (ATP) from adenosine diphosphate (ADP). In ischemic conditions, PCr can act as a temporary buffer providing an ATP production without oxygen until PCr reserves are depleted. To understand how long ATP can be produced without reconstituting PCr through the decomposition of ATP, we can look at the reaction rate for the forward reaction, k_f. In the calf muscle of humans this rate is 0.29 ± 0.06 s-1[31] and for mice 0.38 ± 0.05 s-1(internal data, seven C57BL/6 mice). Therefore, in the absence of the reverse reaction, k_r, one can expect that in about 10 seconds the majority of the PCr levels would be depleted under basal ATP demand. While this is only a simplistic view it demonstrates the limited effectiveness of PCr as a long term buffer. The creatine system has a much more complicated role still being investigated with genetically altered mice for selective creatine kinase knockouts.[32] Additionally, with creatine kinase deficient mice it has been shown that the forward reaction rate can be longer than the limit of MRS detection (0.05 to 10 s-1)[33,34] showing an almost completely metabolically inactive PCr using standard saturation transfer experiments.[35,36]

Bottomley et al.[29] have recently introduced a four angle saturation transfer (FAST) method for determining the creatine kinase reaction rates, up to seven times faster than the current method. To gauge the impact of such a reduction in time one must consider that using the standard satu-

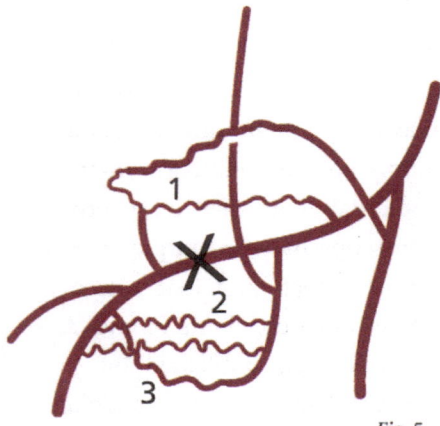

Fig. 5

*Representative image of the arterial vascula-
ture of the adductor and quadriceps muscula-
ture region. The x marks the site of femoral
artery occlusion for experiments presented in
this chapter.*

ration transfer technique it takes about 90 minutes to obtain ten spectra needed to calculate the exchange rates in a mouse calf muscle and twice this time if additional spectra are acquired to determine losses due to radio frequency bleedover during the saturation. The FAST method can acquire all the information needed in four spectra in comparison to twenty required for the previous method. Which ultimately means that about 20 different mouse muscles can be done in ten hours or more if a greater degree of error is accepted.

In addition to measuring the reaction rate additional information can be derived from MRS to give an almost complete picture of the metabolism. The most obvious being the concentration of the metabolites by ^{1}H (phosphorylated and unphosphorylated creatine[37-40]) and ^{31}P (PCr, ATP, inorganic phosphate) spectroscopy. Additionally, local pH[41] and Mg^{2+}[42] can be determined by the chemical shift of the peaks. While ADP and AMP are part of the spectrum it has been suggested that the best way to determine the very low concentration is by the equilibrium equations defining the reaction.[25]

Why not just rely on concentrations determined by freeze clamping? While this method can provide extensive information of metabolites in mice[41], the relevance may be in question since the fast forward and reverse reaction rates can change the concentration before the reactions can be quenched by freezing. These can be seen in the *Scholz*[43] data where the creatine phosphate to ATP levels are considerably lower than the expected 3:1 found in MRS. Controversy over the correctness of either method has arisen. Those in favor of the MRS method argue that the majority of the metabolites are in solution and unbound resulting in narrow observable linewidths and accurate determination of the reaction rate and concentrations[44,45], while others argue that additional metabolites may be bound and the local environment and subcellular structures lead to mis-

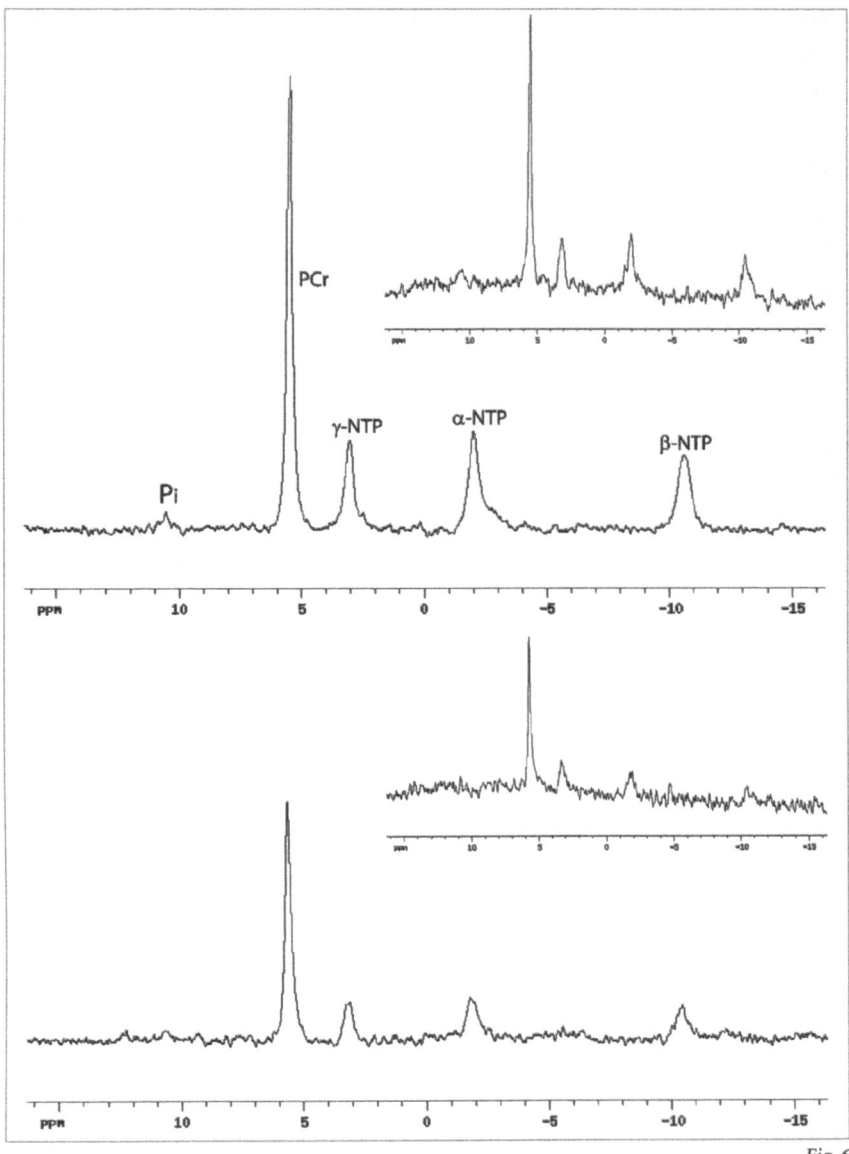

Fig. 6

Mouse skeletal muscle 31p spectra. The top two spectra were obtained with a 60 degree flip angle and a 1 sec repetition time; 512 repetitions for the larger spectrum and 64 repetitions for the inset. The lower spectra were obtained identically but with a 15 degree flip angle. The signal-to-noise ratio for the spectra are 26, 53, 47, 158 for 1 minute 15° and 60° and 8 minute 15° and 60°, respectively. Spectra were obtained in a 7T animal scanner equipped with a broadband low frequency channel using a Helmholtz coil with a Q of 300 (diameter; 1.4 cm, length; 2.3 cm) leading information[46]. The feasibility of mouse studies of hind limb ischemia is a much simpler question to answer. A simple ^{31}P spectrum obtained in 16 minutes with long repetition times shows that the concentration in a C57BL/6 mouse is about 3 mmol/kg which is considerably higher than the threshold previously reported of 0.5 mmol/kg[28] for experiments. We currently have experiments underway, which utilize the complete saturation transfer technique, however, this is very time consuming and limits the number of mice that can be studied. For large studies it is interesting to know if the fast partial saturation technique is effective in mice. Figure 4 shows four spectra obtained using the 15 and 60 degree flip angles described by Bottomley et al.[40] The signal-to-noise ratio in both, the 1 minute and 8 minute scans, are likely high enough to obtain accurate determination of the forward reaction rate by saturation transfer, therefore, experiments in ischemic mouse tissue should be obtainable in less than 30 minutes per mouse making data acquisition for large mouse groups possible in less than 1 day.

References

1. AMANO K, MATSUBARA H, IBA O, OKIGAKI M, FUJIYAMA S, IMADA T, KOJIMA H, NOZAWA Y, KAWASHIMA S, YOKOYAMA M, IWASAKA T. Enhancement of ischemia-induced angiogenesis by eNOS overexpression. *Hypertension.* 2003;41:156-62.
2. ABE M, SATA M, NISHIMATSU H, NAGATA D, SUZUKI E, TERAUCHI Y, KADOWAKI T, MINAMINO N, KANGAWA K, MATSUO H, HIRATA Y, NAGAI R. Adrenomedullin augments collateral development in response to acute ischemia. *Biochem Biophys Res Commun.* 2003;306:10-5.
3. TAMARAT R, SILVESTRE JS, KUBIS N, BENESSIANO J, DURIEZ M, deGASPARO M, HENRION D, LEVY BI. Endothelial nitric oxide synthase lies downstream from angiotensin II-induced angiogenesis in ischemic hind limb. *Hypertension.* 2002;39:830-5.
4. SILVESTRE JS, TAMARAT R, SENBONMATSU T, ICCHIKI T, EBRAHIMIAN T, IGLARZ M, BESNARD S, DURIEZ M, INAGAMI T, LEVY BI. Antiangiogenic effect of angiotensin II type 2 receptor in ischemia-induced angiogenesis in mice hind limb. *Circ Res.* 2002;90:1072-9.
5. SCHOLZ D, ZIEGELHOEFFER T, HELISCH A, WAGNER S, FRIEDRICH C, PODZUWEIT T, SCHAPER W. Contribution of arteriogenesis and angiogenesis to postocclusive hind limb perfusion in mice. *J Mol Cell Cardiol.* 2002;34:775-87.
6. SATA M, HIRATA Y, NAGAI R. Role of Fas/Fas ligand interaction in ischemia-induced collateral vessel growth. *Hypertens Res.* 2002;25:577-82.
7. HEIL M, ZIEGELHOEFFER T, PIPP F, KOSTIN S, MARTIN S, CLAUSS M, SCHAPER W. Blood monocyte concentration is critical for enhancement of collateral artery growth. *Am J Physiol Heart Circ Physiol.* 2002;283:H2411-9.
8. COUFFINHAL T, SILVER M, ZHENG LP, KEARNEY M, WITZENBICHLER B, ISNER JM. Mouse model of angiogenesis. *Am J Pathol.* 1998;152:1667-79.
9. TERJUNG RL, ENGBRETSON BM. Blood flow to different rat skeletal muscle fiber type sections during isometric contractions *in situ. Med Sci Sports Exerc.* 1988;20:S124-30.
10. MAXWELL AJ, SCHAUBLE E, BERNSTEIN D, COOKE JP. Limb blood flow during exercise is dependent on nitric oxide. *Circulation.* 1998;98:369-74.
11. HOEFER IE, van ROYEN N, RECTENWALD JE, BRAY EJ, ABOUHAMZE Z, MOLDAWER LL, VOSKUIL M, PIEK JJ, BUSCHMANN IR, OZAKI CK. Direct evidence for tumor necrosis factor-alpha signaling in arteriogenesis. *Circulation.* 2002;105:1639-41.
12. GILLIES RJ, ED. *NMR in Physiology.* San Diego: Academic Press, Inc.; 1994.
13. MATTHAEI D, HAASE A, MERBOLDT KD, HANICKE W, DEIMLING M. ECG-triggered arterial FLASH-MR flow measurement using an external standard. *Magn Reson Imaging.* 1987; 5:325-30.
14. STAHLBERG F, HENRIKSEN O, THOMSEN C, STUBGAARD M, PERSSON B. Determination of flow velocities from magnetic resonance multiple spin- echo images. A phantom study. *Acta Radiol.* 1987;28:643-8.
15. PONCELET BP, WEISSKOFF RM, WEDEEN VJ, BRADY TJ, KANTOR H. Time-of-flight quantification of coronary flow with echo-planar MRI. *Magnc Reson Med* 1993;30:447-57.
16. PEARLMAN JD, HIBBERD MG, CHUANG ML, HARADA K, LOPEZ JJ, GLADSTONE SR, FRIEDMAN M, SELLKE FW, SIMONS M. Magnetic resonance mapping demonstrates benefits of VEGF induced myocardial angiogenesis. *Nature Med.* 1995;1:1085-1089.
17. HEESCHEN C, JANG JJ, WEIS M, PATHAK A, KAJI S, HU RS, TSAO PS, JOHNSON FL, COOKE JP. Nicotine stimulates angiogenesis and promotes tumor growth and atherosclerosis. *Nature Med.* 2001;7:835-841.
18. WAGNER S, HELISCH A, BACHMANN G, SCHAPER W. Time-of-flight Quantitative Measurements of Blood Flow in Mouse Hindlimbs. *J Magn Reson Imaging.* 2004;19:468-474.

19. SNELL PG, MARTIN WH, BUCKEY JC, BLOMQVIST CG. Maximal vascular leg conductance in trained and untrained men. *J Appl Physiol.* 1987;62:606-10.

20. SINOWAY LI, MUSCH TI, MINOTTI JR, ZELIS R. Enhanced maximal metabolic vasodilatation in the dominant forearms of tennis players. *J Appl Physiol.* 1986;61:673-8.

21. STREIF JU, HILLER KH, WALLER C, NAHRENDORF M, WIESMANN F, BAUER WR, ROMMEL E, HAASE A. *In vivo* assessment of absolute perfusion in the murine skeletal muscle with spin labeling MRI. *J Magn Reson Imaging.* 2003;17:147-52.

22. WOLF C, CAI WJ, VOSSCHULTE R, KOLTAI S, MOUSAVIPOUR D, SCHOLZ D, AFSAH-HEDJRI A, SCHAPER W, SCHAPER J. Vascular remodeling and altered protein expression during growth of coronary collateral arteries. *J Mol Cell Cardiol.* 1998;30:2291-305.

23. QU Z, LIEBLER JM, POWERS MR, GALEY T, AHMADI P, HUANG XN, ANSEL JC, BUTTERFIELD JH, PLANCK SR, ROSENBAUM JT. Mast cells are a major source of basic fibroblast growth factor in chronic inflammation and cutaneous hemangioma. *Am J Pathol.* 1995;147:564-73.

24. BUTTERFIELD JH, WEILER DA, HUNT LW, WYNN SR, ROCHE PC. Purification of tryptase from a human mast cell line. *J Leukoc Biol.* 1990;47:409-19.

25. FEOKTISTOV I, RYZHOV S, GOLDSTEIN AE, BIAGGIONI I. Mast cell-mediated stimulation of angiogenesis: cooperative interaction between A2B and A3 adenosine receptors. *Circ Res.* 2003;92:485-92.

26. BESSELMANN M, LIU M, DIEDENHOFEN M, FRANKE C, HOEHN M. MR angiographic investigation of transient focal cerebral ischemia in rat. *NMR Biomed.* 2001;14:289-96.

27. REESE T, BOCHELEN D, SAUTER A, BECKMANN N, RUDIN M. Magnetic resonance angiography of the rat cerebrovascular system without the use of contrast agents. *NMR Biomed.* 1999; 12:189-96.

28. BECKMANN N, STIRNIMANN R, BOCHELEN D. High-resolution magnetic resonance angiography of the mouse brain: application to murine focal cerebral ischemia models. *J Magn Reson.* 1999;140:442-50.

29. WAGNER S, HELISCH A, ZIEGELHOEFFER T, BACHMANN G, SCHAPER W. Magnetic resonance angiography of collateral vessels in a murine femoral artery ligation model. *NMR Biomed.* 2004;17:21-27.

30. HEERSCHAP A, HOUTMAN C, IN 'T ZANDT HJ, VAN DEN BERGH AJ, WIERINGA B. Introduction to *in vivo* 31P magnetic resonance spectroscopy of (human) skeletal muscle. *Proc Nutr Soc.* 1999;58:861-70.

31. BOTTOMLEY PA, OUWERKERK R, LEE RF, WEISS RG. Four-angle saturation transfer (FAST) method for measuring creatine kinase reaction rates *in vivo. Magn Reson Med.* 2002;47:850-63.

32. IN 'T ZANDT HJ, OERLEMANS F, WIERINGA B, HEERSCHAP A. Effects of ischemia on skeletal muscle energy metabolism in mice lacking creatine kinase monitored by *in vivo* 31P nuclear magnetic resonance spectroscopy. *NMR Biomed.* 1999;12:327-34.

33. RUDIN M, SAUTER A. Measurement of reaction rates *in vivo* using magnetisation transfer techniques. *NMR: Basic Principles and Progress.* 1992;27:257-293.

34. MEYER RA, KUCHMERICK MJ, BROWN TR. Application of 31P-NMR spectroscopy to the study of striated muscle metabolism. *Am J Physiol.* 1982;242:C1-11.

35. IN 'T ZANDT HJ, OERLEMANS F, WIERINGA B, HEERSCHAP A. Dipolar coupling of teh creatine and twurine in proton MRS of the mouse skeletal muscle. *Proc Internat Soc Magn Reson Med* 1999;7:193.

36. STEEGHS K, BENDERS A, OERLEMANS F, DE HAAN A, HEERSCHAP A, RUITENBEEK W, JOST C, VAN DEURSEN J, PERRYMAN B, PETTE D, BRUCKWILDER M, KOUDIJS J, JAP P, VEERKAMP J,

WIERINGA B. Altered Ca^{2+} responses in muscles with combined mitochondrial and cytosolic creatine kinase deficiencies. *Cell.* 1997;89:93-103.

37. MICHAELIS T, MERBOLDT KD, BRUHN H, HANICKE W, FRAHM J. Absolute concentrations of metabolites in the adult human brain *in vivo*: quantification of localized proton MR spectra. *Radiology.* 1993;187:219-27.

38. KREIS R, ERNST T, ROSS BD. Development of the human brain: *in vivo* quantification of metabolite and water content with proton magnetic resonance spectroscopy. *Magn Reson Med.* 1993;30:424-37.

39. BOTTOMLEY PA, WEISS RG. Non-invasive magnetic-resonance detection of creatine depletion in non-viable infarcted myocardium. *Lancet.* 1998;351:714-8.

40. BOTTOMLEY PA, LEE Y, WEISS RG. Total creatine in muscle: imaging and quantification with proton MR spectroscopy. *Radiology.* 1997;204:403-10.

41. MOON RB, RICHARDS JH. Determination of intracellular pH by 31P magnetic resonance. *J Biol Chem.* 1973;248:7276-8.

42. GUPTA RK, MOORE RD. 31P NMR studies of intracellular free Mg2+ in intact frog skeletal muscle. *J Biol Chem.* 1980;255:3987-93.

43. SCHOLZ D, THOMAS S, SASS S, PODZUWEIT T. Angiogenesis and myogenesis as two facets of inflammatory post-ischemic tissue regeneration. *Mol Cell Biochem.* 2003;246:57-67.

44. WISEMAN RW, KUSHMERICK MJ. Creatine kinase equilibration follows solution thermodynamics in skeletal muscle. 31P NMR studies using creatine analogs. *J Biol Chem.* 1995; 270:12428-38.

45. KUSHMERICK MJ. Bioenergetics and muscle cell types. *Adv Exp Med Biol.* 1995;384:175-84.

46. WALLIMANN T. 31P-NMR-measured creatine kinase reaction flux in muscle: a caveat! *J Muscle Res Cell Motil.* 1996;17:177-81.

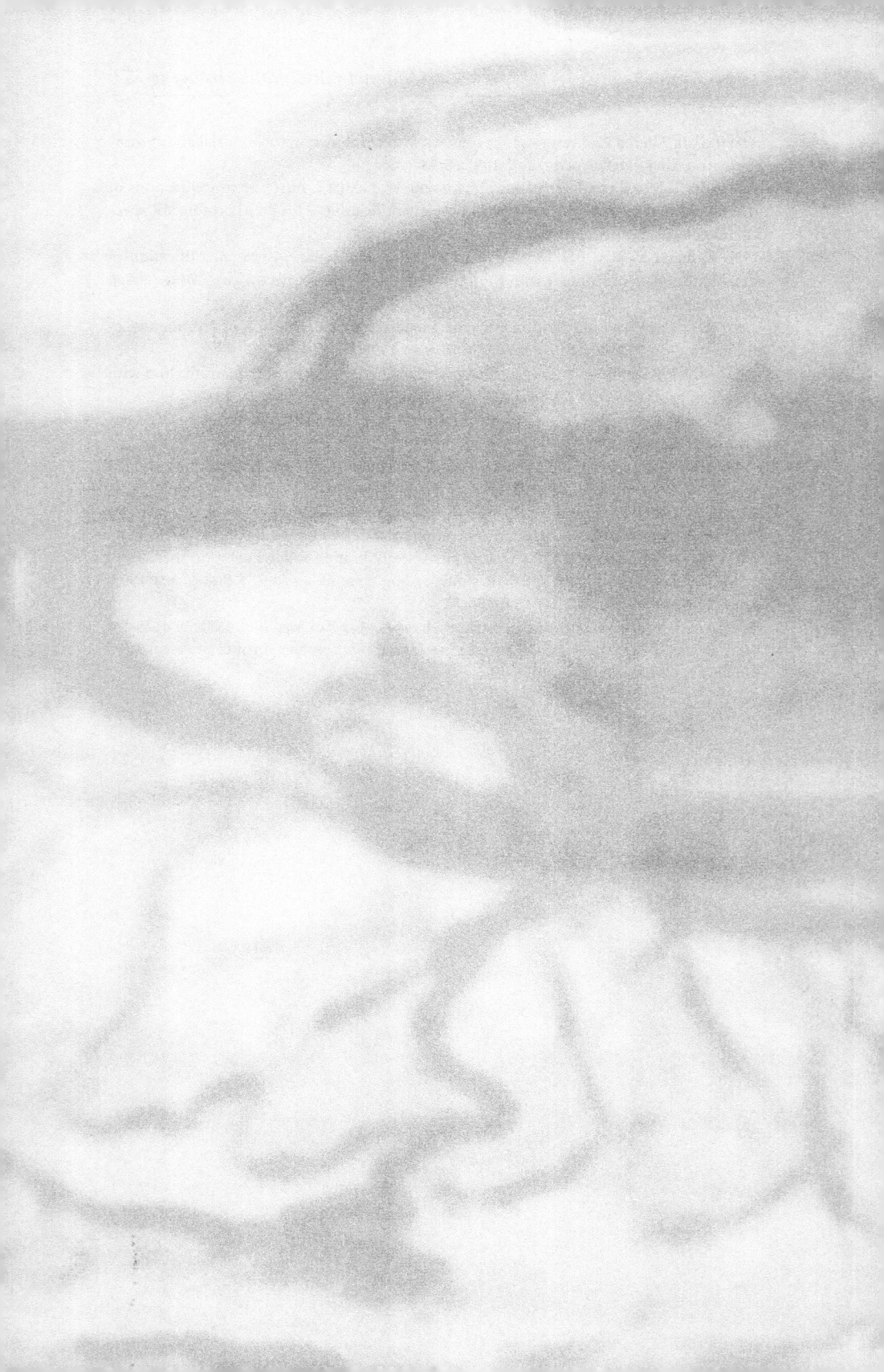

Chapter 5

Physical Forces and their Translation into Molecular Mechanisms

Wolfgang Schaper, Frederic Pipp, Dimitri Scholz,
Stefanie Boehm, Elisabeth Deindl, Miroslaw Barancik,
Inka Eitenmueller, Tibor Ziegelhoeffer, Alexander Kluge
and Thomas Schmitz-Rixen

Blood vessels are constantly subjected to the strain of pressure and flow where a high steady level is superimposed by cyclic variations. The structure of blood vessels is able to adapt to changes of these forces: the thin-walled leg vein becomes arterialized when interposed into an arterial circuit as in an aortic-coronary bypass, the umbilical vessels regress when blood flow ceases after birth, the feeder artery enlarges when part of a high flow system like in an arteriovenous (AV)-fistula, the contralateral carotid artery enlarges when the ipsilateral artery is occluded, the arterial wall thickens in hypertension and - most spectacular of all - the intercostal arteries enlarge in aortic isthmus stenosis and are potentially able to supply the entire body below the head with blood. The forces "felt" by the arteries are the pressure-related stresses (circumferential, radial and longitudinal) and the fluid shear stress (FSS). The circumferential wall stress (CWS) is defined by the intravascular pressure (P), the thickness of the wall (h) and the radius (R):

$$CWS = P\frac{R}{2h}$$

This relationship is known as the Law of Laplace where CWS is proportional to the pressure and the diameter and inversely proportional to the wall thickness, i.e., high values for CWS are obtained with high pressures, large diameters and thin walls. The longitudinal stress is also called the "tethering" force (F) that stretches the vessel between two anchoring points [1,2]. R_I is the original radius of the collateral vessel and P = pressure:

$$F = \frac{P}{2}\,(\pi R_I^2)$$

It becomes evident that F increases markedly with increasing pressure that distends the artery and reduces wall thickness. It can be argued that increase in F exerts a morphogenic influence by inducing the artery to increases its length, which tends to reduce F. Length increase between two fixed points leads to tortuosity, and tortuous collaterals have lost most of their tethering force [3]. This may be interpreted as another example for Murray's law, i.e., that changes in physical strains lead to structural adaptation that restore physiological levels. The disadvantage of tortuosity is its increase in resistance to flow, which is formulated in the Dean number (De). Originally, the Dean number was developed as a correction for the Reynolds number for curvature flows. Although turbulence does not occur in small mammals because the critical Reynolds numbers are not reached, the Dean number is nevertheless useful because it allows an estimation of the influence of tortuosity on collateral blood flow.

$$De = \left(\frac{DV\rho}{\eta}\right) \times \left(\frac{L}{2R}\right)^{0.5}$$

D = diameter	R = radius of curvature of bend
L = length	ρ = density
η = viscosity	V = velocity

Capillaries can afford thin walls because their diameter is small and they have to withstand only low pressures. Veins can remain thin-walled despite their large diameter because of their low intravascular pressure. Arteries must maintain a substantial wall thickness because they have to withstand high pressures at large diameters. From these examples it could be concluded that CWS is the most important physical molding force for blood vessels.

However, the influence of CWS, a strong force, is modified by a much weaker force, the fluid shear stress (τ), which is imposed by the viscous drag of flowing blood on the endothelial lining. FSS has a powerful influence on the diameter of the vessel: chronic changes in blood flow (Q) as cited above lead to structural changes in vessel size. FSS is proportional to blood flow and blood viscosity (η) and inversely related to the cube of the radius (R) of the vessel:

$$\tau = \frac{4\eta Q}{R^3 \pi}$$

As blood flow is proportional to the 4th power of vessel diameter, chronic vasodilatation and therewith increased blood flow along collateral arteries enhances fluid shear stress though FSS itself is inversely proportional to the vessel radius.

$$Q = \frac{R^4 \pi \Delta P}{8\eta l} \, (ml/min)$$

Thus, a more stimulating than an attenuating impact of vasodilatation on FSS can be assumed. However, the exact molecular mechanisms how a weak force, acting only on the endothelial lining, shapes the structure and size of a multi-layered thick-walled artery are not fully elucidated. Nevertheless, one can safely assume that the two forces cooperate in such a way that the weak force amplifies the strong force in analogy to the weak grid voltage of a triode causing large swings of currents through the valve (or the field effect transistor). The difference between these forces is indeed considerable: the circumferential wall stress is 2500-fold higher than the fluid shear stress. At first sight it is difficult to imagine that the weak force is of any importance at all. Scheel states in the conclusion from his computer model[4] experiments of the coronary collateral circulation: "…in the light of this study the shear stresses exerted on vascular walls are negligible compared to all the stresses to which a collateral vessel is exposed". The Scheel model also questioned the morphogenic influence of FSS because the modeling first showed an increase of FSS followed by a decline when auto-regulation and thereafter a new steady state on a higher level was again reached. If, Scheel reasoned, FSS is a molding force, collateral growth should go on until the FSS level had normalized which did not occur. However, one can argue that the new steady state is normal for the size-class of the vessel, which had grown out of the class of resistance vessels into the class of conductance vessels. It remains difficult to understand how fluid shear stress and circumferential shear stress cooperate, since the cells they act upon have no direct means of communication: no tight junctions exist between on the one hand and the smooth muscle layers on the other. Furthermore, not even the smooth muscle cells exhibit tight junctions. The barrier to communication is, however, rapidly broken down by the invasion of monocytes and by smooth muscle cells which develop connexins.

Signals that are elicited from stressed endothelium are NO[5], prostacyclin[6] and hyperpolarizing factor (EDHF)[7] with NO being the most likely candidate for a signal that is transmitted to the smooth muscle cells (SMCs)[8]. Relaxation of the smooth muscle layers causing increases in vascular diameter and wall thinning would invoke Laplace's Law and increase circumferential wall stress, which, if lasting long enough, would lead to structural changes. If this occurs in the class of resistance vessels, to which preexistent collateral arterioles belong, the intravascular pressure will increase (because the pressure fall in this class of vessels is inversely related to diameter and any increase in size by growth will increase pressure) thereby boosting the CWS.

Although prostacyclin is also a potent endothelium-derived relaxing factor, its role as a structural amplifier is dubious because in most blood vessels its contribution to endothelium-dependent relaxation is not major as judged from the limited effects of cyclooxygenase inhibitors on these responses[9]. However, the promoter of the prostacyclin synthase contains the putative shear stress response element (SSRE) GAGACC. EDHF may be of some importance because it is expressed in resistance vessels[10], i.e., the substrate of collateral growth, and its release is triggered by shear stress and cyclical strain[7]. One must bear in mind, though, that hyperpolarized SMCs cannot migrate, a prerequisite for collateral growth. Our experiments aimed at changing eNOS activity arrived at the conclusion that a significant part of the arteriogenic process proceeds in the absence of NO.

Endothelial chloride channels and shear stress signaling*

Despite the increasing evidences that fluid shear stress is the main arteriogenic trigger, the precise molecular mechanisms induced by shear stress remain unclear. Volume-regulated endothelial chloride channels (VRACs) have been shown to be involved in the initiation of the shear stress signaling process[11,12] followed by transcription factor activation, flow responsive genes expression, cytoskeletal reorganization, and alignment of endothelial cells in the direction of shear stress[13]. Similar morphological changes including endothelial cell swelling were previously observed in the early phases of collateral artery growth[14].

Maintenance and regulation of cell volume is crucial for homeostasis in living organisms. Upon a sudden increase in cell volume a cascade of events starts in order to return the cell volume to its original state. Our current knowledge about the mechanisms of volume-sensing and volume-regulation is still rather fragmentary. Nevertheless, activation of anion channels, particularly VRACs seems to be an important event in this scenario. Thus, considering the role of VRACs in endothelial cell-volume regulation and their sensitivity to shear stress it is very likely that the activation of VRACs will participate in the arteriogenic cascade.

Mibefradil, originally developed as a selective T-type calcium channel blocker, was associated with a facilitation of the endothelium-derived NO- and eicosanoic production, and prevention of neointima formation after vascular injury[15-19]. The effect on neointima formation was assumed to be exclusively due to its effect on T-type voltage-operated calcium channels. However, in subsequent studies the very effective blockade of the volume-regulated chloride channels by mibefradil was discovered[20]. Recently, various blockers of volume-activated chloride current, including mibefradil, with completely different physiochemical properties were shown to inhibit cell proliferation of rat microglia, macro- and microvascular endothelial cells, fibroblasts, glioma cells, melanoma cells, lymphocytes, several neuron types, liver cells, etc.[21,22]. Thus, a correlation of cell proliferation and VRAC activation was established[23]. However, because of

---

* Tibor Ziegelhoeffer was the principal investigator of this study

the lack of selective inhibitors a complete block for anion channels is rarely achieved and up to now, no drug has been found to selectively block VRACs and be usable *in vivo*. Nevertheless, although T-type calcium channels were found to be expressed in early mouse embryos [24] and its transient expression in cultured SMCs (SMC) parallels cell proliferation [25,26], the effect of mibefradil on cell proliferation is most probably due to blockade of VRACs. This hypothesis is supported by the fact that overexpression of T-type calcium channels in HEK-293 cells increased basal intracellular calcium concentration without inducing any change in proliferation or cell cycle kinetics [27]. Moreover, four different structurally unrelated agents including mibefradil (mibefradil, NPPB, tamoxifen and clomiphene) with VRAC-inhibition being their only common property, were shown to inhibit *angiogenesis* in a matrigel tube-formation assay, fibrin gel assay, rat aorta-ring assay and chorioallantoic membrane assay [28].

Cell proliferation is an essential aspect of collateral vessel growth. Thus, association of cell proliferation and VRAC activation provides further evidence that activation of VRACs may be involved in the mechanisms of *arteriogenesis*. In order to test this hypothesis, we unilaterally ligated the femoral arteries in mice and implanted osmotic micro-pumps, delivering either the chloride channel blocker mibefradil dissolved in PBS or only PBS intra-arterially. Seven days after the surgery we found a decrease in density of angiographically visible collateral arteries, and significantly impaired perfusion recovery (Fig. 1) and hemoglobin oxygenation (Fig. 2) in the hind limbs of mibefradil-treated mice in comparison to the PBS-treated control animals. In accordance with these functional data, morphometric measurements of the collateral artery diameters showed a decrease in arteriogenic response in the mibefradil-treated group (Fig. 3). Additionally, our electron microscopic studies confirmed the previous findings indicating that endothelial cell swelling is one of the first events in the activated collateral artery (Fig. 4). Interestingly, endothelial cell swelling has been shown to be a hallmark in the activation of the embryonic endocardium leading to endocardial cushion

1) Representative Laser-Doppler images of the distal hind limb: a = immediately (PBS); b = seven days (PBS); c = immediately (MIB); d = seven days (MIB) after right femoral artery ligation. e: Quantification of right-to-left (R/L) flux ratios in the feet: post = immediately after surgery; 7d = seven days after the surgery; MIB = mibefradil.

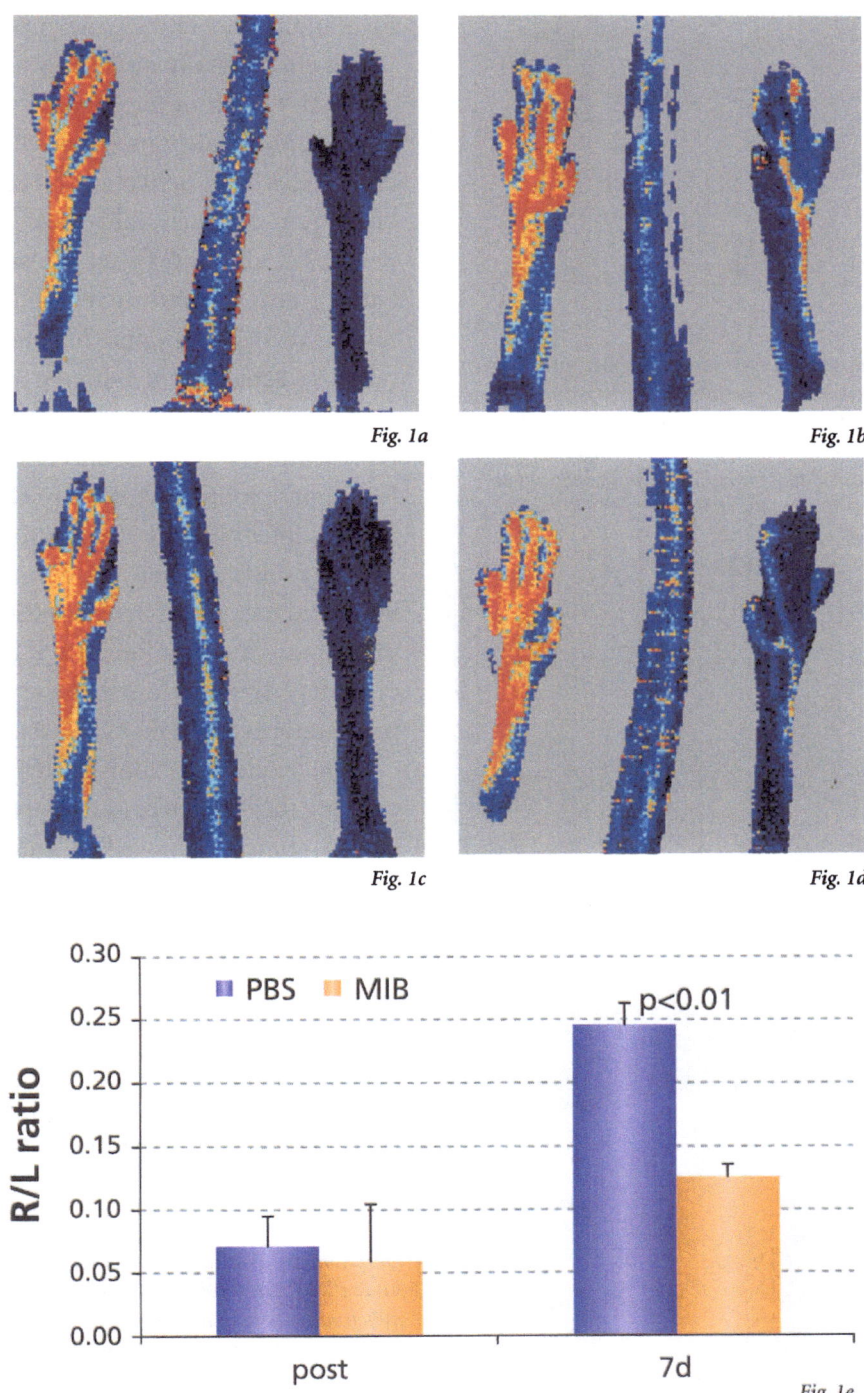

Fig. 1a

Fig. 1b

Fig. 1c

Fig. 1d

Fig. 1e

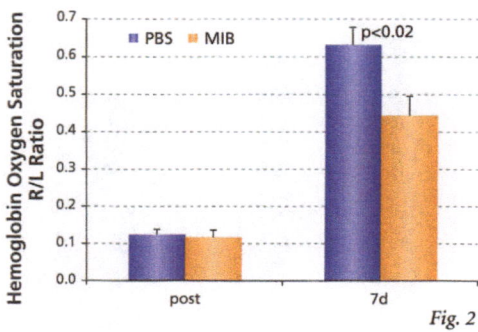

Fig. 2

Hemoglobin oxygen saturation measurements in the mice feet immediately after (post) and one week (7d) after right femoral artery ligation. The right-to-left (R/L), i.e., ligated-to-non-ligated side, ratios were calculated for each mouse and the results expressed as mean ± SEM.

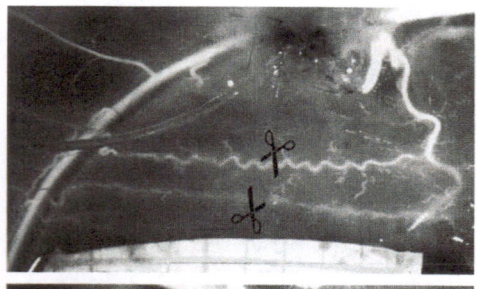

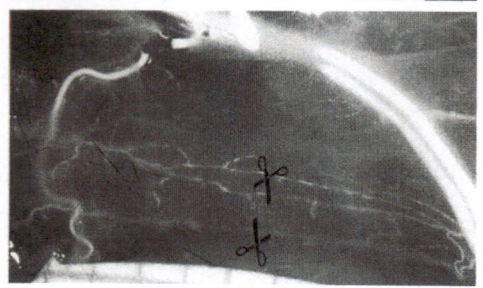

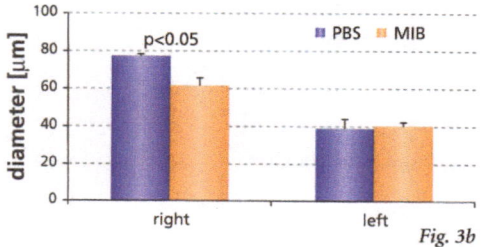

Fig. 3b

formation[29], an embryonic process which shares many structural characteristics with *arteriogenesis* (see chapter 3). In response to swelling, endothelial cells activate the cation and anion channels, and VRACs in particular, allow an efflux of osmolytes in order to return cell volume toward its original value. As a result of VRAC activation, the driving force for Ca^{2+} entry into the cell increases, representing a possible mechanism for the antiproliferative effect of chloride channel blockade[28,30]. Additionally, the blockade of VRACs may induce an increase in the intracellular pH-value. This may inhibit the cell-cycle dependent kinases and trap the proliferating cells in the G_0/G_1 stage[30].

In conclusion, chloride channel opening may be a necessary reaction to FSS-related cell swelling and its inhibition interferes with arteriogenesis.

3) Quantification of collateral vessel diameters by histomorphometry. a: Superficial adductor muscle collateral arteries connecting the deep femoral artery with the saphenous artery as visualized under the stereomicroscope. Semithin cross-sections from the mid-zone of these collaterals were used for histomorphometry (indicated with scissors). b: Inner diameters of collateral arteries in the mibefradil- (MIB) and PBS-treated groups of mice seven days after femoral artery ligation: left = non-occluded side; right = occluded side. Results are expressed as mean ± SEM.

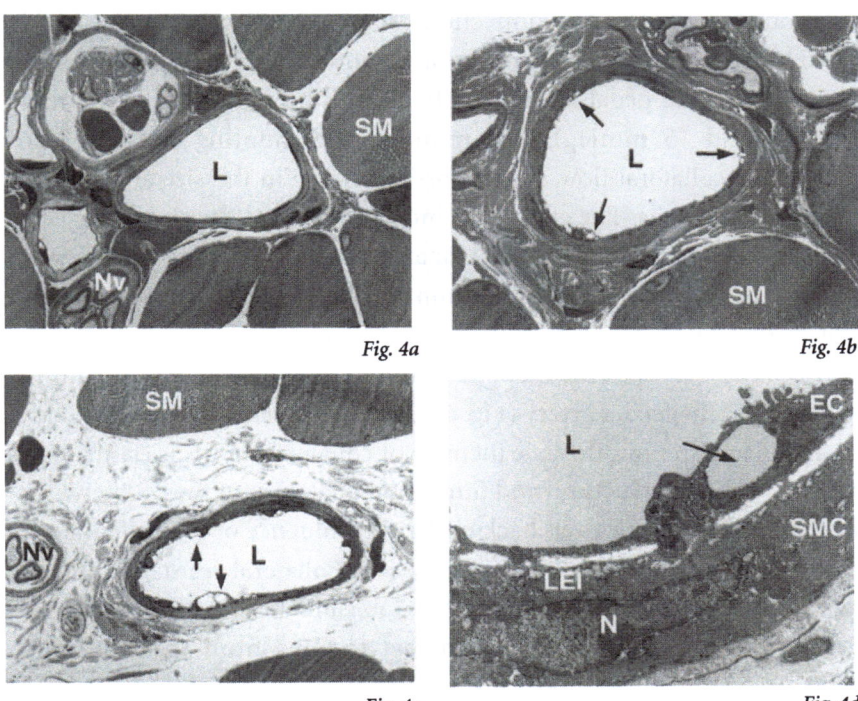

Fig. 4a

Fig. 4b

Fig. 4c

Fig. 4d

*Light and electron microscopy of mouse collateral arteries. a: Normal vessel (x1250);
b: Perinuclear vacuolization (arrows) of activated endothelial cells 4 hours after occlusion
(x1250); c: Progression of endothelial cell swelling 24 hours after femoral artery ligation,
perinuclear edema (arrows) (x1250); d: Electron microscopy showing perinuclear vacuolization (arrow) of an activated endothelial cell 4 hours after surgery (x8800). EC = endothelial
cell; LEI = lamina elastica interna; L = lumen; N = nucleus; Nv = nerve; SM = skeletal
muscle; SMC = smooth muscle cell.*

Studies interrogating the causative role of shear stress[*]

The controversies regarding the causative role of the weak force "fluid
shear stress" encouraged us to design experiments that are capable to
establish a cause-and-effect relationship by stepwise increasing FSS without simultaneously increasing CWS. In a first series of experiments we
occluded both femoral arteries in domestic pigs and, one week later,
established an AV-shunt between the distal stump of one of the occluded
arteries and the accompanying vein. In this way a large and permanent
pressure gradient was created that forced most of the collateral flow to
empty into the vein and only a smaller portion enters the peripheral cir-

[*] Frederic Pipp, Thomas Schmitz-Rixen and Wolfgang Schaper were the principal investigators of this study

culation (Fig. 5). The AV-connection prevented, at least at first, a rise in CWS because the low-pressure region extended well into the arterial bed (pressures in the pedal artery in rabbits with partial collateral shunting were around 15 mmHg). The result of the shunting was a marked increase in collateral flow and a drastic increase in the size and number of collateral vessels. The enormous increase in shunt flow became visible in contrast-enhanced magnetic resonance angiography where the average increase of iliac vein flow of the shunt-ligated side over that of the control-ligated side was 2.5 fold. (Fig. 6a). Digital subtractive angiography (DSA) clearly showed the increased number of collateral vessels and the widening of the feeder artery (Fig. 6b). Since collateral flow is only a fraction of iliac vein flow, the true increase of collateral flow was estimated as up to 5-fold. The structural and functional dilatation of the collateral vessels had brought the vessels back under the influence of CWS. The steady increase in pressure, due to the decrease of collateral resistance and the finite size of the AV-fistula and the re-establishment of auto-regulation in the periphery, amplified the strain that resulted from the increase in diameter. Shear stress falls because of the rise in diameter but not back to control levels because the increase in radius is potentially able to increase flow to the 4th power. Finally, the arteriogenic process ends, when the resistance of the AV-fistula is equal to the (markedly reduced) peripheral and collateral resistances. Interestingly, arteries that feed into the collateral network also increased their diameter significantly and arterial growth continued for at least two weeks.

The species pig was chosen for these experiments because of surgical feasibility. However, the logistic problems of obtaining fresh and viable vascular tissue from growing collateral vessels that are buried deep in the gluteal muscles were considerable. The size of the animal and the difficulty in handling precluded meaningful drug studies. Therefore we established a similar model of AV-shunted femoral collaterals in the rabbit which was much more difficult from the surgical point of view but more rewarding from the experimental point, i.e., tissue harvesting and drug treatment were much more feasible. Like in the pig the AV-shunt between the distal stump of the occluded femoral artery and its accompanying vein drastically increased collateral blood flow, which increased collateral artery growth. This was evidenced by computer tomography (CT) (Fig. 8). In

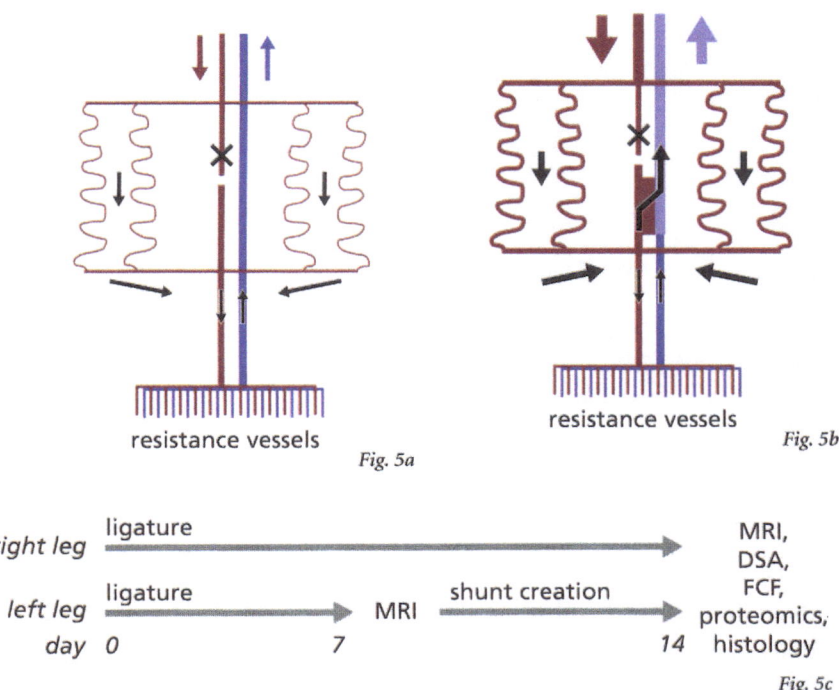

Schema presenting the hemodynamic situation after ligation (a) and ligation + shunt (b) and the experimental timetable (c) of the pig study, e.g., the onset of shunt-related high FSS after seven days of femoral ligation. FCF = fractional collateral flow

this model, hind leg blood flow could be quantitatively measured by MR angiography, which was compared with that measured by Flowmeter-probes positioned at the proximal femoral stump upstream from the feeder branches of the collateral network (Fig. 9). Both methods agreed well. The Flowmeter method had the advantage that the dilatory reserve could be tested (with the AV-shunt closed again at the time of the terminal experiment) under the influence of maximally tolerated doses of adenosine, which is an accepted method to induce maximal vasodilatation[31]. Flow values thus obtained divided by the pressure gradient across the collateral bed result in conductance units. Since the normal maximal arterial conductance is known, these conductance units provide an indication of the degree of adaptation by collateral arteries. The physiological conductance of the unoccluded femoral artery down-stream from the profunda branch is around 450 ml/min/100mmHg. Acutely after femoral occlusion it falls to about 50 ml/min/100mmHg and a few weeks later and without

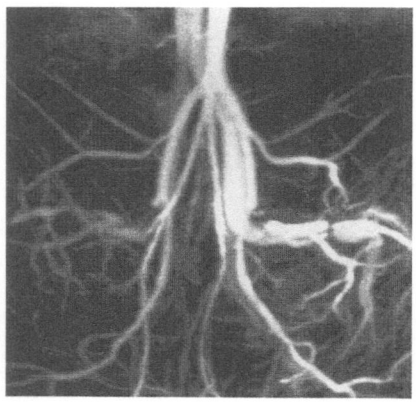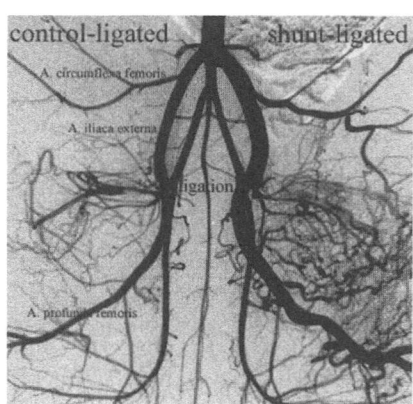

Fig. 6a   Fig. 6b

Angiography of the porcine hind limb collateral circulation by MRI (a) and by DSA (b) one week after shunt creation and two weeks after femoral ligature. Increased blood flow to the shunt-ligated leg is visible by MRI-angiogram by the early venous filling and its arteriogenic effect is obvious by DSA as the diameter of feeding arteries and the number of collaterals are increased.

treatment about 110 ml/min/100mmHg are reached. The AV-shunt resulted, after 4 weeks in place and acutely occluded for the terminal experiment, in an almost complete adaptation, i.e., 380 ml/min/100mmHg were obtained (Fig. 10). Such a result was never observed before although maximally tolerated doses of VEGF, PlGF and MCP-1 were tested in the same model. Growth factor treatment never exceeded 50 % of the normal maximal conductance. The shunt experiments show that it is indeed possible to obtain complete restitution of the maximal conductance by collateral artery growth and that this is obtained primarily by increasing fluid shear stress. **Complete restoration of maximal conductance by collateral vessels is therefore the new benchmark for therapeutic trials, at least in experimental animals.**

The mechanism for enhanced growth caused by increased fluid shear stress through venous drainage of collateral flow is again dominated by the monocyte system: a much stronger attraction, adherence and penetration of monocytes occurred and all layers of the collateral vessels were invaded by them and the perivascular space was particularly infested. This was caused by the FSS-induced strong upregulation of the adhesion molecules ICAM-1 and VCAM-1. The latter was not only overexpressed in the endothelium but also in the adventitia and media (see Fig. 7a). This suggests a correlation (probably a causal relationship) between the degree of fluid

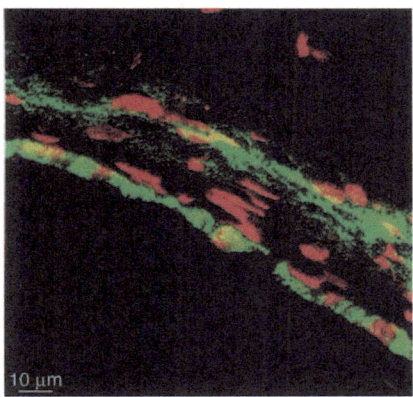

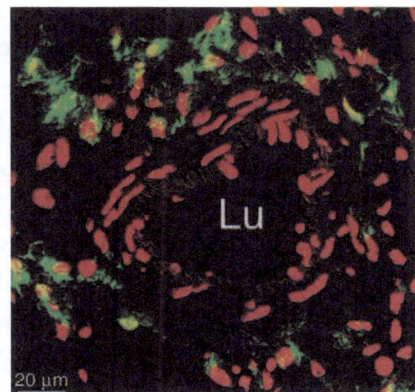

Fig. 7a

Fig. 7b

Immunoconfocal microscopic picture of VCAM labeling in endothelium and the adventitia. Specific labeling is green, nuclei are red.

Immunoconfocal micrograph of a growing collateral artery under chronic high fluid shear stress. Note the large number of monocytes/ macrophages (yellow/green) in the adventitia.

shear stress and the number of invading monocytes (Fig. 7b). As a result of increased monocyte influx the proliferative activity was switched on again in the pig where it had almost completely subsided during the week that was interposed between the ligature and the creation of the venous drainage. In the rabbit where the shunt had to be created simultaneously with the ligature (shunts created later caused acute cardiac failure due to volume overload) the mitotic index was much higher in venous drainage collaterals than on the control side (same animal) where the femoral artery was simply ligated. The angiographic images of the collateral system of fluid shear stressed collateral vessels also suggest that the process of elimination of most small collaterals to the advantage of a few large ones ("pruning") is delayed. Furthermore it appears that the degree of tortuosity is also lesser compared to collateral vessels that were not shear stressed.

The concept of vasodilatory reserve of the collateral dependent coronary vascular bed in the dog heart (after ameroid occlusion of 2 of the 3 coronary arteries), as a measure of adaptation by collateral vessels was introduced by our group in 1976[32]. It describes the range of blood flows during adenosine-induced vasodilation over a range of pump-induced pressures and arrives as an expression of conductance. Typical values, expressed in conductance ratios (normal zone over collateral dependent zones) are 0.35 ± 0.10. These were reached about 8 to 12 weeks after occlusion.

Unger's group [33,34] used a modification of our method (only one coronary artery occluded, no pressure variations, chromonar instead of adenosine) and arrived at slightly higher values (0.40 to 0.50). Similar values were also obtained in ameroid-occluded left circumflex coronary arteries (the smallest) of the pig by the laboratory with the widest experience in pig collaterals [35,36]. However, differences between two forms of vasodilatation were noted: higher conductances were obtained after adenosine compared to severe exercise. These results in pigs were possible only by also remodeling of the microvascular bed in addition to the interconnecting thin-walled non-muscle "collaterals": a massive angiogenic response had resulted in a decrease of the microvascular resistance as shown by Roth et al. [36] and by Goerge et al. [37]: pump perfusion of the collateral dependent vascular bed via the distal stump of the occluded artery resulted in higher flows at any given pressure compared to normally-perfused regions. In

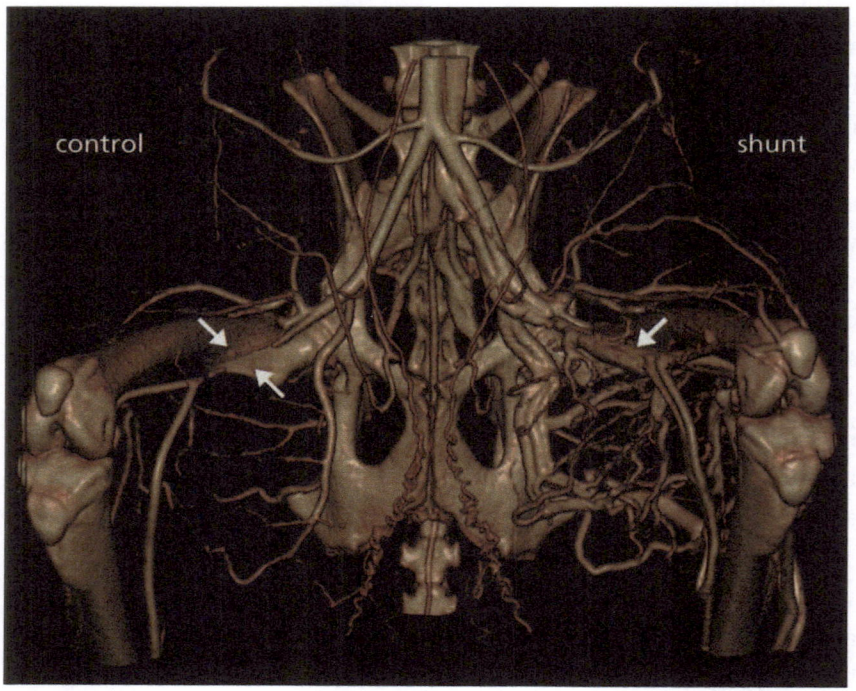

Fig. 8

CT-imge of rabbit hind limb vasculature after one week of AV-shunt and femoral ligation. The patent shunt between the distal femoral stump and its accompanying vein is clearly visible. Note: the number and size of collaterals spanning from the deep femoral to the caudal femoral artery. Arrow – site of shunt, Double arrow – site of occlusion without shunt.

our experiments with a wide range of aortic perfusion pressures the plot of peripheral pressure versus collateral flow was shifted towards much higher flow values compared to the plot of aortic pressure versus normal flow.

In other species like the rabbit and in certain mouse strains similar results for the degree of adaptation to femoral artery occlusion were reported (always under maximal vasodilatation). Only about 40% of maximal flow values were restored by collaterals.

From these and other observations we conclude that growing collaterals only provide a fraction of the maximal flow reserve (maximal conductance) in all animal species that we have studied. Only a drastic increase in shear stress can improve the degree of adaptation.

Reduction of fluid shear stress*

Intima formation is a regular feature of collateral artery growth in animals larger than the mouse. It is always present, usually as a subendothelial layer of dedifferentiated SMCs surrounded by increased amounts of matrix material. Sometimes the intima mass totally occludes the lumen. We have speculated that this is the process of natural selection that takes place among the many preexistent collaterals that initially participate in the growth process after arterial occlusion, and which is survived

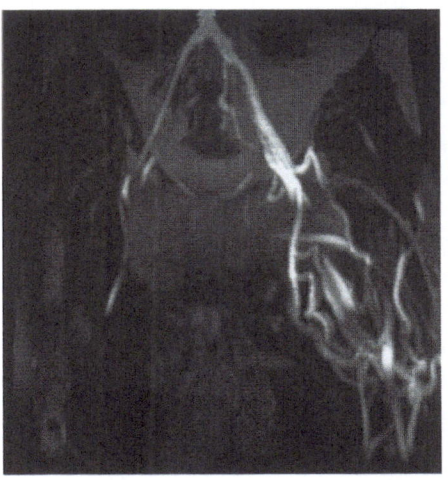

Fig. 9

MRI angiography of the rabbit hind limb after four weeks of AV-shunt and femoral ligation. The increased number and size of the collateral arteries spanning the ligature is evident in comparison to ligation only. Besides, the feeding arteries show enlarged diameters indicating an enhanced blood flow through the collateral circulation. The collateral flow directly entering the venous system is 10-fold higher than the contralateral normal collateral flow.

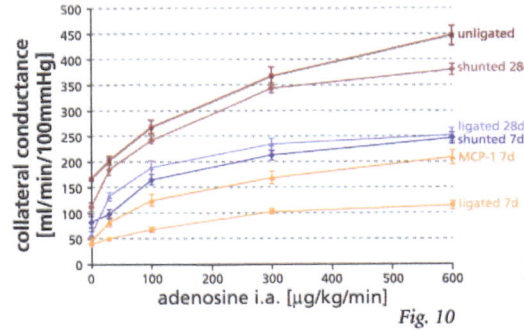

Fig. 10

Adenosine dose response curves for collateral conductance values in the rabbit hind limb after one week of shunting or ligation only (control). Hemodynamic measurements were performed after acute shunt ligation. Results are presented as mean ± SEM. Maximal vasodilatation was obtained at infusion of 600 μg adenosine/kg/min into the terminal aorta.

---

*Dimitri Scholz and Wolfgang Schaper were the principal investigators of this study

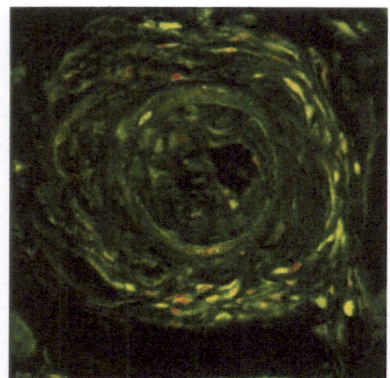

Fig. 11

Immunohistochemistry of a murine collateral artery at 3 days after femoral artery occlusion followed by 14 days of femoral artery reperfusion. The animal received BrdU immediately after onset of reperfusion. Note the thick occlusive intima and numerous BrdU positive cells (yellow). Reduction of shear stress in the collateral vessel by restoration of antegrade flow had resulted in inward remodeling.

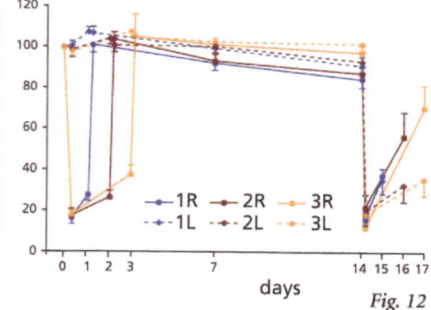

Fig. 12

Effect of femoral artery occlusion, - reperfusion and - reocclusion on recovery of pedal blood flow. The femoral artery was occluded for 1, 2 or 3 days before reperfusion and both femoral arteries were occluded, resp. re-occluded, at day 14. Recovery of blood flow was much faster on the re-occluded side when the primary occlusion had lasted for 2 days and longer. Values in % of control, R –right, L – left.

only by a few large-calibre ones. Mild forms of intima formation were considered as signaling the reduction of shear stress that comes with the increase of the vessel size by growth: the repellent action of NO is no longer dominating and cells having migrated into the intima complete the cell cycle and remain there. Another hypothesis is that the intima may serve as an "incubator" for SMC proliferation: the activated endothelium produces the chemoattractants and mitogens for SMCs. Under the influence of the repellent action of endothelial NO the new cells leave the intima and participate in the outward remodeling of the vessel or they undergo apoptotic death while still in the intimal space. We tested this hypothesis in mice. This species is not prone to intimal formation in growing collaterals, probably because the one-layer-SMC-media needs only one cell division to double its diameter and thereafter remains a one-to-two-layered media without the need of an "incubator". When, the femoral artery ligature is removed after two to three days and antegrade flow has resumed (monitored by LDI), cell proliferation continues for some time in the collateral vessels (now deprived of NO production because of the drastic reduction of flow) and the new cells occlude the lumen (Fig. 11). If the femoral artery is again occluded two weeks after reperfusion, pedal blood flow drops to the same low levels as with the first occlusion but the recovery of flow is much faster than before (Fig. 12): the intimal cells were apparently able to rapidly rearrange under the influence of the restored fluid shear stress, much faster than possible by cell division. Two days after re-occlusion the collateral diameters were indeed wider than expected and only small clusters of intimal cells were visible (Fig. 13). We call this process "medialization" of the intima (Scholz). The rapidity of structural dilatation was sufficient to prevent ischemia,

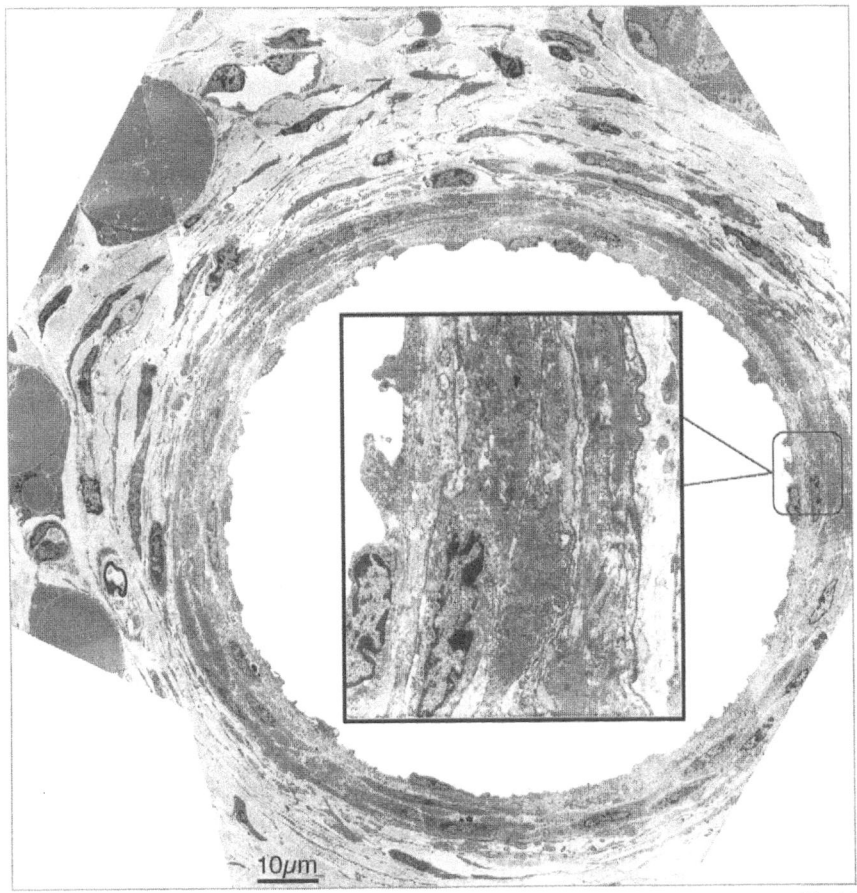

Fig. 13

Electron microscopy of a collateral artery after 3 days of femoral artery occlusion, followed by 14 days of femoral reperfusion, followed by 2 days of femoral re-occlusion. Note the rapid outward remodeling resulting in a vessel with a much larger diameter than after primary occlusion. Former intimal cells were incorporated into the media ("medialization"), a process occurring much faster than by re-entry into the cell cycle.

necrosis of the lower leg muscles, and subsequent activation of satellite cells, all typical consequences of the first occlusion. These experiments support our hypothesis that (1.) indeed intima formation is a function of shear stress, that (2.) the intima is an incubator for SMC proliferation, and (3.) it may serve a valuable function during outward remodeling, and (4.) that it is the process of eliminating small and inefficient collaterals in favor of few large ones.

The role of NO*

Shear stress was demonstrated to upregulate eNOS expression *in vitro*[39] and increased levels of eNOS mRNA and protein were found in localized areas of high shear stress *in vivo*[40]. The mechanism underlying shear stress induced eNOS expression includes mediators like tyrosine kinase cSrc, Raf, Ras and PKC, etc.[41].

Since we know that FSS is increased immediately after femoral occlusion, and since the result of that is increased NO release, it may be assumed that NO plays a significant role in arteriogenesis. Indeed, Terjung's group[42] has published elegant studies showing that NO is particularly relevant for arteriogenesis but to a lesser degree in angiogenesis. Matsunaga et al. propose that NO is critical for arteriogenesis. They based it on the observation that collateral artery formation in the peripheral circulation was impaired in eNOS-knockout mice[43]. Our own studies in the femoral-occluded rabbit hind limb and in coronary collateral arteries in the canine heart showed a marked intimal upregulation of eNOS. FSS-related endothelial NO release leads to relaxation of the underlying SMCs and this could, by increasing tangential wall tension, indirectly lead to proliferation of the vascular smooth muscle cells. We performed several experiments to test the hypothesis of NO involvement in arteriogenesis.

1. Our studies with N-Methyl-L-Arginine-Acetate (L-NNA) treated mice after femoral artery occlusion initially showed poor recovery of pedal blood flow but cessation of treatment led to quick recovery within two days to normal values. This is too fast to explain the return to expected levels by a new wave of cell proliferation. However, even continuous treatment showed a convergence of the flow values toward the end of the experiment: at three weeks of occlusion plus L-NNA treatment the same result was obtained as with no NO-inhibition, which

---

*Dimitri Scholz carried out the mouse studies, Miroslav Barancik was responsible for the signaling studies

possibly means that only the initial stages of the arteriogenic process were inhibited. The explanation for these findings is that collateral growth had occurred uninhibited but its effect was obscured by the increased vascular tone that had reduced pedal blood flow, i.e., the readout was imperfect and did not reflect collateral artery growth.

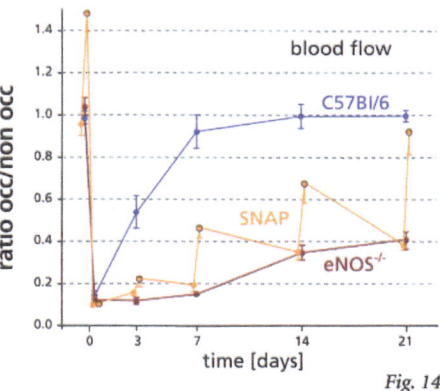

Fig. 14

Influence of targeted disruption of the eNOS gene on the recovery of blood flow after femoral artery occlusion in mice. Quantitative analysis of Laser-Doppler-based pedal blood flow measurement illustrating the poor recovery of the eNOS⁻/⁻ mice. Exogenous application of the NO- donor SNAP could completely rescue blood flow at day 21.

2. Another experiment was performed in mice with targeted disruption of the eNOS gene. These mice showed a very poor recovery of pedal blood flow after femoral artery occlusion but blood flow could be rescued by application of NO donors like SNAP (Fig. 14). This again suggests that the overriding influence of vasoconstriction had obscured the adaptation of the collateral resistance which had indeed taken place: morphometric studies revealed that the collateral vessels diameter were slightly wider compared to wildtypes, but had significantly thinner walls (Fig. 15).

3. We found that in the rabbit model the expression of neural NOS (nNOS) was strongly upregulated in growing collateral vessels as detected by microarray studies and confirmed by Northern-blot-analysis. However, nNOS knockout mice did not differ from wildtypes with regard to blood flow recovery following femoral artery occlusion.

These experimental results would argue against a significant primary contribution of the NO system to arteriogenesis. It is furthermore difficult to see a direct role of NO as a mitogen for SMCs because it is a known anti-mitogen [44,45] and SMCs under the influence of NO remain in the differentiated state by regulating the transcription of smooth muscle specific myosin heavy chain (MHC) [46].

NO also inhibits migration of vascular SMCs, but promotes endothelial cell migration and tube formation. It is further reported that NO protects the endothelium against platelet aggregation and leukocyte adherence.

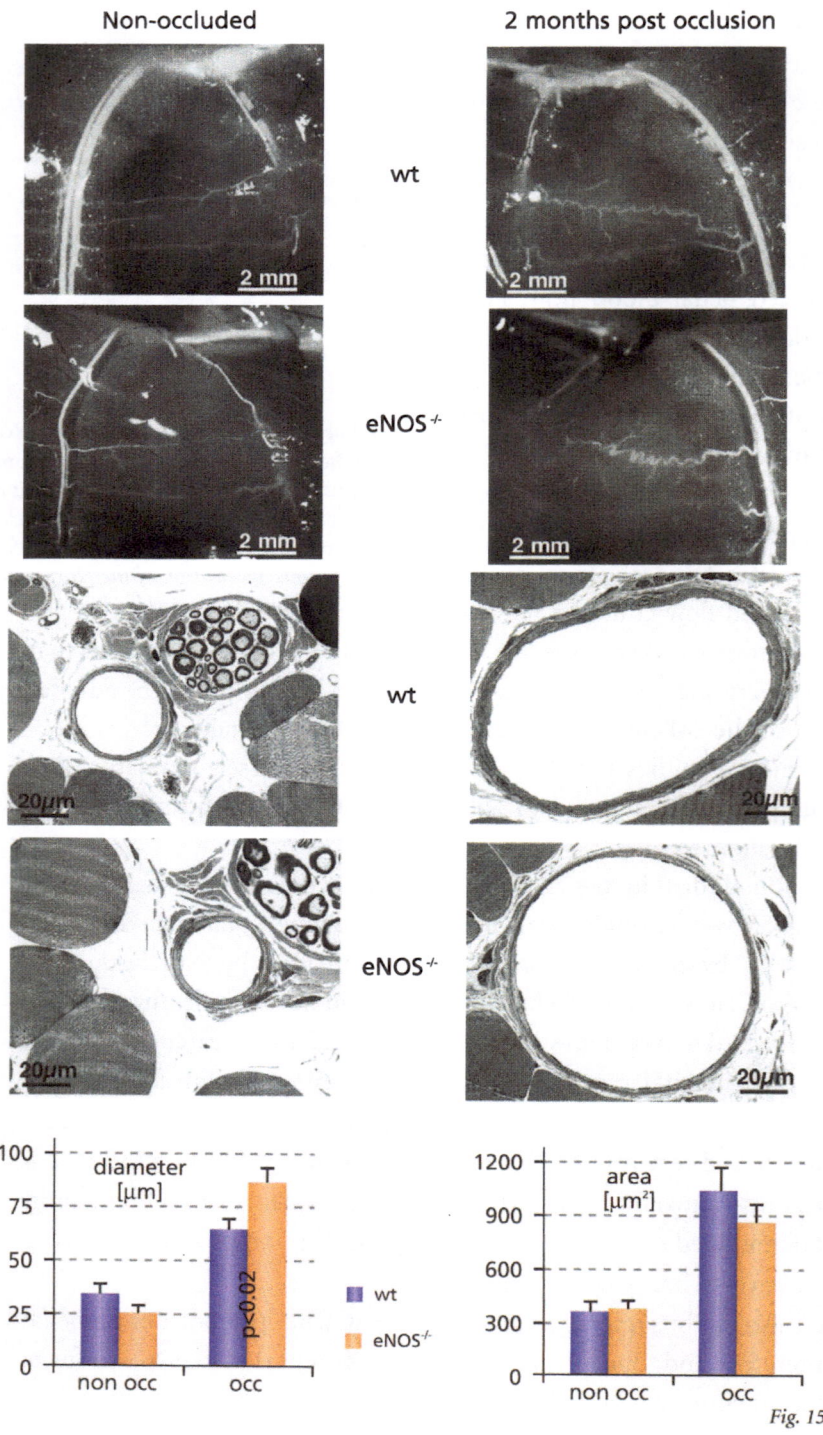

Fig. 15

However, the latter is of critical importance for collateral development. Furthermore, NO inhibits MMP-2 and MMP-9 activity, i.e., factors essential for arteriogenesis. Our studies have shown that in normal collateral arterioles endothelial cells express MMP-2 and MMP-9 and exhibit weak eNOS signals, but that in growing collateral vessels endothelial cells contain high eNOS and low MMP levels. This is different in SMCs of growing collateral vessels, where the MMPs are upregulated. Other studies showed that eNOS gene transfer inhibits smooth muscle cell migration and MMP-2 and MMP-9 activity[47]. These observations make it difficult to accept a direct positive influence of NO on arteriogenesis, except perhaps for a structuring effect based on the repellent action of endothelial NO upon SMCs in the intima: in the presence of insulin NO has a pro-migratory effect[48-50].

In our experiments in rabbits, where a large part of the collateral flow was shunted into the venous system, an upregulation of eNOS was also observed. To test the significance of this observation, which was, however, not quantitatively different from the degree of marked upregulation in non-shunted collaterals, the shunt-operated animals were treated with oral L-NAME. Indeed, L-NAME significantly (but not totally) inhibited the shunt effect, i.e., fewer and smaller collaterals on the angiograms and lower maximal conductances were observed. The causal role of NO seemed to be established. However, when testing the signaling chain in excised collateral vessels, we found that the Ras-ERK-1,-2 cascade was constitutively active (about 2.5-fold over control) in the shunt collateral vessels but only half as much in shunt vessels under L-NAME treatment (Pipp, 2003 unpublished; table 1). Constitutive MAPKinase activity is an expression of continuing proliferation and, since the tissue under study is mainly composed of smooth muscle, we must assume that the Ras activity primarily reflects SMC proliferation. The FGF- and PDGF-family of growth factors is known to signal through these pathways. A reduction of SMC proliferation by eNOS inhibition is puzzling because

15) *Collateral arteries in eNOS[-/-] mice. Upper 2 panels: Contrast medium injected femoral arteries and collateral vessels before and after femoral occlusion showing collateral growth but no difference between eNOS[-/-] and wildtype mice. Middle 2 panels: Histology of collateral arteries show no obvious differences in vessel width but significant collateral growth after femoral occlusion in both groups. Note the thinner wall of the eNOS[-/-] collateral. Lower panels: Morphometric determination of collateral diameter and area. The diameter in eNOS[-/-] collaterals is larger but the total vascular area is not different from wildtype mice.*

NO proper inhibits SMC proliferation. Treatment with eNOS inhibitors should therefore lead to SMC proliferation which obviously did not occur.

NO inhibition leads to vasoconstriction but the effect on shear stress can be complex: vasoconstriction tends to increase shear stress because of the diameter change, but it simultaneously reduces flow, which has the opposite effect. In fact, velocity is related to the square of the radius, so in the presence of an unchanged pressure gradient, as it exists in the shunt circuit, fluid shear stress and circumferential wall stress decrease. The reduction of FSS would mean that other shear stress signaling pathways that are independent of NO (integrins, Rho) are also affected.

$$V = \frac{\Delta P \cdot R^2}{4l \cdot \mu}$$

$$Tw = \frac{4 \cdot \mu \cdot V}{R}$$

V	= velocity
R	= radius
P	= pressure
L	= length
μ	= viscosity
Tw	= Fluid shear stress

Decreased Ras/ERK activity by L-NAME could also be the result of a direct anti-proliferative effect of that drug, which, however, was reported not to be signalled via Ras[51]. Smooth muscle relaxation by NO increases the pressure related strain because the fully relaxed smooth muscle is much more stretched by the pulsatile pressure than the contracted SMC, which may change the transcriptional activity. The results from the L-NAME experiments can also be explained by assuming an uncoupling of the eNOS (produced in excess and phosphorylated) in such a way that O_2^--radicals are produced rather than NO[48-50].

Western blot analysis of collateral artery signaling proteins						
	ERK1/2	p-ERK1/2	H-Ras	Akt	p-SEK	p-eNOS
Control artery		-	-			
Untreated shunt compared to control collateral	nc	+250%	+230%	nc	nc	nc
Shunt L-NAME compared to untreated shunt	nc	-50%	-50%	nc	nc	nc

nc - not changed

Table 1

Oxygen-based free radicals are known to stimulate SMC proliferation. L-NAME would inhibit NO- as well as O_2^--production. The free radical-hypothesis is strengthened by our observation that the Akt pathway, which is involved in NO signaling, was not activated in shear stressed collateral vessels. The hypothesis of an "uncoupling" of eNOS by excessive shear stress is supported by our finding that VCAM is markedly overexpressed in shunt-stimulated collaterals and that this overexpression is not restricted to the intima (see Fig. 7a). To differentiate between NO and ROS the level of soluble cGMP in collateral vessels could be decisive. In conclusion, we can say that the shear-stress-related overexpression of eNOS influences collateral artery growth, especially under extremely high shear stress, which may lead to the production of oxygen-based radicals. The unforced development of collateral vessels does proceed without involvement of NO.

Gene transcription under the influence of high fluid shear stress*

The search for flow-dependent genes had begun more than 10 years ago, when the expression of individual endothelial genes was tested and compared under static or shear stress conditions *in vitro*.

More than 40 genes were reported to be upregulated by laminar shear stress (LSS) and their expression level varied in response to flow[52-55]. Promoter sequences, mediating shear stress transcriptional responses were defined and termed shear stress responsive elements (SSREs).

Shear stress was found to increase the activities of a number of kinases to modulate the phosphorylation of many signaling proteins in endothelial cells, e.g., the proteins in focal adhesion sites and the proteins in the mitogen-activated protein kinase pathways. Downstream to such signaling cascades, multiple transcription factors such as AP-1, NF-κB, the cAMP-responsive element-binding protein CREB, SMAD-proteins, Sp-1, and Egr-1 are activated. The actions of these transcription factors on the corresponding *cis*-elements result in the induction of genes encoding for vasoactivators, adhesion molecules, monocyte chemoattractants, and growth factors in endothelial cells, thus modulating vascular structure, function and growth.

Several genes are reported to be induced by shear stress[56,57]; among these are genes which are also involved in the process of arteriogenesis or atherosclerosis, e.g. transforming growth factor-β_1 (TGF-β_1)[58,59], the early

*Elisabeth Deindl was the principal investigator of this study

growth response factor Egr-1 [60,61] and the monocyte chemoattractant protein-1 (MCP-1) [58,62,63]. However, it also should be mentioned that the shear stress-induced increase in NO production may eventually dampen this response [62,64,65].

The finding that gene transcription can be modulated by fluid shear stress prompted investigators to search for conserved *cis*-elements in the promoters of shear stress-inducible genes. Such *cis*-elements have been identified, suggesting that several regulatory sequences may be involved in the regulation of transcription in cells exposed to shear stress. For example, functional analyses have indicated that a tetra-decanoyl phorbol acetate responsive element (TRE, TPA-responsive element, AP-1 binding site, respectively) with the sequence TGACTACA, as well as a divergent TRE (TGACTCC) is important for the induction of MCP-1 in bovine endothelial cells by shear stress [66,67]. Furthermore, a recent study has also demonstrated that reporter gene activity driven by the glucocorticoid response element was enhanced in endothelial cells exposed to shear stress [68].

The regulatory element GAGACC was initially identified as a SSRE on the basis of analyses performed on the platelet-derived growth factor B chain (PDGF-B) promoter following the application of fluid shear stress [69]. The same sequence has also been found in the 5'-flanking regions of other shear stress-sensitive genes such as TGF-β_1, MCP-1 and endothelial nitric oxide synthase, eNOS [70]. NF-κB was demonstrated to bind the core SSRE within a 20 bp oligonucleotide derived from the PDGF-B promoter implicating a role for NF-κB in the shear stress-induced activation of gene expression [71].

Many of the published results on shear stress and SSRE are *in vitro* results obtained from ECs that were cultured under static conditions with a subsequent exposition to high shear stress for a short period. However, this does not necessarily reflect physiological conditions where vascular cells are constantly exposed to physiological levels of flow-related stress. A shift from low flow to high flow might elicit different biological responses than a shift from static conditions to high levels of flow. For example, when endothelial cells are cultured under static conditions and exposed to fluid shear stress for a short period, there is an initial stress response that includes a Ca^{2+} transient [72], the pronounced activation of NF-κB, and the expression of adhesion molecules such as E-selectin and the chemokine MCP-1. Over the next 4 to 8 hours any further increase in shear stress does not necessarily elicit a second Ca^{2+} transient nor reactivate NF-κB[73]. Moreover, a number of changes take place. One good example is an increase in the expression of eNOS[74-76], and the increased production of NO from cells exposed to shear stress then counteracts the activation of NF-κB and, as a consequence, adhesion molecule and chemokine expression[62,64,77]. Therefore, to avoid a generalized stress response and to avoid false positive results concerning shear stress, it is advisable to precondition endothelial cells with low shear stress before applying high shear stress.

Our results on applying high levels of shear stress (12 dynes cm^{-2}) to bovine aortic endothelial cells (BAECS) preconditioned with low shear stress (3 dynes cm^{-2}) showed that the shear stress responsive element GAGACC is not generally valid for the mediation of transcriptional activity in response to shear stress. The data indicated that the nucleotides adjacent to the SSRE rather than the GAGACC core element itself are important in mediating the response. The results showed that a putative CREB-like protein is part of a protein-complex binding to the novel identified SSRE with the sequence $ACC^G/_T AGACCAG$[78]. Furthermore, our *in vivo* results in the mouse and rabbit model of arteriogenesis never pointed to a role of NF-κB in mediating shear stress induced collateral artery growth (unpublished data, E. Deindl).

However, our data on preconditioned BAECs showed that application of high shear stress results in an increased expression of the reporter gene β-galactosidase driven by a shortened Egr-1 promoter fragment (-425 to +12bp)[78]. The promoter contained 5 serum response elements (SRE), each composed of a serum response factor binding site (SRF, CC [A/T]6GG box, also known as CArG box), and one cAMP-response site (CRE, TGACGTCA). This is in agreement with previous results showing enhanced CAT activity driven by a similar Egr-1 promoter fragment (-425bp to + 65bp) in shear stress-stimulated HeLa cells[60]. The deletion of an AP-1 site and an EBS site (Egr-1 binding site, CG[C]5GC) 5' to the SRE sites did not prevent shear stress activation[60]. In contrast, we found that Egr-1 downregulates its own promoter by binding to an upstream EBS[79]. Although it has been reported that the activator protein-1, AP-1, is involved in shear stress mediated signal transduction[80], our own results did not point to a functional role of the c-jun/c-jun c-fos/c-jun dimer for collateral artery growth (unpublished data, E. Deindl).

Egr-1 is a nuclear transcription factor of the zinc-finger class that has been implicated in SMC migration and proliferation. Our studies in the mouse model of arteriogenesis showed that Egr-1, which is expressed in arteriolar ECs and SMCs, is strongly upregulated on the RNA- and protein level during the early phase of arteriogenesis indicating that the transcription factor is strongly implicated in the initiation of collateral artery growth (E. Deindl, unpublished). Transcriptional activation of Egr-1 is responsible for the coordinated expression of vascular proteins such as tissue factor (TF), TGF-β_1 and urokinase-plasminogen activator (chapter 6). All of them are involved in vascular remodeling and arteriogenesis [59,81,82]. Based on the fact that the consensus recognition sequences of Egr-1 and the specificity protein 1 (Sp1) are overlapping, it has been proposed that the rapid shear stress mediated trans-activation of genes like TF is achieved by replacement of Sp1 by Egr-1 [60].

The fluid shear stress mediated induction of Egr-1 itself is processed via the Ras-MEK-ERK pathway involving as downstream target beside the transcription factor SRF the transcription factor Elk-1 that binds to its consensus sequence Ets (GGAA). Previous results have shown that Ets containing promoters can also be activated by growth factors like FGF-2 [60,83]. However, it is likely that during arteriogenesis the action of FGF-2, which itself induces the Ras/Raf-MEK-ERK pathway upon binding to FGFR receptor-1, (chapter 11, Fig. 2) is mediated by shear stress. Involving the integrin – Rho – cofilin pathway, fluid shear stress induces the release of FGF-2 [84], which is necessary for ligand induced dimerization and activation of the high affinity receptor resulting in signal transduction through the Ras/Raf-MEK-ERK pathway.

The MADS box transcription factor SRF controls a wide range of genes involved in cell proliferation and differentiation. The SRE (CArG-box motif) and a TGF-β_1 control element are present in the promoters of virtually all SMC differentiation marker genes characterized to date including smooth muscle alpha actin, smooth muscle myosin heavy chain, telokin, and SM22 alpha. The control elements are required for expression of these genes *in vivo* and *in vitro* (for review see Owens [85]).

The TGF-β_1 promoter bearing an SRE element and TGF-β_1 proper have been shown to be upregulated due to fluid shear stress *in vitro*[86]. However, our *in vivo* data did not reveal an increased expression of TGF-β_1 on the RNA level but clearly showed an activation of TGF-β_1 during arteriogenesis. Furthermore, arteriogenesis was stimulated by infusion of TGF-β_1 in rabbits[59]. The signal transduction cascade associated with TGF-β_1 – dependent transcription involves SMAD transcription factors and a CREB-binding protein as cofactor[87]. Our results showed that TGF-β_1 induces enhanced expression of carp (cardiac ankyrin repeat protein), a co-transcription factor identified to be involved in arteriogenesis[88].

Several publications have shown that fluid shear stress activates multiple signal transduction molecules, such as the Ras/extracellular-regulated kinase (ERK1/2)[89,90], phophatidylinositol 3-kinase (PI3)/Akt[91,92], and p38 MAPK[93,94]. However, since deviations of arterial levels of fluid shear stress can result in positive (arteriogenesis) but also in negative (atherosclerosis) remodeling of arteries and arterioles, it is obvious that distinct physiological levels of blood flow do not result in a general induction of all pathways, but that individual signal transduction pathways are differentially regulated and induced. **Our own *in vivo* results on collateral artery growth have shown that the integrin/Rho/LIMK pathway and the Ras-Raf/ERK1/2 pathway but not the p38 or Akt pathway are responsible for arteriogenesis.**

Proteins expressed under the influence of high fluid shear stress*

The AV-shunt model provided tissue for a study of high fluid shear stress-induced protein expression using 2D gel elecrophoresis (2D-PAGE). More than 1000 proteins were detected (Fig. 16). About 50 of these were differentially expressed in collateral artery samples. So far we could identify 20 proteins with altered expression, among which is a relatively large group of proteins which are known to take part in the regulation of the actin cytoskeleton (cofilin-destrin family). Actin filaments (F-actin) constitute a dynamic component of the cytoskeleton of eukaryotic cells. Processes of cellular motility[95] and cell division are dependent upon a pool of actin subunits capable of rapid assembly and disassembly in response to extracellular signals. The interaction of actin with the cell membrane, and changes in actin organization, both bases of cell movement, are reg-

---

* Stefanie Boehm is the first author of this paragraph

ulated by actin-binding proteins such as destrin/actin depolymerizing factor (ADF) and both cofilins [96-99]. These actin-binding proteins are essential for the rapid turnover of filamentous actin [100,101] and possess a nuclear transport sequence. Thus, they may be responsible for the nuclear import of actin [102,103].

The three members of the destrin/cofilin family with a molecular weight of about 19 kD serve different functions and differ in their relative abundance [104,105]. They are affected by pH-value [106] and their activity is regulated by phosphorylation [107,108].

Until now, nothing is known about the promoter or regulatory elements of either destrin or the cofilins. Only the regulation of the activity of destrin and cofilin has been described to be regulated by phosphorylation of a single serine residue. LIMK1, 2 [108,109] and TESK 1, 2 [107] can phosphorylate destrin and cofilin. LIMK1 is regulated by the small GTPase rac, whereas LIMK2 is regulated by cdc42 and rho but not by rac [110,111]. The half-life period of phosphorylated destrin is very short depending on energy level or oxidative stress.

In locomoting cells, pAC (phospho-ADF/cofilin) is localized within the cell body but is depleted from the lamellipodium itself. In non-migrating fibroblasts pAC is detectable in both the cell body and the lamellipodium. G-actin concentration is limited to the lamellipodium of migrating cells, and the recycling of actin is the limiting step for membrane protrusion in such cells [112].

The protein slingshot (SSH) is an actin-binding phosphatase. It suppresses LIMK1-induced actin reorganization and dephosphorylates phospho-cofilin [113]. Another protein called 14-3-3 protein prevents destrin and cofilin phosphorylation and activitation [114].

Downregulation of destrin/ADF in growing collateral arteries

In humans, the mRNA of destrin [96,98] with a size of 1.8 kb is expressed in most organs but not in skeletal muscle.

mRNA of destrin with a size of 1.9 kb is detectable in normal arteries from pigs. Destrin expression in our experiments markedly decreased in growing collateral arteries from both, shunt and non-shunted sides (Fig. 17). Shortly after femoral artery ligation the destrin mRNA was no longer detectable.

Cofilin1 and Cofilin2 are reciprocally expressed

Two different cofilin isoforms have been identified. Cofilin1 is the non-muscle isoform and the intermediate between cofilin2 and destrin. Cofilin1 is highly expressed in brain and liver, moderately in heart, spleen, lung, kidney and testis. Almost no expression can be detected in skeletal muscle. In humans, the mRNA of cofilin1 has a size of 1.4 kb. Cofilin2 is the muscle specific isoform of both cofilins[115,116]. Cofilin2 is expressed in skeletal muscle and possesses two transcripts of 1.8 and 3 kb. Both, mRNA and protein can also be found in SMCs and in other organs[117].

In Northern blot analysis, both cofilins showed a reciprocal expression pattern. In collateral arteries after AV-shunting, cofilin1 mRNA was upregulated, whereas cofilin2 mRNA was downregulated (Fig. 17). Comparing this expression of cofilin2 with that in control arteries, we found an increase in growing collateral arteries two weeks after ligation. This is consistent with the results found in the rabbit model of femoral occlusion[118].

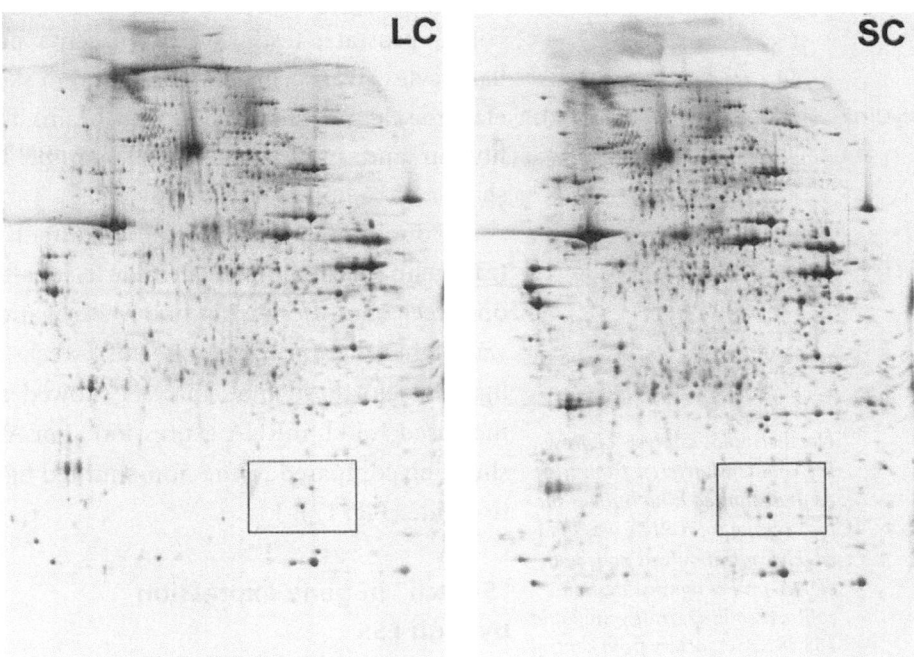

Fig. 16

2D-PAGE of proteins obtained from isolated collateral arteries from the control-ligated (LC) and the shunt-ligated (SC) side. One hundred µg protein were separated and silver stained. Framed region shows differentially expressed proteins.

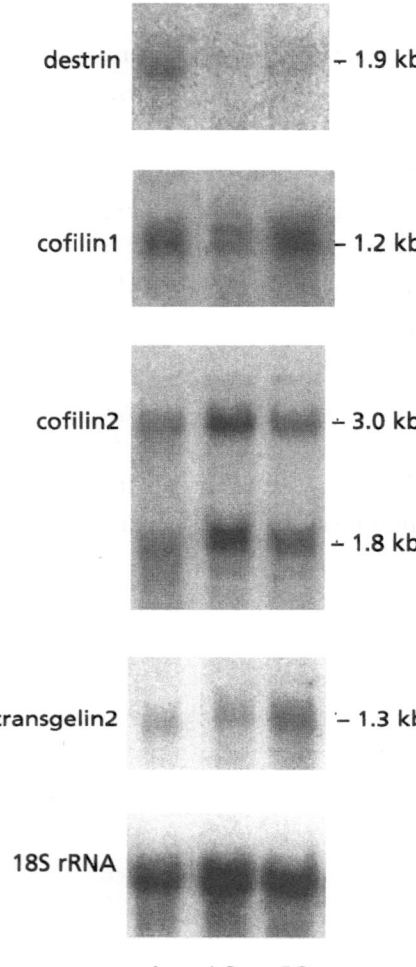

destrin — 1.9 kb

cofilin1 — 1.2 kb

cofilin2 — 3.0 kb

— 1.8 kb

transgelin2 — 1.3 kb

18S rRNA

A   LC   SC

Fig. 17

Northern blot analysis of growing collateral arteries from ligated and shunted hind limb of the pig. Ten µg total RNA was loaded. Hybridization was done with cDNA-probes against destrin, cofilin1, cofilin2, transgelin2 and 18S rRNA. A, artery from control pig; LC, collateral artery after 2 weeks of ligation; SC, collateral artery after 2 weeks of ligation including one week of shunting.

Transgelin2 is expressed in smooth muscle cells

Only little information about transgelin2 is available but more is known about transgelin, also called SM22-alpha. Transgelin is expressed in SMCs, mesenchymal cells and fibroblasts [119]. It is one of the earliest markers of differentiated SMCs in adults and transiently expressed in embryonic skeletal and cardiac tissue. Transgelin is highly conserved, binds F-actin (1:6, transgelin:G-actin) and causes gelatination.

Transgelin2 is also called KIAA0120 or "SM22-alpha homologue". It shares 69.7% amino acid sequence homology with NP25 (rat neuronal protein). It is expressed in lung, liver, kidney, spleen, thymus, small intestine, colon, prostate, testis, ovary, placenta and leukocytes. Transgelin2 can be found in skeletal muscle, pancreas, heart and brain. The human and mouse cDNAs of transgelin2 share a 95% homology.

In our proteomic studies the content of transgelin2 protein in collateral arteries after one week shunt following one week ligation was higher than in vessels after two weeks of ligation. Northern blot analysis showed an increased 1.3 kb mRNA expression after AV-shunting compared to the non-shunted ligation side (Fig. 17).

"Switch" in gene expression by high FSS

The increased expression of transgelin2 and the expression pattern of the destrin-cofilin family lead us to postulate a "switch" of the arteriogenesis program after AV-shunting following ligation. First, the induction of cofilin2 mRNA expression may play a role in the dedifferentiation of the SMCs, in the process of changing from the contractile to the synthetic phenotype. Secondly, the ongoing arteriogenesis program seems to be arrested in SMCs, and to be reversed, as the cells increased the expression of transgelin2 (which may be a differentiation marker like SM22-alpha) and decreased the expression of cofilin2 (depolymerization of actin is reduced). In contrast to cofilin2 expression, the non-muscle specific isoform cofilin1 is upregulated. Cofilin1 again starts to depolymerize actin, thereby changing the cytoskeleton of the cells to restart the program of proliferation and arteriogenesis. Cofilin was found in the contractile ring during the late stages of proliferation, thus cofilin is involved in the reorganization during cytokinesis[120].

The strong and prolonged change of the expression of cytoskeletal genes (and those regulating proliferation) that we observed in our shunt experiments is a repitition of expression changes that already occurred with the first wave of collateral growth following the original femoral artery occlusion, but with lower intensity. During the ensuing week between occlusion and shunt operation these changes had stopped, only to be restarted more pronouncedly by the high shear forces created by the shunt. Because of the promptness and magnitude of the response we refer to these changes as the "arteriogenic switch".

The role of blood viscosity as part of the shear stress response*

Blood viscosity is linearly related to shear stress and manipulations of viscosity should become an interesting tool for testing the shear stress hypothesis of arteriogenesis because, at least in theory, it would be an isolated change without altering pressure-related stresses.

The viscosity of flowing blood is dependent on the hematocrit, which is drastically increased in transgenic erythropoietin overexpressing mice. The strain of mice that we studied (a kind gift by Prof. Max Gassmann, Zurich, Switzerland) was generated by pronuclear microinjection of human EPO cDNA, which was driven by the human PDGF B-chain promoter. After backcrossing of the transgene into a C57BL/6 background for 7-10 generations, we studied 12-14 weeks old male mice in the femoral artery occlusion model. The recovery of blood flow, usually very quick in this

---

*Dimitri Scholz was the principal investigator of this study

wildtype strain, was very slow in the transgenic animals which exhibited hematocrits of over 90 % (Fig. 18), and at first sight it looked as if our working hypothesis was refused. However, the morphometry of perfusion fixed collateral vessels showed a significant increase in the diameter and wall thickness of the collateral vessels over and above that of wildtype mice with femoral occlusion (Fig. 19). The retardation of blood flow recovery was thus not caused by defective vascular growth but by the decrease of blood flow velocity below the critical Farräus-Lindhquist threshold.

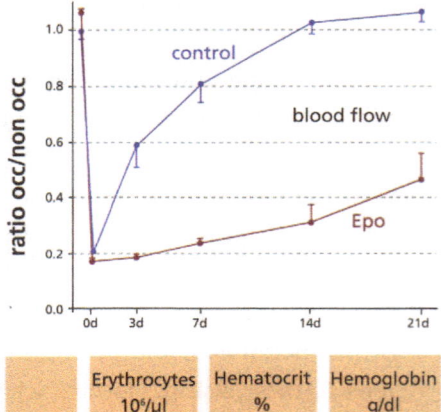

	Erythrocytes $10^6/\mu l$	Hematocrit %	Hemoglobin g/dl
Control	6.7±1.7	37.2±6.7	10.6±2.4
EPO	16.8±0.7	91.6±3.5	23.9±0.6
	p<0.001	p<0.001	p<0.001

Fig. 18

Laser-Doppler images of pedal blood flow in transgenic mice overexpressing human erythropoetin under the control of the PDGF-B promoter. Note the rapid recovery of pedal blood flow in the wildtype mice and the virtually absent recovery in the transgenic mice (left panel). Upper right panel: Quantitative analysis of blood flow recovery. Lower panel right: Quantitative analysis of erythrocytosis and hematocrit. Note the excessively high hematocrit of 92 %.

This is one of the two occasions where the measurement of pedal blood flow by the Laser-Doppler imaging method was misleading (the other was the failure to reflect collateral development in eNOS knockout mice). In conclusion, we can say that the experiments with increased shear stress by increased blood viscosity again confirm the morphogenic force of shear stress which had indeed produced wider collateral vessels.

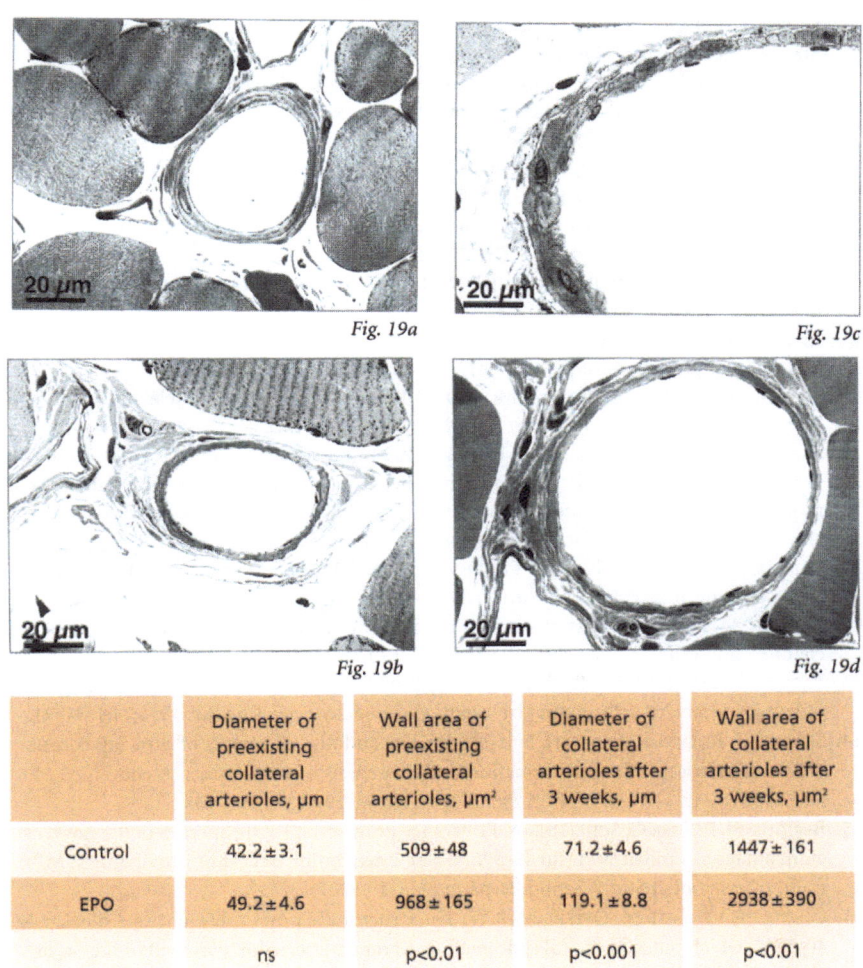

	Diameter of preexisting collateral arterioles, μm	Wall area of preexisting collateral arterioles, μm²	Diameter of collateral arterioles after 3 weeks, μm	Wall area of collateral arterioles after 3 weeks, μm²
Control	42.2±3.1	509±48	71.2±4.6	1447±161
EPO	49.2±4.6	968±165	119.1±8.8	2938±390
	ns	p<0.01	p<0.001	p<0.01

Collateral vessels 3 weeks after femoral artery occlusion in EPO-overexpressing transgenic mice. Note the thicker walls in the preexisting transgenic collateral vessel (a) as compared to control (b) and the larger diameter and thicker walls of the transgenic collaterals 3 weeks after femoral artery occlusion (c) in comparison to wildtype mice (d). The table shows the morphometric data of control and EPO collateral vessels. In spite of the higher shear stress resulting in wider collateral vessels, the blood flow did not recover to levels seen in wildtype mice.

References

1. SCHAPER W. *The Pathophysiology of Myocardial Perfusion.* Amsterdam, New York, Oxford: Elsevier/North-Holland Biomedical Press;1979.
2. LANGILLE BL, O'DONNELL F. Reductions in arterial diameter produced by chronic decreases in blood flow are endothelium-dependent. *Science.* 1986;231:405-7.
3. JACKSON ZS, GOTLIEB AI, LANGILLE BL. Wall tissue remodeling regulates longitudinal tension in arteries. *Circ Res.* 2002;90:918-25.
4. SCHEEL KW, FITZGERALD EM, MARTIN RO, LARSEN RA. The Possible Role of Mechanical Stresses on Coronary Collateral Development during Gradual Coronary Occlusion, in Schaper W (eds.): *The Pathophysiology of Myocardial Perfusion.* Amsterdam, New York, Oxford: Elsevier/North-Holland Biomedical Press; 1979:
5. AWOLESI MA, SESSA WC, SUMPIO BE. Cyclic strain upregulates nitric oxide synthase in cultured bovine aortic endothelial cells. *J Clin Invest.* 1995;96:1449-54.
6. GRABOWSKI EF, JAFFE EA, WEKSLER BB. Prostacyclin production by cultured endothelial cell monolayers exposed to step increases in shear stress. *J Lab Clin Med.* 1985;105:36-43.
7. FISSLTHALER B, POPP R, MICHAELIS UR, KISS L, FLEMING I, BUSSE R. Cyclic stretch enhances the expression and activity of coronary endothelium-derived hyperpolarizing factor synthase. *Hypertension.* 2001;38:1427-32.
8. ARNAL JF, DINH-XUAN AT, PUEYO M, DARBLADE B, RAMI J. Endothelium-derived nitric oxide and vascular physiology and pathology. *Cell Mol Life Sci.* 1999;55:1078-87.
9. VANHOUTTE PM, BOULANGER CM, MOMBOULI JV. Endothelium-derived relaxing factors and converting enzyme inhibition. *Am J Cardiol.* 1995;76:3E-12E.
10. BRANDES RP, SCHMITZ-WINNENTHAL FH, FELETOU M, GODECKE A, HUANG PL, VANHOUTTE PM, FLEMING I, BUSSE R. An endothelium-derived hyperpolarizing factor distinct from NO and prostacyclin is a major endothelium-dependent vasodilator in resistance vessels of wildtype and endothelial NO synthase knockout mice. *Proc Natl Acad Sci USA.* 2000;97:9747-52.
11. BARAKAT AI, LEAVER EV, PAPPONE PA, DAVIES PF. A flow-activated chloride-selective membrane current in vascular endothelial cells. *Circ Res.* 1999;85:820-8.
12. BARAKAT AI. Responsiveness of vascular endothelium to shear stress: potential role of ion channels and cellular cytoskeleton (review). *Int J Mol Med.* 1999;4:323-32.
13. BARBEE KA, DAVIES PF, LAL R. Shear stress-induced reorganization of the surface topography of living endothelial cells imaged by atomic force microscopy. *Circ Res.* 1994;74:163-171.
14. SCHAPER J, KOENIG R, FRANZ D, SCHAPER W. The endothelial surface of growing coronary collateral arteries: Intimal margination and diapedesis of monocytes.; A combined SEM and TEM study. *Virchows Arch A Pathol Anat Histol.* 1976;370:193-205.
15. BERNINK PJ, PRAGER G, SCHELLING A, KOBRIN I. Antihypertensive properties of the novel calcium antagonist mibefradil (Ro 40-5967): a new generation of calcium antagonists? Mibefradil International Study Group. *Hypertension.* 1996;27:426-32.
16. CLOZEL JP, VENIANT M, OSTERRIEDER W. The structurally novel Ca2+ channel blocker Ro 40-5967, which binds to the [3H] desmethoxyverapamil receptor, is devoid of the negative inotropic effects of verapamil in normal and failing rat hearts. *Cardiovasc Drugs Ther.* 1990;4:731-6.
17. GRAY GA, CLOZEL M, CLOZEL JP, BAUMGARTNER HR. Effects of calcium channel blockade on the aortic intima in spontaneously hypertensive rats. *Hypertension.* 1993;22:569-576.

18. SCHMITT R, CLOZEL JP, IBERG N, BUHLER FR. Mibefradil prevents neointima formation after vascular injury in rats. Possible role of the blockade of the T-type voltage-operated calcium channel. *Arterioscler Thromb Vasc Biol.* 1995;15:1161-5.

19. ROUX S, BUHLER M, CLOZEL JP. Mechanism of the antiischemic effect of mibefradil, a selective T calcium channel blocker in dogs: comparison with amlodipine. *J Cardiovasc Pharmacol.* 1996;27:132-9.

20. NILIUS B, PRENEN J, KAMOUCHI M, VIANA F, VOETS T, DROOGMANS G. Inhibition by mibefradil, a novel calcium channel antagonist, of Ca(2+)- and volume-activated Cl- channels in macrovascular endothelial cells. *Br J Pharmacol.* 1997;121:547-55.

21. NILIUS B. Chloride channels go cell cycling. *J Physiol.* 2001;532:581.

22. VOETS T, SZUCS G, DROOGMANS G, NILIUS B. Blockers of volume-activated Cl- currents inhibit endothelial cell proliferation. *Pflugers Arch.* 1995;431:132-4.

23. WONDERGEM R, GONG W, MONEN SH, DOOLEY SN, GONCE JL, HOUSER M, ECAY TW, FERSLEW KE. Blocking swelling-activated chloride current inhibits mouse liver cell proliferation. *J Physiol.* 2001;532:661-672.

24. DAY ML, JOHNSON MH, COOK DI. Cell cycle regulation of a T-type calcium current in early mouse embryos. *Pflugers Arch.* 1998;436:834-842.

25. KUGA T, KOBAYASHI S, HIRAKAWA Y, KANAIDE H, TAKESHITA A. Cell cycle-dependent expression of L- and T-type Ca2+ currents in rat aortic smooth muscle cells in primary culture. *Circ Res.* 1996;79:14-19.

26. RICHARD S, NEVEU D, CARNAC G, BODIN P, TRAVO P, NARGEOT J. Differential expression of voltage-gated Ca(2+)-currents in cultivated aortic myocytes. *Biochim Biophys Acta.* 1992; 1160:95-104.

27. CHEMIN J, MONTEIL A, BRIQUAIRE C, RICHARD S, PEREZ-REYES E, NARGEOT J, LORY P. Overexpression of T-type calcium channels in HEK-293 cells increases intracellular calcium without affecting cellular proliferation. *FEBS Letters.* 2000;478:166-172.

28. MANOLOPOULOS VG, LIEKENS S, KOOLWIJK P, VOETS T, PETERS E, DROOGMANS G, LELKES PI, DE CLERCQ E, NILIUS B. Inhibition of angiogenesis by blockers of volume-regulated anion channels. *Gen Pharmacol.* 2000;34:107-16.

29. PEXIEDER T. Prenatal development of the endocardium: a review. *Scan Electron Microsc.* 1981;2:223-253.

30. NILIUS B, EGGERMONT J, VOETS T, DROOGMANS G. Volume-activated Cl- channels. *Gen Pharmacol.* 1996;27:1131-40.

31. PIPP F, HEIL M, ISSBRUCKER K, ZIEGELHOEFFER T, MARTIN S, VAN DEN HEUVEL J, WEICH H, FERNÁNDEZ B, GOLOMB G, CARMELIET P, SCHAPER W, CLAUSS M. VEGFR-1-selective VEGF homologue PlGF is arteriogenic: evidence for a monocyte-mediated mechanism. *Circ Res.* 2003;92:378-85.

32. SCHAPER W, FLAMENG W, WINKLER B, WUESTEN B, TUERSCHMANN W, NEUGEBAUER G, CARL M, PASYK S. Quantification of collateral resistance in acute and chronic experimental coronary occlusion in the dog. *Circ Res.* 1976;39:371-377.

33. BANAI S, JAKLITSCH MD, SHOU M, LAZAROUS DF, SCHEINOWITZ M, BIRO S, EPSTEIN SE, UNGER EF. Angiogenic-induced enhancement of collateral blood flow to ischemic myocardium by vascular endothelial growth factor in dogs. *Circulation.* 1994;89:2183-2189.

34. UNGER EF, BANAI S, SHOU M, LAZAROUS DF, JAKLITSCH MT, SHEINOWITZ M, CORREA R, KLINGBEIL C, EPSTEIN SE. Basic fibroblast growth factor enhances myocardial collateral flow in a canine model. *Am J Physiol.* 1994;266:H1588-H1595.

35. WHITE FC, CARROLL SM, MAGNET A, BLOOR CM. Coronary collateral development in swine after coronary artery occlusion. *Cir Res.* 1992;71:1490-1500.

36. ROTH DM, MARUOKA Y, ROGERS J, WHITE FC, LONGHURST JC, BLOOR CM. Development of coronary collateral circulation in left circumflex ameroid-occluded swine myocardium. *Am J Physiol.* 1987;253:H1279-H1288.

37. GOERGE G, SCHMIDT T, ITO BR, PANTELY GA, SCHAPER W. Microvascular and collateral adaptation in swine hearts following progressive coronary artery stenosis. *Basic Res Cardiol.* 1989;84:524-535.

38. SCHOLZ D, ZIEGELHOEFFER T, HELISCH A, WAGNER S, FRIEDRICH C, PODZUWEIT T, SCHAPER W. Contribution of arteriogenesis and angiogenesis to postocclusive hind limb perfusion in mice. *J Mol Cell Cardiol.* 2002;34:775-787.

39. SESSA W. The nitric oxide synthase family of proteins. *J Vasc Res.* 1994;31:131-143.

40. POPPA V, MIYASHIRO JK, CORSON MA, BERK BC. Endothelial NO synthase is increased in regenerating endothelium after denuding injury of the rat aorta. *Arterioscler Thromb Vasc Biol.* 1998;18:1312-1321.

41. WEDGWOOD S, BEKKER JM, BLACK SM. Shear stress regulation of endothelial NOS in fetal pulmonary arterial endothelial cells involves PKC. *Am J Physiol Lung Cell Mol Physiol.* 2001;281:490-498.

42. YANG HT, REN J, LAUGHLIN MH, TERJUNG RL. Prior exercise training produces NO-dependent increases in collateral blood flow after acute arterial occlusion. *Am J Physiol Heart Circ Physiol.* 2002;282:H301-10.

43. MUROHARA T, ASAHARA T, SILVER M, BAUTERS C, MASUDA H, KALKA C, KEARNEY M, CHEN D, SYMES JF, FISHMAN MC, HUANG PL, ISNER JM. Nitric oxide synthase modulates angiogenesis in response to tissue ischemia. *J Clin Invest.* 1998;101:2567-78.

44. OKAZAKI J, KOMORI K, KAWASAKI K, EGUCHI D, ISHIDA M, SUGIMACHI K. L-arginine inhibits smooth muscle cell proliferation of vein graft intimal thickness in hypercholesterolemic rabbits. *Cardiovasc Res.* 1997;36:429-36.

45. CHEN C, HANSON SR, KEEFER LK, SAAVEDRA JE, DAVIES KM, HUTSELL TC, HUGHES JD, KU DN, LUMSDEN AB. Boundary layer infusion of nitric oxide reduces early smooth muscle cell proliferation in the endarterectomized canine artery. *J Surg Res.* 1997;67:26-32.

46. ITOH S, KATOH Y, KONISHI H, TAKAYA N, KIMURA T, PERIASAMY M, YAMAGUCHI H. Nitric oxide regulates smooth-muscle-specific myosin heavy chain gene expression at the transcriptional level-possible role of SRF and YY1 through CArG element. *J Mol Cell Cardiol.* 2001;33:95-107.

47. GURJAR MV, SHARMA RV, BHALLA RC. eNOS gene transfer inhibits smooth muscle cell migration and MMP-2 and MMP-9 activity. *Arterioscler Thromb Vasc Biol.* 1999;19:2871-7.

48. CAI H, HARRISON DG. Endothelial dysfunction in cardiovascular diseases. The role of oxidant stress. *Circ Res.* 2000;87:840-844.

49. DIXIT M, ZHUANG D, CEACAREANU B, HASSID A. Treatment with insulin uncovers the motogenic capacity of nictric oxide in aortic smooth muscle cells. *Circ Res.* 2003;93:e113-e123.

50. WILCOX CS. Redox regulation of the afferent arteriole and tubuloglomerular feedback. *Acta Physiol Scand.* 2003;179:217-223.

51. EL MABROUK M, SINGH A, TOUYZ RM, SCHIFFRIN EL. Antiproliferative effect of L-NAME on rat vascular smooth muscle cells. *Life Sci.* 2000;67:1613-23.

52. CHIEN S, LI S, SHYY YJ. Effects of mechanical forces on signal transduction and gene expression in endothelial cells. *Hypertension.* 1998;31:162-9.

53. GIMBRONE MA, JR., TOPPER JN, NAGEL T, ANDERSON KR, GARCIA-CARDENA G. Endothelial dysfunction, hemodynamic forces, and atherogenesis. *Ann NY Acad Sci.* 2000;902:230-9; discussion 239-40.

54. RESNICK N, YAHAV H, KHACHIGIAN LM, COLLINS T, ANDERSON KR, DEWEY FC, GIMBRONE MA, JR. Endothelial gene regulation by laminar shear stress. *Adv Exp Med Biol.* 1997;430:155-164.

55. RESNICK N, YAHAV H, SCHUBERT S, WOLFOVITZ E, SHAY A. Signaling pathways in vascular endothelium activated by shear stress: relevance to atherosclerosis. *Curr Opin Lipidol.* 2000;11:167-77.

56. BROOKS AR, LELKES PI, RUBANYI GM. Gene expression profiling of human aortic endothelial cells exposed to disturbed flow and steady laminar flow. *Physiol Genomics.* 2002;9:27-41.

57. GARCIA-CARDENA G, COMANDER JI, BLACKMAN BR, ANDERSON KR, GIMBRONE MA. Mechanosensitive endothelial gene expression profiles: scripts for the role of hemodynamics in atherogenesis? *Ann NY Acad Sci.* 2001;947:1-6.

58. NEGISHI M, LU D, ZHANG YQ, SAWADA Y, SASAKI T, KAYO T, ANDO J, IZUMI T, KURABAYASHI M, KOJIMA I, MASUDA H, TAKEUCHI T. Upregulatory expression of furin and transforming growth factor-beta by fluid shear stress in vascular endothelial cells. *Arterioscler Thromb Vasc Biol.* 2001;21:785-90.

59. VAN ROYEN N, HOEFER I, BUSCHMANN I, HEIL M, KOSTIN S, DEINDL E, VOGEL S, KORFF T, AUGUSTIN H, BODE C, PIEK JJ, SCHAPER W. Exogenous application of transforming growth factor beta 1 stimulates arteriogenesis in the peripheral circulation. *FASEB J.* 2002;16:432-4.

60. SCHWACHTGEN JL, HOUSTON P, CAMPBELL C, SUKHATME V, BRADDOCK M. Fluid shear stress activation of Egr-1 transcription in cultured human endothelial and epithelial cells is mediated via the extracellular signal-related kinase 1/2 mitogen-activated protein kinase pathway. *J Clin Invest.* 1998;101:2540-9.

61. MCCAFFREY TA, FU C, DU B, EKSINAR S, KENT KC, BUSH H, JR., KREIGER K, ROSENGART T, CYBULSKY MI, SILVERMAN ES, COLLINS T. High-level expression of Egr-1 and Egr-1-inducible genes in mouse and human atherosclerosis. *J Clin Invest.* 2000;105:653-62.

62. SHYY YJ, HSIEH HJ, USAMI S, CHIEN S. Fluid shear stress induces a biphasic response of human monocyte chemotactic protein 1 gene expression in vascular endothelium. *Proc Natl Acad Sci USA.* 1994;91:4678-4682.

63. ITO WD, ARRAS M, WINKLER B, SCHOLZ D, HTUN P, SCHAPER W. Angiogenesis but not collateral growth is associated with ischemia after femoral artery occlusion. *Am J Physiol.* 1997;273:H1255-H1265.

64. ZEIHER AM, FISSLTHALER B, SCHRAY-UTZ B, BUSSE R. Nitric oxide modulates the expression of monocyte chemoattractant protein 1 in cultured human endothelial cells. *Circ Res.* 1995;76:980-6.

65. BAO X, LU C, FRANGOS JA. Temporal gradient in shear but not steady shear stress induces PDGF-A and MCP-1 expression in endothelial cells: role of NO, NF kappa B, and Egr-1. *Arterioscler Thromb Vasc Biol.* 1999;19:996-1003.

66. SHYY JY, LI YS, LIN MC, CHEN W, YUAN S, USAMI S, CHIEN S. Multiple *cis*-elements mediate shear stress-induced gene expression. *J Biomech.* 1995;28:1451-7.

67. SHYY JY, LIN MC, HAN J, LU Y, PETRIME M, CHIEN S. The *cis*-acting phorbol ester "12-O-tetradecanoylphorbol 13-acetate"-responsive element is involved in shear stress-induced monocyte chemotactic protein 1 gene expression. *Proc Natl Acad Sci USA.* 1995;92:8069-73.

68. JI JY, JING H, DIAMOND SL. Shear stress causes nuclear localization of endothelial gluco-corticoid receptor and expression from the GRE promoter. *Circ Res.* 2003;92:279-85.

69. RESNICK N, COLLINS T, ATKINSON W, BONTHRON DT, DEWEY CF, JR., GIMBRON MA, JR. Platelet-derived growth factor B chain promoter contains a *cis*-acting fluid shear-stress-responsive element. *Proc Natl Acad Sci USA.* 1993;90:7908.

70. BRADDOCK M, SCHWACHTGEN JL, HOUSTON P, DICKSON MC, LEE MJ, CAMPBELL CJ. Fluid Shear Stress Modulation of Gene Expression in Endothelial Cells. *News Physiol Sci.* 1998; 13:241-246.

71. KHACHIGIAN LM, RESNICK N, GIMBRONE MA, JR., COLLINS T. Nuclear factor-kappa B inter-acts functionally with the platelet-derived growth factor B-chain shear-stress response ele-ment in vascular endothelial cells exposed to fluid shear stress. *J Clin Invest.* 1995;96:1169-75.

72. PRASAD AR, LOGAN SA, NEREM RM, SCHWARTZ CJ, SPRAGUE EA. Flow-related responses of intracellular inositol phosphate levels in cultured aortic endothelial cells. *Circ Res.* 1993; 72:827-36.

73. AYAJIKI K, KINDERMANN M, HECKER M, FLEMING I, BUSSE R. Intracellular pH and tyrosine phosphorylation but not calcium determine shear stress-induced nitric oxide production in native endothelial cells. *Circ Res.* 1996;78:750-8.

74. NISHIDA K, HARRISON DG, NAVAS JP, FISHER AA, DOCKERY SP, UEMATSU M, NEREM RM, ALEXANDER RW, MURPHY TJ. Molecular cloning and characterization of the constitutive bovine aortic endothelial cell nitric oxide synthase. *J Clin Invest.* 1992;90:2092-6.

75. XIAO Z, ZHANG Z, RANJAN V, DIAMOND SL. Shear stress induction of the endothelial nitric oxide synthase gene is calcium-dependent but not calcium-activated. *J Cell Physiol.* 1997;171:205-11.

76. ZIEGLER T, SILACCI P, HARRISON VJ, HAYOZ D. Nitric oxide synthase expression in endothe-lial cells exposed to mechanical forces. *Hypertension.* 1998;32:351-5.

77. TSAO PS, LEWIS NP, ALPERT S, COOKE JP. Exposure to shear stress alters endothelial adhe-siveness. Role of nitric oxide. *Circulation.* 1995;92:3513-9.

78. FISSLTHALER B, BOENGLER K, FLEMING I, SCHAPER W, BUSSE R, DEINDL E. Identification of a *cis*-element regulating transcriptional activity in response to fluid shear stress in bovine aortic endothelial cells. *Endothelium.* 2003;10:267-275.

79. CAO X, MAHENDRAN R, GUY GR, TAN YH. Detection and characterization of cellular Egr-1 binding to its recognition site. *J Biol Chem.* 1993;268:16949-57.

80. NAGEL T, RESNICK N, DEWEY CF, JR., GIMBRONE MA, JR. Vascular endothelial cells respond to spatial gradients in fluid shear stress by enhanced activation of transcription factors. *Arterioscler Thromb Vasc Biol.* 1999;19:1825-34.

81. KHACHIGIAN LM, LINDNER V, WILLIAMS AJ, COLLINS T. Egr-1-induced endothelial gene ex-pression: a common theme in vascular injury. *Science.* 1996;271:1427-31.

82. DEINDL E, ZIEGELHOFFER T, KANSE SM, FERNÁNDEZ B, NEUBAUER E, CARMELIET P, PREISSNER KT, SCHAPER W. Receptor-independent role of the urokinase-type plasminogen activator during arteriogenesis. *FASEB J.* 2003;17:1174-6.

83. SPENCER JA, MAJOR ML, MISRA RP. Basic fibroblast growth factor activates serum re-sponse factor gene expression by multiple distinct signaling mechanisms. *Mol Cell Biol.* 1999;19:3977-88.

84. GLOE T, SOHN HY, MEININGER GA, POHL U. Shear stress-induced release of basic fibrob-last growth factor from endothelial cells is mediated by matrix interaction via integrin alpha(v)beta3. *J Biol Chem.* 2002;277:23453-8.

85. OWENS GK. Molecular control of vascular smooth muscle cell differentiation. *Acta Physiol Scand.* 1998;164:623-35.

86. OHNO M, COOKE JP, DZAU VJ, GIBBONS GH. Fluid shear stress induces endothelial transforming growth factor beta-1 transcription and production. Modulation by potassium channel blockade. *J Clin Invest.* 1995;95:1363-9.

87. RODRIGUEZ-PASCUAL F, REDONDO-HORCAJO M, LAMAS S. Functional cooperation between SMAD proteins and activator protein-1 regulates transforming growth factor-beta-mediated induction of endothelin-1 expression. *Circ Res.* 2003;92:1288-95.

88. BOENGLER K, PIPP F, FERNÁNDEZ B, ZIEGELHOEFFER T, SCHAPER W, DEINDL E. Arteriogenesis is associated with an induction of the cardiac ankyrin repeat protein (carp). *Cardiovasc Res.* 2003;59:573-81.

89. BUTLER PJ, TSOU TC, LI JY, USAMI S, CHIEN S. Rate sensitivity of shear-induced changes in the lateral diffusion of endothelial cell membrane lipids: a role for membrane perturbation in shear-induced MAPK activation. *FASEB J.* 2002;16:216-8.

90. NI CW, WANG DL, LIEN SC, CHENG JJ, CHAO YJ, HSIEH HJ. Activation of PKC-epsilon and ERK1/2 participates in shear-induced endothelial MCP-1 expression that is repressed by nitric oxide. *J Cell Physiol.* 2003;195:428-34.

91. BOYD NL, PARK H, YI H, BOO YC, SORESCU GP, SYKES M, JO H. Chronic shear induces caveolae formation and alters ERK and Akt responses in endothelial cells. *Am J Physiol Heart Circ Physiol.* 2003;285:H1113-22.

92. JIN ZG, UEBA H, TANIMOTO T, LUNGU AO, FRAME MD, BERK BC. Ligand-independent activation of vascular endothelial growth factor receptor 2 by fluid shear stress regulates activation of endothelial nitric oxide synthase. *Circ Res.* 2003;93:354-63.

93. ILLI B, NANNI S, SCOPECE A, FARSETTI A, BIGLIOLI P, CAPOGROSSI MC, GAETANO C. Shear stress-mediated chromatin remodeling provides molecular basis for flow-dependent regulation of gene expression. *Circ Res.* 2003;93:155-61.

94. AZUMA N, AKASAKA N, KITO H, IKEDA M, GAHTAN V, SASAJIMA T, SUMPIO BE. Role of p38 MAP kinase in endothelial cell alignment induced by fluid shear stress. *Am J Physiol Heart Circ Physiol.* 2001;280:H189-97.

95. CARLIER M-F, RESSAD F, PANTALONI D. Control of actin dynamics in cell motility. Role of ADF/cofilin. *J Biol Chem.* 1999;274:33827-33830.

96. MAEKAWA S, NISHIDA E, OHTA Y, SAKAI H. Isolation of low molecular weight actin-binding proteins from porcine brain. *J Biochem.* 1984;95:377-385.

97. NISHIDA E, MAEKAWA S, SAKAI H. Cofilin, a protein in porcine brain that binds to actin filaments and inhibits their interactions with myosin and tropomyosin. *Biochemistry.* 1984;23:5307-5313.

98. MORIYAMA K, NISHIDA E, YONEZAWA N, SAKAI H, MATSUMOTO S, IIDA K, YAHARA I. Destrin, a mammalian actin-depolymerizing protein, is closely related to cofilin. Cloning and expression of porcine brain destrin cDNA. *J Biol Chem.* 1990;265:5768-73.

99. MACIVER SK, HUSSEY PJ. The ADF/cofilin family: actin-remodeling proteins. *Genome Biol.* 2002;3:reviews3007.

100. THERIOT JA. Accelerating on a treadmill: ADF/cofilin promotes rapid actin filament turnover in the dynamic cytoskeleton. *J Cell Biol.* 1997;136:1165-8.

101. BAMBURG JR, BRAY D. Distribution and cellular localization of Actin Depolymerizing Factor. *J Cell Biol.* 1987;105:2817-2825.

102. ABE H, NAGAOKA R, OBINATA T. Cytoplasmic localization and nuclear transport of cofilin in cultured myotubes. *Exp Cell Res.* 1993;206:1-10.

103. ONO S, ABE H, NAGAOKA R, OBINATA T. Colocalization of ADF and cofilin in intranuclear actin rods of cultured muscle cells. *J Muscle Res Cell Motil.* 1993;14:195-204.

104. ARIMA K, IMANAKA M, OKUZONO S, KAZUTA Y, KOTANI S. Evidence for structural differences between the two highly homologous actin-regulatory proteins, destrin and cofilin. *Biosci Biotech Biochem.* 1998;62:215-220.

105. VARTIAINEN MK, MUSTONEN T, MATTILA PK, OJALA PJ, THESLEFF I, PARTANEN J, LAPPALAINEN P. The three mouse actin-depolymerizing factor/cofilins evolved to fulfill cell-type-specific requirements for actin dynamics. *Mol Biol Cell.* 2002;13:183-194.

106. YONEZAWA N, NISHIDA E, SAKAI H. pH control of actin polymerization by cofilin. *Journal of Biological Chemistry.* 1985;260:14410-14412.

107. TOSHIMA J, TOSHIMA JY, AMANO T, YANG N, NARUMIYA S, MIZUNO K. Cofilin Phosphorylation by Protein Kinase Testicular Protein Kinase 1 and Its Role in Integrin-mediated Actin Reorganization and focal Adhesion Formation. *Molecular Biology of the Cell.* 2001;12:1131-1145.

108. ARBER S, BARBAYANNIS FA, HANSER H, SCHNEIDER C, STANYON C, BERNARD O, CARONI P. Regulation of actin dynamics through phosphorylation of cofilin by LIM-kinase. *Nature.* 1998;393:805-809.

109. AIZAWA H, WAKATSUKI S, ISHII A, MORIYAMA K, SASAKI Y, OHASHI K, SEKINE-AIZAWA Y, SEHARA-FUJISAWA A, MIZUNO K, GOSHIMA Y, YAHARA I. Phosphorylation of cofilin by LIM kinase is necessary for semaphorin 3A-induced growth cone collapse. *Nat Neurosci.* 2001; 4:367-373.

110. EDWARDS DC, SANDERS LC, BOKOCH GM, GILL GN. Activation of LIM-kinase by Pak1 couples Rac/Cdc42 GTPase signaling to actin cytoskeletal dynamics. *Nature Cell Biol.* 1999;1:253-259.

111. AMANO T, TANABE K, ETO T, NARUMIYA S, MIZUNO K. LIM-kinase 2 induces formation of stress fibres, focal adhesions and membrane blebs, dependent on its activation by Rho-associated kinase-catalysed phopshorylation at threonine-505. *Biochem J.* 2001;354:149-159.

112. DAWE HR, MINAMIDE LS, BAMBURG JR, CRAMER LP. ADF/cofilin controls cell polarity during fibroblast migration. *Current Biology.* 2003;13:252-257.

113. NIWA R, NAGATA-OSHI K, TAKEICHI M, MIZUNO K, UEMURA T. Control of Actin Reorganization by Slingshot, a Family of Phosphatases that Dephosphorylate ADF/cofilin. *Cell.* 2002;108:233-246.

114. GOHLA A, BOCKOCH M. 14-3-3 regulates actin dynamics by stabilizing phosphorylated cofilin. *Curr Biol.* 2002;12:1704-1710.

115. ONO S, MINAMI N, ABE H, OBINATA T. Characterization of a novel cofilin isoform that is predominantly expressed in mammalian skeletal muscle. *J Biol Chem.* 1994;269:15280-15286.

116. THIRION C, STUCKA R, MENDEL B, GRUHLER A, JAKSCH M, NOWAK KJ, BINZ N, LAING NG, LOCHMULLER H. Characterization of human muscle type cofilin (CFL2) in normal and regenerating muscle. *Eur J Biochem.* 2001;268:3473-3482.

117. BOENGLER K, PIPP F, SCHAPER W, DEINDL E. Rapid identification of differentially expressed genes by combination of SSH and MOS. *Lab Invest.* 2003;83:759-61.

118. BOENGLER K, PIPP F, BROICH K, FERNÁNDEZ B, SCHAPER W, DEINDL E. Identification of differentially expressed genes like cofilin2 in growing collateral arteries. *Biochem Biophys Res Commun.* 2003;300:751-756.

119. LAWSON D, HARRISON M, SHAPLAND C. Fibroblast transgelin and smooth muscle SM22alpha are the same protein, the expression of which is down-regulated in many cell lines. *Cell Motil Cytoskel.* 1997;38:250-257.

120. NAGAOKA R, ABE H, KUSANO K, OBINATA T. Concentration of cofilin, a small actin-binding protein, at the cleveage furrow during cytikinesis. *Cell Motil Cytoskel.* 1995;30:1-7.

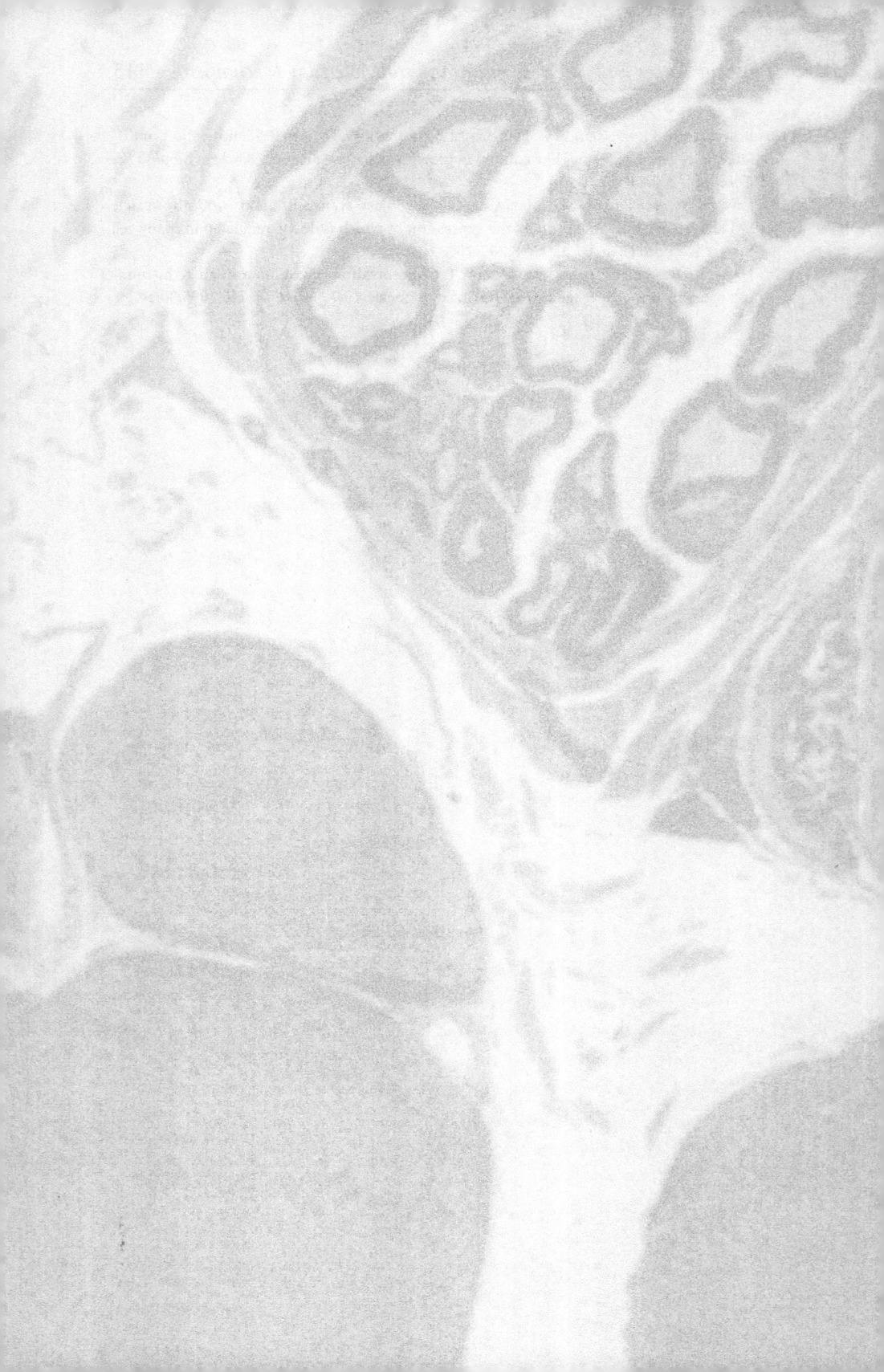

Role of Hypoxia/Ischemia/VEGF-A, and Strain Differences

Elisabeth Deindl, Armin Helisch, Dimitri Scholz,
Matthias Heil, Shawn Wagner and Wolfgang Schaper

Hypoxia and ischemia are the most important stimuli for angiogenesis. With severe stenoses, the reduced oxygen and metabolite supply is recognized in the affected muscle tissue by an intracellular sensing system triggering diverse biological emergency steps. Energy shortage leads to a breakdown of the high energy phosphates, increased concentrations of lactate as a consequence of anaerobic glycolysis and the activation of hypoxia inducible factors, e.g. hypoxia inducible factor 1-α (HIF-1α). Binding of the transcription factor to consensus sequences on corresponding promoters in turn results in an increased expression of genes like vascular endothelial growth factor-A (VEGF-A). The gene products are released from the hypoxic cell resulting in a concentration gradient highest in the hypoxic tissue. Upon binding of VEGF-A to its receptors expressed on endothelial cells, which do not express VEGF-A *in vivo*, endothelial cells start to proliferate and migrate in direction of the concentration gradient. Capillary sprouting starts, resulting in a network of capillaries surrounding and invading the ischemic and hypoxic tissue. However, since SMCs are not a target for VEGF-A, VEGF-A cannot be part of the interaction between endothelial cells and SMCs, the main players in arteriogenesis. Only muscular collateral arteries and not capillaries are able to supply enough blood from outside the risk region to prevent the consequences of severe ischemia. Collateral artery growth does not necessarily take place within hypoxic tissue. The arterial tissue itself, constantly bathed in oxygen-rich blood, never gets hypoxic. Since it has never been analyzed whether there exists a causal relation between ischemia and colateral artery growth, we investigated the role of hypoxia in our rabbit model of arteriogenesis. As described below, we therefore determined the level of metabolites indicative for ischemia and monitored the expression level of diverse hypoxia inducible genes such as HIF-1α, lactate dehydrogenase A (LDH A), heme oxygenase-1 (HO-1), and VEGF-A.

VEGF-A (for a review see Neufeld[1]) was shown to be upregulated under hypoxic and ischemic conditions *in vitro*[2] and *in vivo*[3], both on the transcriptional and translational level[4]. Hypoxia induced transcription of VEGF-A is mediated via the binding of HIF-1 (alpha/beta heterodimer) to a HIF-1 binding site located in the VEGF-A promoter[5,6]. Furthermore, hypoxia promotes the stabilization of the VEGF-A mRNA by proteins that bind to sequences located in the 3' untranslated region (UTR) of VEGF-A. In addition, under unfavorable stress conditions like hypoxia/ischemia, an efficient cap-independent translation of VEGF-A is maintained via the use of an internal ribosome entry site (IRES) at the 5' UTR[7,8].

The temporal and spatial correlation of VEGF-A overexpression with angiogenesis during tumor growth[9], inflammation[10-12], and wound healing[10-12] provides strong evidence for a functional role of VEGF-A as a key regulator of angiogenesis. The growth factor stimulates vascular endothelial proliferation[13-16], macrophage migration[17] and increases microvessel permeability[18-20] to macromolecules. The effects of VEGF-A are mediated via two distinct high affinity receptors, flt-1 (fms-like tyrosine kinase)[21] and flk-1 (fetal liver kinase)[22,23]. These are almost exclusively expressed on endothelial cells rendering VEGF-A, an endothelial cell specific mitogen.

Although the role of VEGF-A in angiogenesis is obvious it is not clear whether VEGF-A is also involved in arteriogenesis and available data are controversial[24-31]. The administration of VEGF-A as a bolus (0.5 to 1 mg) into the iliac artery of an ischemic rabbit limb was described to result in an increased development of collateral arteries[24]. However, the evidence was based solely on the change of cuff pressure measured in the lower legs of rabbits. Cuff pressure is compounded by several factors that are in need of definition, in particular because VEGF increases tissue pressure and higher flows across collateral resistance vessels cause lower pressures in the lower leg.

To characterize whether adaptive collateral artery growth is associated with an increased expression of VEGF-A, we analyzed the abundance of the transcript directly in growing collateral arteries in the rabbit as a function of time in the m. quadriceps, which consistently harbors collaterals. Northern blot results displayed a significant downregulation of the VEGF-A mRNA in the m. quadriceps of the experimental tissue. However, a similar downregulation was also seen in sham operated animals, indicating that the altered mRNA level of VEGF-A in experimental animals was not due to arteriogenesis, but due to the experimental procedure. In growing collaterals we found no change of the mRNA level of VEGF-A compared to control or sham operated animals, however, the mRNA abundance of VEGF-A in collateral arteries was very low compared to the surrounding muscle tissue. Our Western blot results showed an almost comparable level of the VEGF-A protein in skeletal muscle tissue and in collateral arteries, but did not show an increased protein level of VEGF-A during arteriogenesis. These data clearly demonstrate that collateral artery growth is neither associated with nor dependent on an increased expression of VEGF-A[32].

Although VEGF-A is well described as a rapidly induced hypoxia-response gene, other growth factors and cytokines can also modulate the expression of VEGF-A. To define clearly whether arteriogenesis is associated with ischemia, we investigated the expression level of LDH A and HO-1, two genes known to be induced by hypoxia and containing a HIF-1 binding-site[33-37]. Furthermore, we analyzed the expression of HIF-1α itself, although the latter might not be regulated on the transcriptional but on the translational or post-translational level[38]. Our results showed that none of the mentioned genes was upregulated during arteriogenesis, representing additional evidence that collateral artery growth is not ischemia dependent[32].

Hypoxia is a condition, which occurs mainly by exposure to high altitude. Hypoxia inducible genes are also upregulated in ischemia. It differs from ischemia in that only the latter leads to catabolism of the high-energy phosphates, i.e., from ATP to ADP and its breakdown products. It causes a decrease of phosphocreatine and an increased concentration of lactate. Analyzing these markers of ischemia, we found no change of any of the described parameters in our rabbit model[32].

Our *in situ* analysis displayed a strong staining for VEGF-A in skeletal muscle cells (m. quadriceps), but not in cells of larger vessels or their close vicinity (Fig. 1). However, our Western blots showed an almost equal abundance of the protein in the m. quadriceps and in collateral arteries (Fig. 2). These data show that VEGF-A protein is produced in skeletal muscle, secreted and taken up by vascular endothelium where it may have maintenance functions[32].

To characterize whether the action of VEGF-A during collateral artery growth is mediated via the availability of its receptor, we evaluated the mRNA level of flt-1 and flk-1; however, we could not find an increased expression of any of the two receptors during arteriogenesis. These data are in keeping with the unchanged expression level of VEGF-A, since it was shown that VEGF itself has the capability to potentiate the expression

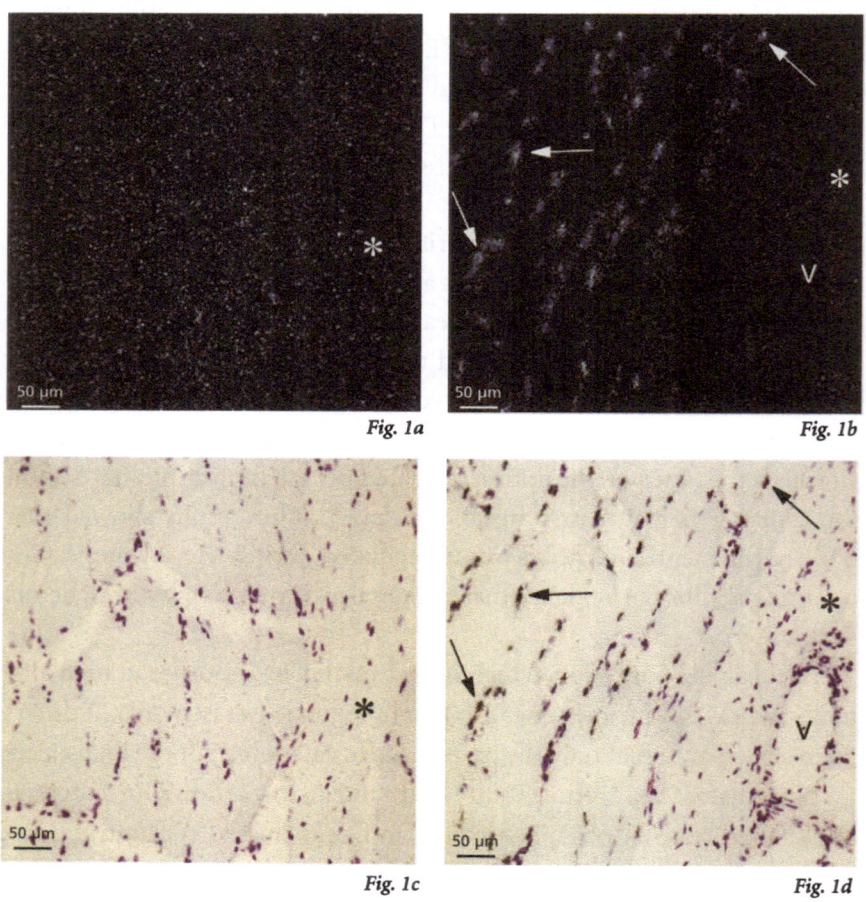

Fig. 1a   *Fig. 1b*

Fig. 1c   *Fig. 1d*

Radioactive in situ hybridization studies of VEGF-A in the m. quadriceps of a rabbit after 3h of collateral artery growth. In 1a and 1c we used sense probes, in 1b and 1d antisense probes. 1a and 1b are dark field pictures of 1c and 1d. Note the density of the labeled antisense probe in the cell nuclei of myocytes (arrows), but not in vessels (v) or in connective tissue (asterisk). (reprinted from [32] with permission) of both its receptors[39-41]. The data confirm furthermore that in our *in vivo* system collateral artery growth occurs independently from ischemia (hypoxia), since it was demonstrated that flt-1, which like VEGF-A contains a HIF-1 consensus binding site, is upregulated under hypoxic conditions on the transcriptional level *in vitro*[42] and *in vivo*[43].

For flk-1 our Northern blot analysis displayed - beside the transcript of about 6 kb - a second one of about 4.6 kb, which has been described before[44], and a third of about 1.6 kb, which showed a slight upregulation in growing collateral arteries. The function of the smaller forms of flk-1 has not been defined yet, however, it is likely that they negatively regulate the bioavailability, and hence the activity of VEGF-A as reported for the soluble form of flt-1[45,46].

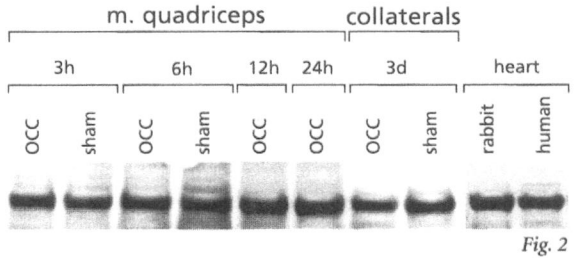

Fig. 2

Western blot showing the protein level of VEGF-A in the m. quadriceps of experimental and sham operated animals at distinct intervals of collateral artery growth, in collateral arteries of experimental and sham operated animals at day 3 of collateral artery growth, and in rabbit and human heart (controls). (reprinted from[32] *with permission)*

To analyze whether we could stimulate collateral artery growth in our rabbit system via application of VEGF-A, we infused the growth factor via osmotic minipump in a concentration more than 30-fold higher than the active concentration of MCP-1. However, the results showed that application of VEGF-A had only modest effects on the diameter of collateral arteries and on collateral conductance compared to MCP-1 that had already been demonstrated before to be a potent inducer of collateral artery growth[47]. VEGF-A has been described to be no direct mitogen for arterial endothelium *in vivo*[48]. Collateral artery growth does not only involve the proliferation of endothelial cells but also of SMCs, however, the receptors for VEGF-A are only expressed on endothelial cells. Therefore, it is likely that the – although minor – effect of VEGF-A was due to an indirect mechanism. It seems reasonable that circulating blood cells, in particular monocytes, are involved as these are the only cells – besides endothelial cells – which express a VEGF-A-receptor (flt-1[49,50]). Furthermore, monocytes have already previously been described to play an important role in arteriogenesis[47]. VEGF-A activates monocytes[17], induces integrin expression on monocytes[51], and promotes monocyte adhesion and migration[17].

The indirect positive effect of VEGF-A on collateral artery growth by recruitment and activation of monocytes[52], however, might be counterbalanced by a feature of VEGF-A itself, as this growth factor has the ability to reduce smooth muscle cell proliferation in arteries[53]. Furthermore, it has recently been shown in a 3-dimensional spheroid coculture model that direct contact with SMCs abrogates the VEGF-A responsiveness of endothelial cells[54]. On the other hand: ECs and SMCs are never in direct contact in collateral vessels in contrast to the situation in the spheroid model.

In a second approach, we investigated whether inhibition of VEGF-A does affect arteriogenesis induced by femoral artery ligation in C57BL/6 mice. Animals were randomized to receive twice a week s.c. injections of VEGF trap$_{R1R2}$25 mg/kg, or solvent starting one day prior to surgery. VEGF trap is composed of the Ig2 domain of VEGFR1 fused with the Ig3 domain of VEGFR2 fused with human Fc and at the stated dose strongly inhibits tumor-growth and -angiogenesis in C57BL/6 mice. Hind-foot perfusion was serially measured in C57BL/6 mice by Laser-Doppler

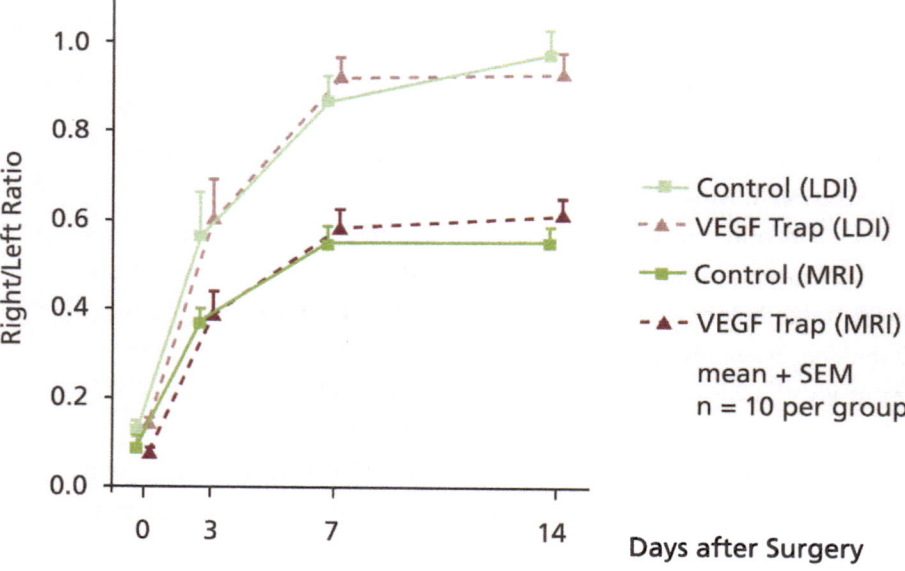

Fig. 3

Influence of a soluble injectable VEGF trap on the recovery of blood flow following femoral artery occlusion in C57/B1 6 mice. Superficial pedal blood flow, measured with Laser-Doppler Imaging (LDI), shows a complete recovery (the right-to-left ratio reaches unity after 14 days) and no influence of the trap (activity was checked on healing of a cutaneous wound). Deep muscular blood flow in the calf was measured with Magnetic Resonance Imaging (MRI), which shows only a <60% recovery and also no influence of the VEGF trap.

imaging (LDI), hemoglobin oxygenation by transcutaneous oxygen spectrometry, calf flow by 2D TOF-MRI. BrdU uptake by collateral arteries was quantified in adductor muscle cross-sections after feeding mice with BrdU since the day before surgery. Our results showed that recovery of hind limb perfusion/flow (Fig. 3) and oxygenation was not significantly different between controls and VEGF trap treated mice. There was also no significant difference between controls and VEGF trap treated mice in the number of BrdU positive adductor muscle collaterals and the relative number of BrdU containing cells in the walls of these vessels, indicating that endogenous VEGF or related factors acting on VEGFR 1 and 2 do not play a major role for collateral growth after femoral artery occlusion.

In summary, our data show that collateral artery growth *in vivo* is associated neither with ischemia nor with an increased expression of VEGF-A. The unchanged expression levels of flt-1 and flk-1 make it unlikely that collateral artery growth is stimulated by VEGF-A mediated by an increased availability of its two high affinity receptors[32]. These results show clearly that VEGF-A is not normally involved in the induction of arteriogenesis. However, arteriogenesis can be promoted artificially by administration of VEGF-A due to its property to activate monocytes, although to a minor extent. Nevertheless, VEGF-A exerts a biological function under normal physiological conditions by acting as a survival factor for endothelial cells in paracrine manner. In conclusion, our data demonstrate that VEGF-A is not a natural agent to induce collateral artery growth *in vivo* and that hypoxia and ischemia are not obligatory for arteriogenesis.

To further evaluate the role of hypoxia and ischemia for arteriogenesis, we investigated different strains of mice. We studied C57BL/6, Balb/C and 129/Sv mice after femoral artery ligation. All mouse strains studied reacted to femoral artery occlusion with growth of collateral arteries. However, the strains differed markedly in the intensity of lower limb ischemia and collateral artery growth in the upper leg. The Balb/C strain developed severe lower leg ischemia with a marked decrease in ATP content and general break-down of high-energy phosphates (Fig. 4), early edema, focal necrosis, and tissue loss. By Laser-Doppler Imaging and monitoring of tissue oxygenation, Balb/C had the most incomplete recovery compared with the other strains. The Balb/C mice showed a strong angiogenic response in the lower leg and a minor arteriogenic response in the upper leg. The C57BL/6 mice, in contrast, exhibited a lesser flow reduction upon

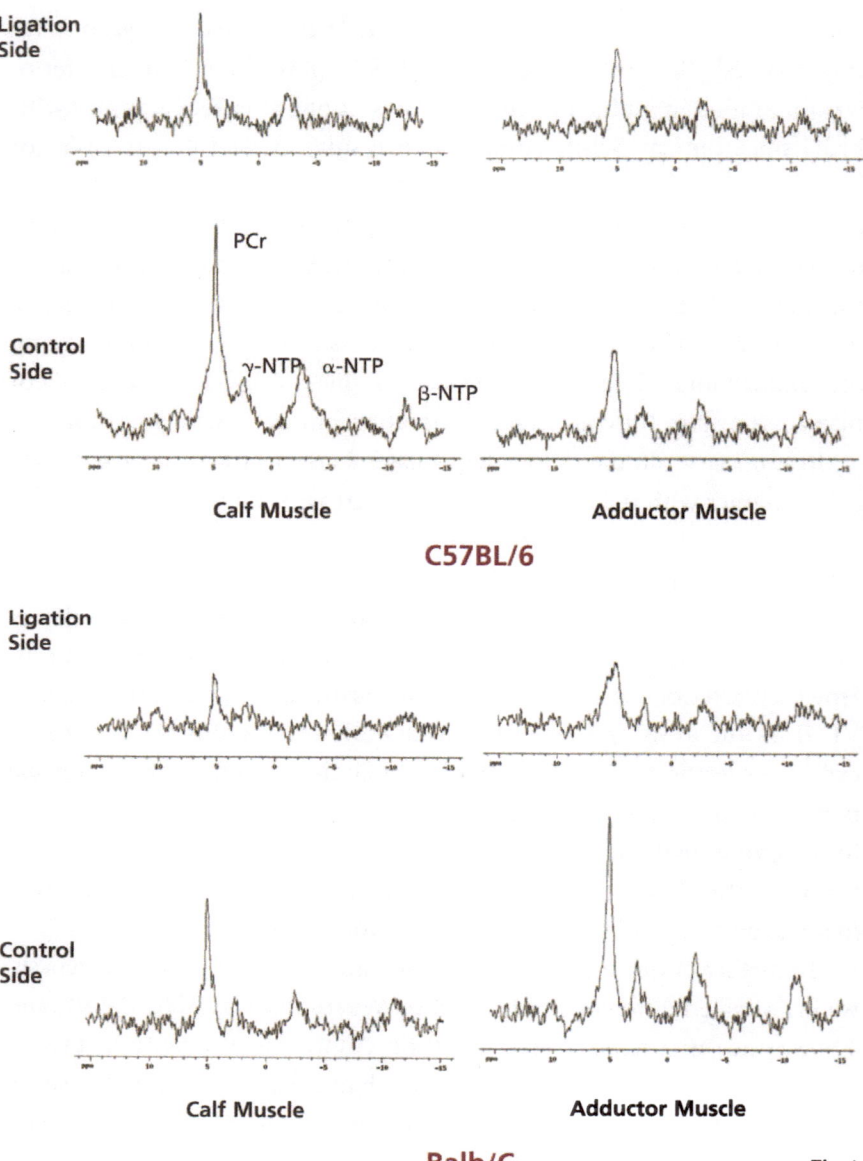

C57BL/6

Balb/C

Fig. 4

31P Magnetic resonance spectra 12 hours after one-sided femoral artery ligation, 512 repetitions. Spectra were obtained in a 7.0 Tesla magnet by placing the region of interest inside the acquisition area of a surface coil with a repetition time 1.5 sec and a flip angle power that maximized the signal acquired. Both mice types show a considerable loss in PCr and NTP in the calf muscle and the Balb/C mice show also ischemic losses in the adductor muscle.

acute femoral occlusion, only a minor brief drop in ATP content and no tissue loss but a strong and fast arteriogenic response with early normalization of blood flow. When further comparing C57BL/6 with Balb/C mice, C57BL/6 mice had larger preexistent collaterals on *in vivo* magnetic resonance angiography and a higher collateral dependent filling index on postmortem x-ray angiography immediately after arterial occlusion. The number of angiographically visible collateral artery vessels was higher in C57BL/6 mice one week after arterial occlusion. Thus, the different degrees of ischemia directly after femoral artery occlusion are likely to be due to the differences in size and number of preexisting collateral arteries.*

Strain-related differences in vascular remodeling have been described before. In a carotid artery ligation model, multiple inbred mouse strains were compared, and significant differences were found[55]. A trend for increased carotid artery luminal areas on the ligated and non-ligated side in C57BL/6J mice compared to 129/SvJ and Balb/CJ mice was observed[55]. In a model of mycoplasma pulmonis induced growth of tracheal microvessels, C57BL/6 mice responded with an increased number of capillaries and venules, while in C3H mice the diameters of arterioles, capillaries and venules increased[56].

The significance of strain-related variations of preexisting collateral arterial networks was highlighted by cerebral ischemia studies. The posterior communicating arteries in the circle of Willis were found to be less often patent in Balb/C than in BDF and CFW mice, and this was associated with an increased risk of infarction after creating focal or multifocal cerebral ischemia[57]. The higher susceptibility of C57BL/6 compared to 129/Sv mice to ischemia by transient bilateral common carotid artery occlusion was associated with poorly developed vascular connections in to the intensity of ischemia[59]. More serve ischemia leads to slower collateral artery growth and to smaller collateral diameters, because tissue loss is a factor that reduces speed and extent of collateral growth, and with it fluid shear stress is less.

Because of their small size, mice offer the unique opportunity to study complete cross sections of hind limb muscle in which collateral arteries develop permitting a non-selective histological approach, which would the circle of Willis of C57BL/6[58]. Interestingly, differences in vasomotor reactivity

---

* The VEGF-trap and the mouse strain studies were carried out by A.H. and S.W.

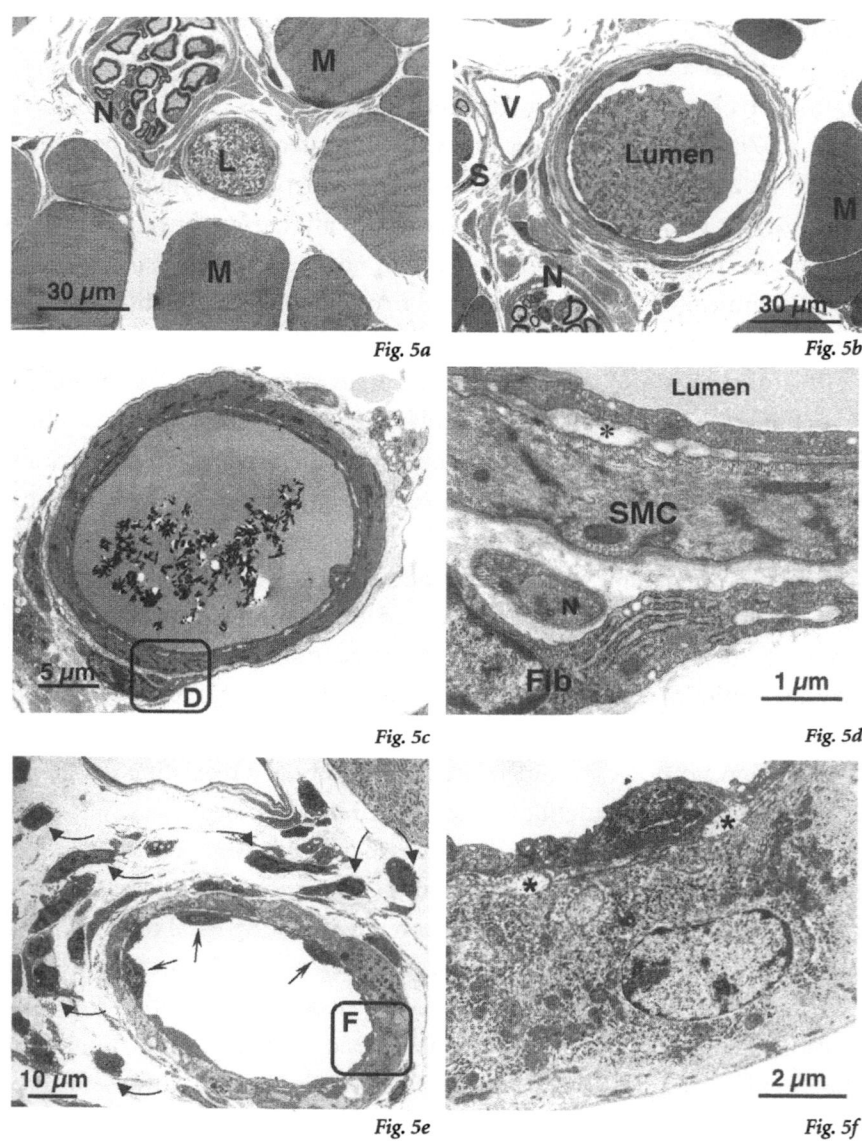

Fig. 5a

Fig. 5b

Fig. 5c

Fig. 5d

Fig. 5e

Fig. 5f

were observed in this study as well: C57BL/6 had a more pronounced vasodilation response of pial vessels to superfusion with acetylcholine than 129/Sv mice.

In summary, our studies contradict the reigning paradigm that predicts the more ischemia, the more vascular (in this case arteriolar) growth. Our studies clearly show that the speed of arteriogenesis is inversely related be too cumbersome in larger animals. By labeling studies with BrdU, we made use of this advantage to define whether collateral artery growth is the result of remodeling of preexisting arteriolar connections or whether they are also formed *de novo*. It was previously hypothesized that collateral arteries may originate from recently sprouted capillaries that recruit SMCs from the surrounding tissue and had thus formed an artery *de novo*.

Cross sections of the adductor muscles of C57BL/6 mice one week after femoral artery ligation revealed no uptake of BrdU by capillaries. However, several arteriolar vessels, as identified by their size (> 10 μm) and presence of a tunica media (α-smooth muscle actin positive), had a large number of BrdU positive nuclei in all of their wall layers. In Balb/C mice, the same histological picture emerged in regions of normal appearing thigh muscle. In areas of tissue necrosis, some capillaries were positive for BrdU. The percentage of BrdU positive cells in growing arteries was identical in both mouse strains. Thus, major strain-dependent differences in preexistent inter-arterial connections exist and may result in very different outcomes after femoral artery ligation, even with identical proliferative activities in growing collateral arteries. Ultrastructural analysis (Fig. 5) showed that veins and nerves accompanied growing collaterals, comparable to the situation of quiescent arteries. Collaterals developed at well-known locations and contained a marker of first origin for a considerable time: remnants of the old lamina elastica. Our labeling studies using BrdU or Ki67 showed that growth occurred by division of existing endothelial cells and SMCs. The wall thickness also increased significantly, indicating that real growth and not passive dilatation of vessels had taken place[59].

Ultrastructure of a preexisting (5a, c, d) collateral vessel and 3 (5e, f) and 7 (5b) days after femoral artery occlusion. 5a: Light microscope image of a preexisting collateral arteriole with barely visible endothelium, thin media consisting of one layer of SMCs and a lumen filled with the contrast medium (L). "M" corresponds to muscle fibers. Semithin section, stained with toluidine blue. Magnification x 625. 5b: Light microscope image of a collateral artery 7 days after occlusion of the femoral artery accompanied by a vein (V), nerve (N) and muscle spindle (S). Semithin section, stained with toluidine blue. Magnification x 625. 5c: Electron microscope image of a preexistent collateral arteriole. Lumen is filled with the contrast medium where crystals of BiCl2 are visible. The frame indicates the part shown in D. Magnification x 2500. 5d: Detail from 5c, showing a SMC of the contractile phenotype, the intact lamina elastica interna (asterisk), fragments of non-activated endothelial cells with typical pinocytic vesicles, a fibroblast (Fib) and a nerve (N). Magnification x 16500. 5e: Growing collateral artery three days after occlusion of the femoral artery. Nuclei of the activated endothelial cells are protruding into the lumen (arrows). Macrophages (curved arrows) are accumulated in the perivascular space. Electron microscopy, magnification x 1000. 5f: Detail from e showing activated thick endothelial and a SMC with a large number of ribosomes indicating increased protein synthesis. The lamina elastica interna (asterisk) appears partially degraded. Electron microscopy, magnification x 9000. (reprinted from [59] with permission)

In summary, our data clearly show that collateral artery growth is the result of remodeling of preexisting vessels and render other hypotheses obsolete that rely on the *de novo* formation of arteries. Furthermore, if angiogenesis was the precursor of arteriogenesis it should happen in the lower leg of the Balb/C strain, a location where collaterals were never recognized after femoral artery occlusion.

As a résumé of this chapter we arrive at the following statements: 1. Collateral artery growth is not associated with an increased expression of VEGF-A or its two high affinity receptors. VEGF-A does not represent a natural agent to induce or promote collateral artery growth. 2. Furthermore, arteriogenesis is neither associated nor promoted by hypoxia or ischemia; on the contrary it is inversely related to the intensity of ischemia. And 3rd, arteriogenesis is a result of the growth of preexisting arteriolar connections and does not rely on the *de novo* formation of arteries.

References

1. NEUFELD G, COHEN T, GENGRINOVITCH S, POLTORAK Z. Vascular endothelial growth factor (VEGF) and its receptors. *FASEB.* 1999;13:9-22.
2. SHWEIKI D, ITIN A, SOFFER D, KESHET E. Vascular endothelial growth factor induced by hypoxia may mediate hypoxia-initiated angiogenesis. *Nature.* 1992;359:843-845.
3. BANAI H, SHWEIKI D, PINSON A, CHANDRA M, LAZAROVICI G, KESHET E. Upregulation of vascular endothelial growth factor expression induced by myocardial ischemia: implications for coronary angiogenesis. *Carciovasc Res.* 1994;28:1176-1179.
4. IKEDA E, ACHEN MG, BREIER G, RISAU W. Hypoxia-induced transcriptional activation and increased mRNA stability of vascular endothelial growth factor in C6 glioma cells. *J Biol Chem.* 1995;270:19761-19766.
5. LIU YX, COX SR, MORITA T, KOUREMBANAS S. Hypoxia regulates vascular endothelial growth factor gene expression in endothelial cells - identification of a 5′ enhancer. *Circ Res.* 1995; 77:638-643.
6. LEVY AP, LEVY NS, WEGNER S, GOLDBERG MA. Transcriptional regulation of the rat vascular endothelial growth factor gene by hypoxia. *J Biol Chem.* 1995;270:13333-13340.
7. STEIN I, ITIN A, EINAT P, SKALITER R, GROSSMAN Z, E. K. Translation of vascular endothelial growth factor mRNA by internal ribosome entry: implications for translation under hypoxia. *Mol Cell Biol.* 1998;18:3112-3119.
8. AKIRI G, NAHARI D, FINKELSTEIN Y, LE S, ELROY-STEIN O, LEVI B. Regulation of vascular endothelial growth factor (VEGF) expression is mediated by internal initiation of translation and alternative initiation of transcription. *Oncogene.* 1998;12:227-236.
9. SENGER DR, PERRUZZI CA, FEDER J, DVORAK HF. A highly conserved vascular permeability factor secreted by a variety of human and rodent tumor cell lines. *Cancer Res.* 1986;46:5629-5632.

10. KOCH AE, HARLOW LA, HAINES GK, AMENTO EP, UNEMORI EN, WONG WL, POPE RM, FERRARA N. Vascular endothelial growth factor. A cytokine modulating endothelial function in rheumatoid arthritis. *J Immunol.* 1994;152:4149-1456.

11. BROWN LF, OLBRICHT SM, BERSE B, JACKMAN RW, MATSUEDA G, TOGNAZZI KA, MANSEAU EJ, DVORAK HF, VAN DE WATER L. Overexpression of vascular permeability factor (VPF/VEGF) and its endothelial cell receptors in delayed hypersensitivity skin reactions. *J Immunol.* 1995;154:1-7.

12. AIELLO L, AVERY RL, ARRIGG PG, KEYT BA, JAMPEL HD, SHAH ST, PASQUALE LR, THIEME H, IWAMOTO MA, PARK JE, NGUYEN HV, AIELLO LM, FERRARA N, KING GL. Vascular endothelial growth factor in ocular fluid of patients with diabetic retinopathy and other retinal disorders. *N Engl J Med.* 1994;331:1480-1487.

13. CONOLLY DT, HEUVELMAN DM, NELSON R, OLANDER JV, EPPLEY BL, DELFINO JJ, SIEGEL NR, LEIMGRUBER RM, FEDER J. Tumor vascular permeability factor stimulates endothelial cell growth and angiogenesis. *J Clin Invest.* 1989;84:1470-1478.

14. FERRARA N, HENZEL WJ. Pituitary follicular cells secrete a novel heparin-binding growth factor specific for vascular endothelial cells. *Biochem Biophys Res Com.* 1989;161:851-858.

15. LEUNG DW, CACHIANES G, KUANG WJ, GOEDDEL DV, FERRARA N. Vascular endothelial growth factor is a secreted angiogenic mitogen. *Science.* 1989;246:1306-1309.

16. GOSPODAROWICZ D, ABRAHAM JA, SCHILLING J. Isolation and characterization of a vascular endothelial cell mitogen produced by pituitary- derived folliculo stellate cells. *Proc Natl Acad Sci USA.* 1989;86:7311-7315.

17. CLAUSS M, GERLACH M, GERLACH H, BRETT J, WANG F, FAMILLETTI PC, PAN YCE, OLANDER JV, CONNOLLY DT, STERN D. Vascular permeability factor: a tumor-derived polypeptide that induces endothelial cell and monocyte procoagulant activity, and promotes monocyte migration. *J Exp Med.* 1990;172:1535-1545.

18. YEO TK, SENGER DR, DVORAK HF, FRETER L, YEO K. Glycosylation is essential for efficient secretion but not for permeability-enhancing activity of vascular permeability factor (vascular endothelial growth factor). *Biochem Biophys Res Com.* 1991;179:1568-1575.

19. SENGER DR, GALLI SJ, DVORAK AM, PERUZZI CA, HARVEY VS, DVORAK HF. Tumor cells secrete a vascular permeability factor that promotes accumulation of ascites fluid. *Science.* 1983; 219:983-985.

20. KECK PJ, HAUSER SD, KRIVI G, SANZO K, WARREN T, FEDER J, CONNOLLY DT. Vascular permeability factor, an endothelial cell mitogen related to PDGF. *Science.* 1989;246:1309-1312.

21. DE VRIES C, ESCOBEDO JA, UENO H, HOUCK K, FERRARA N, WILLIAMS LT. The fms-like tyrosine kinase, a receptor for vascular endothelial growth factor. *Science.* 1992;255:989-991.

22. MATTHEWS W, JORDAN CT, GAVIN M, JENKINS NA, COPELAND NG, LEMISCHKA IR. A receptor tyrosine kinase cDNA isolated from a population of enriched primitive hemapoietic cells and exhibiting close genetic linkage to c-kit. *Proc Natl Acad Sci USA.* 1991;88:9026-9030.

23. MILLAUER B, WIZIGMANN-VOOS S, SCHNUERCH H, MARTINEZ R, MOELLER NPH, RISAU W, ULLRICH A. High affinity VEGF binding and developmental expression suggest flk-1 as a major regulator of vasculogenesis and angiogenesis. *Cell.* 1993;72:835-846.

24. TAKESHITA S, ROSSOW ST, KEARNEY M, ZHENG LP, BAUTERS C, BUNTING S, FERRARA N, SYMES JF, ISNER JM. Time course of increased cellular proliferation in collateral arteries after administration of vascular endothelial growth factor in a rabbit model of lower limb vascular insufficiency. *Am J Pathol.* 1995;147:1649-1660.

25. ISNER JM, PIEZCEK A, SCHAINFELD R, BLAIR R, HALEY L, ASAHARA T, ROSENFIELD K, RAZVI S, WALSH K, SYMES JF. Clinical evidence of angiogenesis after arterial gene transfer of phVEGF165 in patients with ischaemic limb. *The LANCET.* 1996;348:370-374.

26. TSURUMI Y, KEARNEY M, CHEN D, SILVER M, TAKESHITA S, YANG J, SYMES JF, ISNER JM. Treatment of acute limb ischemia by intramuscular injection of vascular endothelial growth factor gene. *Circulation.* 1997;96:382-388.

27. FINE JT, BAJAMANDE A, McCLUSKEY ER, HENRY TD, SPERTUS JA. Unexplained improvement in health-related quality of life in the vascular endothelial growth factor and ischemia for vascular angiogenesis trial. *Circulation.* 1999;100:2062(Abstract).

28. HENRY TD, ANNEX BH, AZRIN MA, McKENDALL GR, WILLERSON JT, HENDEL RC, GIORDANO FJ, KLEIN R, GIBSON CM, BERMAN DS, LUCE CA, McCLUSKEY ER. Double blind, placebo controlled trial of recombinant human vascular endothelial growth factor - the VIVA trial. *J Am Coll Cardiol.* 1999;33 A:384(Abstract).

29. SCHWARZ ER, KLONER RA. Direkte Applikation der DNA für vascular endothelial growth factor (VEGF) in die Randbereiche infarzierten Myokards induziert Angiogenese ohne Verbesserung der regionalen Myokardperfusion bei Ratten. Z Kardiol. 1999;88:675 (Abstr.).

30. SCHWARZ ER, SPEAKMAN MT, PATTERSON M, HALE SS, ISNER JM, KEDES LH, KLONER RA. Evaluation of the effects of intramyocardial injection of DNA expressing vascular endothelial growth factor (VEGF) in a myocardial model in the rat-angiogenesis and angioma formation. *J Am Coll Cardiol.* 2000;35:1323-1330.

31. HERSHEY JC, BASKIN EP, GLASS JD, HARTMAN HA, GILBERTO DB, ROGERS IT, COOK JJ. Revascularization in the rabbit hind limb: dissociation between capillary sprouting and arteriogenesis. *Cardiovasc Res.* 2001;49:618-625.

32. DEINDL E, BUSCHMANN I, HOEFER IE, PODZUWEIT T, BOENGLER K, VOGEL S, VAN ROYEN N, FERNÁNDEZ B, SCHAPER W. Role of ischemia and hypoxia-inducible genes in arteriogenesis after femoral artery occlusion in the rabbit. *Circ Res.* 2001;89:779-786.

33. LEE PJ, JIANG BH, CHIN BY, IYER NV, ALAM J, SEMENZA GL, Choi AM. Hypoxia-inducible factor-1 mediates transcriptional activation of the heme oxygenase-1 gene in response to hypoxia. *J Biol Chem.* 1997;272:5375-5381.

34. FIRTH JD, EBERT BL, PUGH CW, RATCLIFFE PJ. Oxygen-regulated control elements in the phosphoglycerate kinase 1 and lactate dehydrogenase A genes: similarities with the erythropoietin 3′ enhancer. *Proc Natl Acad Sci USA.* 1994;91:6496-6500.

35. FIRTH JD, EBERT BL, RATCLIFFE PJ. Hypoxic regulation of lactate dehydrogenase A: interaction between hypoxia inducible factor 1 and cAMP response elements. *J Biol Chem.* 1995;270:21021-21027.

36. SEMENZA GL, ROTH PH, FANG HM, WANG GL. Transcriptional regulation of genes encoding glycolytic enzymes by hypoxia-inducible factor 1. *J Biol Chem.* 1994;269:23757-23763.

37. SEMENZA GL, JIANG BH, LEUNG SW, PASSANTINO R, CONCORDET JP, GIALLONGA A. Hypoxia response elements in aldolase A, enolase and lactate dehydrogenase A gene promotor contain essential binding sites for hypoxia-inducible factor 1. *J Biol Chem.* 1996;271:32529-32537.

38. GLEADLE MJ, RATCLIFFE PJ. Hypoxia and the regulation of gene expression. *Mol Med Today.* 1998;4:122-129.

39. SHEN B-Q, LEE DY, GERBER H-P, KEY BA, FERRARA N, ZIONCHECK TF. Homologous up-regulation of kdr/flk-1 receptor expression by vascular endothelial growth factor *in vitro.* *J Biol Chem.* 1998;273:29979-29985.

40. WILTING J, BIRKENHAEGER R, EICHMANN A, KURZ H, MARTINY-BARON G, MARMÉ D, McCARTHY JEG, CHRIST B, WEICH HA. VEGF121 induces proliferation of vascular endothelial cells and expression of flk-1 without affecting lymphatic vessels of the chorioallantoic membrane. *Devel Biol.* 1996;176:76-85.

41. BARLEON B, SIEMEISTER G, MARTINY-BARON G, WEINDEL K, HERZOG K, MARME D. Vascular endothelial growth factor up-regulates its receptor fms-like tyrosine kinase 1 (flt-1) and soluble variant of flt-1 in human vascular endothelial cells. Cancer Res. 1997;57:5421-5425.

42. GERBER HP, CONDRELLI F, PARK J, FERRARA N. Differential transcriptional regulation of the two vascular endothelial growth factor receptor genes. Flt-1, but not flk-1/kdr, is upregulated by hypoxia. *J Biol Chem.* 1997;272:23659-23667.

43. MARTI HH, RISAU W. Systemic hypoxia changes the organ-specific distribution of vascular endothelial growth factor and its receptors. *Proc Natl Acad Sci USA.* 1998;95:15809-15814.

44. WEN Y, EDELMAN JL, KANG T, ZENG N, SACHS G. Two functional forms of vascular endothelial growth factor receptor-2/flk-1 mRNA are expressed in normal rat retina. *J Biol Chem.* 1998;273:2090-2097.

45. HORNIG C, BEHN T, BARTSCH W, YAYON A, WEICH HA. Detection and quantification of complexed and free soluble human vascular endothelial growth factor receptor-1 (sVEGFR-1) by ELISA. *J Immunol Methods.* 1999;226:169-177.

46. TANAKA K, YAMAGUCHI S, SAWANAO A, SHIBUYA M. Characterization of the extracellular domain in vascular endothelial growth factor receptor-1 (flt-1 tyrosine kinase). *Jap J Cancer Res.* 1997;88:867-876.

47. ITO WD, ARRAS M, WINKLER B, SCHOLZ D, SCHAPER J, SCHAPER W. Monocyte chemotactic protein-1 increases collateral and peripheral conductance after femoral artery occlusion. *Circ Res.* 1997;80:829-837.

48. LINDNER V, REIDY M. Expression of VEGF receptors in arteries after endothelial injury and lack of increased endothelial regrowth in response to VEGF. *Arterioscler Thromb Vasc Biol.* 1996;16:139-1405.

49. BARLEON B, SOZZANI S, ZHOU D, WEICH HA, MANTOVANI A, MARME D. Migration of human monocytes in response to vascular endothelial growth-factor (VEGF) is mediated via the VEGF receptor flt-1. *Blood.* 1996;87:3336-3343.

50. CLAUSS M, WEICH H, BREIER G, KNIES U, ROECKL W, WALTENBERG J, RISAU W. The vascular endothelial growth factor receptor flt-1 mediates biological activities. *J Biol Chem.* 1996; 271:17629-17634.

51. HEIL M, CLAUSS M, BUSCHMANN I, KATZER E, HOEFER I, DEINDL E, VAN ROYEN N, SCHAPER W. VEGF induces integrin expression and L-selectin shedding in human monocytes. *Eur Heart J.* 1999;20:213(Abstract).

52. HEIL M, CLAUSS M, SUZUKI K, BUSCHMANN IR, WILLUWEIT A, FISCHER S, SCHAPER W. Vascular endothelial growth factor (VEGF) stimulates monocyte migration through endothelial monolayers via increased integrin expression. *Europ J Cell Biol.* 2000;79:850-857.

53. LAITINEN M, ZACHARY I, BREIER G, PAKKANEN T, HAKKINEN T, LUOMA J, ABEDI H, RISAU W, SOMA M, LAAKSO M, MARTIN JF, YLA-HERTTUALA S. VEGF gene transfer reduces intimal thickening via increased production of nitric oxide in carotid arteries. *Hum Gene Ther.* 1997;8:1737-1744.

54. KORFF T, KIMMINA S, MARTINY-BARON G, AUGUSTIN HG. Blood vessel maturation in a 3-dimensional spheroidal coculture model: direct contact with smooth muscle cells regulates endothelial cell quiescence and abrogates VEGF responsiveness. *FASEB J.* 2001;15:447-457.

55. HARMON KJ, COUPER LL, LINDNER V. Strain-dependent vascular remodeling phenotypes in inbred mice. *Am J Pathol.* 2000;156:1741-1748.

56. THURSTON G, MURPHY TJ, BALUK P, LINDSEY JR, McDONALD DM. Angiogenesis in mice with chronic airway inflammation: strain-dependent differences. *Am J Pathol.* 1998;153:1099-1112.

57. BARONE FC, KNUDSEN DJ, NELSON AH, FEUERSTEIN GZ, WILLETTE RN. Mouse strain differences in susceptibility to cerebral ischemia are related to cerebral vascular anatomy. *J Cereb Blood Flow Metab.* 1993;13:683-692.

58. FUJII M, HARA H, MENG W, VONSATTEL JP, HUANG Z, MOSKOWITZ MA. Strain-related differences in susceptibility to transient forebrain ischemia in SV-129 and C57black/6 mice. *Stroke.* 1997;28:1805-1810.

59. SCHOLZ D, ZIEGELHOEFFER T, HELISCH A, WAGNER S, FRIEDRICH C, PODZUWEIT T, SCHAPER W. Contribution of arteriogenesis and angiogenesis to postocclusive hind limb perfusion in mice. *J Mol Cell Cardiol.* 2002;34:775-787.

Chapter 7

Monocytes and Cytokines

Matthias Heil and Elisabeth Deindl

The importance of attachment of circulating blood cells to the endothelium of growing collateral blood vessels was described for the first time in 1976[1]. Data from further studies[2] contributed to the development of the hypothesis that the invasion of the arteriolar wall by monocytes might be a key feature of arteriogenesis. Monocytes from the blood are attracted to the collateral vessel endothelium and after their adhesion at the vessel wall they transmigrate through the endothelium and invade the perivascular space. The regulation of this recruitment process is triggered by the local appearance of attracting and activating factors and by increased expression of a panel of adhesion molecules, thus guiding circulating cells to and through the collateral vascular wall.

Adhesion mechanisms

Under physiological conditions, monocytes and other leukocytes are patrolling in the blood stream in a quiescent state with a low adhesion tendency. Their conversion into an active state occurs by binding of stimulatory factors such as cytokines, chemokines and other cell-derived molecules. Monocyte adhesion to activated endothelium including that of collateral vessels is mediated by a group of specific adhesion molecules on monocytes termed integrins, and by intercellular adhesion molecules (ICAM-1 and ICAM-2) and vascular cell adhesion molecules (VCAM-1) on endothelial cells. Activation of the collateral vessel endothelium is initiated after the occlusion of a major artery which leads to a passive redis-tribution of blood flow. Preexisting collateral arterioles are now recruited and exposed to mechanical forces. These forces are the initial triggers for activation of collateral endothelial cells (role of shear stress and other mechanical forces are described in detail in chapter 5). During the early phase of arteriogenesis additional triggers like cytokines (i.e. TNF-α) modulate activation state of endothelial cells and lead to sustained expression of adhesion proteins on the endothelial cell surface (details on upregulation of cell adhesion molecules in this chapter).

Integrin expression on monocytes

Integrins are a group of heterodimers comprising of a variable α-chain and a non-variable β-chain (see also chapter 9). The β_2-subfamily represents leukocyte-specific integrins, e.g. LFA-1 (leukocyte function associated antigen-1; $\alpha_L\beta_2$ integrin; CD11a/CD18) and Mac-1 ($\alpha_M\beta_2$ integrin; CD11b/CD18). Activation of monocytes by agonists triggers ligand binding to β_2 integrins[3,4]. In a process called "inside-out signaling" or "integrin activation", integrins undergo a conformational change. Mediated by a small GTPase termed Rho, surface expression of LFA-1 and Mac-1 is enhanced upon the activation process[5]. A rapid presentation of integrins on the cell surface is based on the release from storage pools and structural changes of the cell membrane. In own experiments using flow cytometry, in which we stimulated monocytes with growth factors such as vascular endothelial growth factor (VEGF) over a period of four hours, we detected in addition to conformation changes an induction of gene expression of β_2 integrins. Furthermore, flow cytometric analysis unraveled an increase in Mac-1 and LFA-1 expression on the monocyte

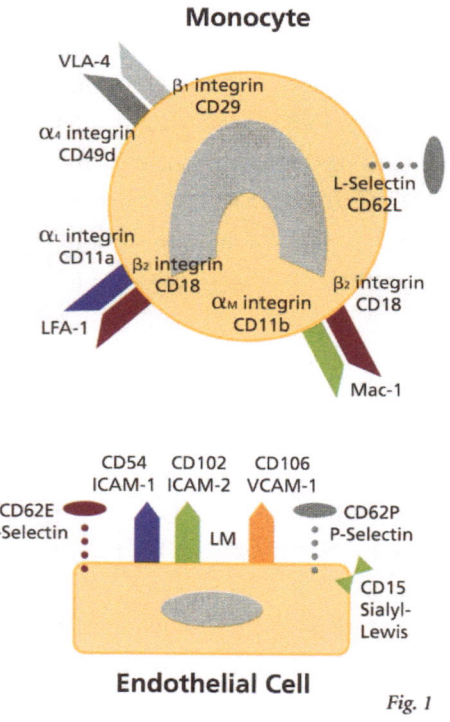

Fig. 1

Monocyte and endothelial cell adhesion molecules involved in arteriogenesis. Abbreviations: ICAM intercellular adhesion molecule; VCAM vascular cell adhesion molecule; P- platelet-; E- endothelial-; L- leukocyte-; LM- luminal side

surface when cells were incubated with other growth factors like TGF-β and bFGF but also after stimulation with chemokines like MCP-1. However, not only receptor presentation on the cell surface was augmented, but conformational changes also modulated affinity and avidity of the integrins. Studies performed *in vitro* using cultured human umbilical endothelial cells (HUVEC) and isolated monocytes demonstrated that these changes in Mac-1 and LFA-1 expression on the monocyte surface stimulated their adhesion on and their transmigration through endothelial monolayers. These data indicate that quiescent monocytes patrolling in the blood stream have the ability to rapidly change their properties upon specific stimulation to highly adhesive cells which then can invade the vascular wall.

Interaction of monocytes and endothelial cells: a multistep process

Invasion of the collateral vessel wall by circulating monocytes is a complex process where several groups of adhesion molecules are involved.

Initially, monocytes travelling in the blood stream have to be slowed down at the vessel wall. This first monocyte-endothelial cell interaction is called tethering or rolling. Monocyte rolling is mainly mediated by a group of adhesion molecules called selectins[6]. L-selectin (CD62L) on monocytes binds to specific non-protein-structures termed Sialyl Lewis(x) antigen (CD15) on the endothelial cell surface. Ligands for E-selectin (CD62E) and P-selectin (CD62P) which are present on the activated endothelium bind to corresponding types of Sialyl Lewis(x) antigen on monocytes. In case of P-selectin these structures are exposed on P-selectin glycoprotein ligand-1 (PSGL-1). Specific chemokines such as MCP-1 rapidly convert initial monocyte rolling on the collateral vessel surface to a firm adhesion via the activation of leukocyte integrins[7]. Monocyte adhesion is basically mediated by two integrin receptors on monocytes, Mac-1 and LFA-1. Their corresponding binding partners on the vascular endothelium are proteins of the Ig gene superfamily, intercellular adhesion molecules, ICAM-1 and ICAM-2. In immunohistological studies we were able to show that expression of ICAM-1 was markedly increased on the endothelium of activated collateral arterioles and (constitutively) on vascular smooth muscle cells[8,9]. In addition, data from a cell culture

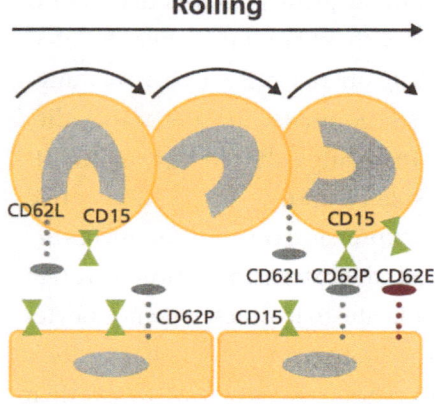

Rolling

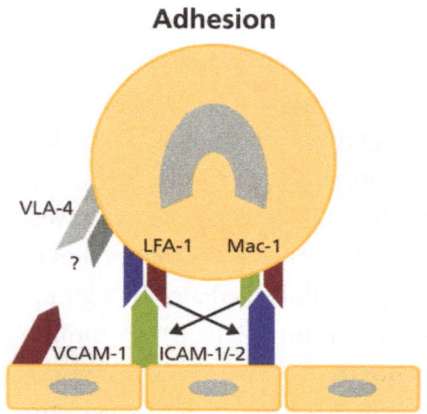

Adhesion

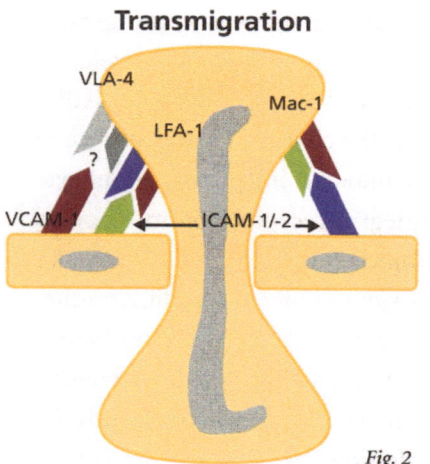

Transmigration

Fig. 2

model suggested that this upregulation of ICAM-1 and ICAM-2 expression was due to mechanical forces: after two hours of fluid shear stress a strong upregulation of ICAM-1 was observed using human umbilical vein endothelial cells[8]. Furthermore, our *in vitro* adhesion assays showed that inhibition of either ICAM-1 or ß₂ integrin by monoclonal antibodies abolished monocyte adhesion to HUVEC[10]. We finally transferred these *in vitro* studies to our rabbit model of femoral artery occlusion. When the monoclonal antibody against ICAM-1 was continuously infused after ligation of the femoral artery in rabbits, collateral artery growth was reduced[11]. However, integrins and ICAMs are not only responsible for monocyte adhesion, they also play a

Multistep process of monocyte-endothelial cell interaction which leads to a monocyte invasion of the activated collateral arteriole. The initial contact between circulating blood monocytes and vascular endothelial cells is mediated by selectins and oligosaccharide structures (sialyl-Lewis X). Monocytes are slowed down from the blood stream by these adhesion molecule interactions in a process called rolling. This is followed by a tight monocyte adhesion at the collateral endothelium which is mediated by two integrins, Mac-1 and LFA-1 on monocytes and intercellular adhesion molecules (ICAM-1 and ICAM-2) on endothelial cells. These adhesion molecules also mediate monocyte transmigration through the collateral vascular wall. The role of VCAM-1 and VLA-4 for this process remains hypothetical.

key role in the transmigration process which finalizes monocyte invasion of the activated collateral vessel. Again, we used monoclonal antibodies against either ICAM-1 or β_2 integrin and were able to successfully inhibit monocyte transmigration through the HUVEC monolayer[10]. Increased expression of a third member of the Ig gene superfamily, vascular cell adhesion molecule-1 (VCAM-1), were also detected in immunohistological investigations on the endothelium of collateral arterioles three days after the occlusion of the femoral artery. Upregulation of VCAM-1 was induced by incubation of endothelial cells with cytokines. Indeed, VCAM-1 was described to be involved in leukocyte-endothelial cell interactions by binding to its counterreceptor, VLA-4 (α_4/β_1 integrin, CD49d/CD29)[12]. However, the role of VLA-4 and VCAM-1 for monocyte adhesion on endothelial cells or for monocyte transmigration through the collateral vessel endothelium during the very initial phases of collateral artery growth remains open. Our *in vitro* adhesion and transmigration studies revealed that blocking of β_2 integrins almost totally abolished interaction between isolated monocytes and HUVEC suggesting that the β_2 integrins are of major importance for the process, thus limiting the impact of β_1 integrins in this process.

In summary, after activation of the endothelium of a preexisting collateral arteriole, monocyte infiltration is regulated by a multistep process with a panel of different adhesion molecule groups being involved. Chemokines such as MCP-1 play an important role in this initial phase of monocyte infiltration, since their release mainly by endothelial cells primes the quiescent circulating monocytes for this process.

Blood monocyte concentration is critical for enhancement of arteriogenesis

Although adherent monocytes were found at the activated endothelium of collateral arteries and both, *in vitro* and *in vivo* studies, indicated the importance of circulating blood monocytes for arteriogenesis, we still had to prove our concept functionally. By using the cytostatic agent 5-fluoruracil (5FU) we could manipulate blood monocyte concentration[13]. Due to its cytotoxic properties, a bolus injection of 5FU in mice led to a depletion of monocytes from the blood (in rabbits, the tolerated 5FU concentration was not sufficient to induce a significant depletion).

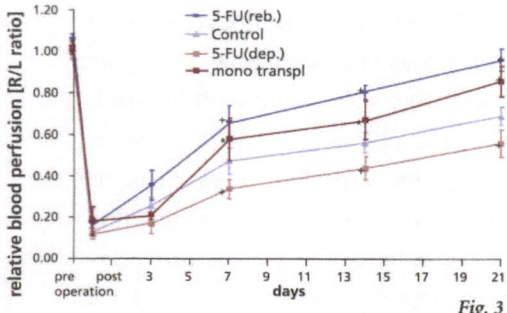

Fig. 3

Blood monocyte concentration is important for arteriogenesis. Right femoral artery of mice was either ligated during pharmacological monocyte depletion (5FU (dep.)) or monocyte rebound (5FU(reb.)). In a third group depleted monocytes were rescued by monocytes isolated from donor mice (mono transpl). * p<0.05, + p<0.01.

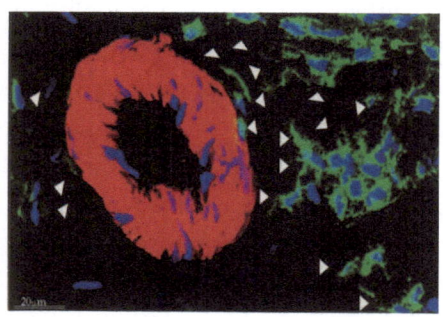

Fig. 4

Accumulation of macrophages in the perivascular space of growing collateral arteries. Immunohistological detection of RAM-11-positive macrophages (green) around the collateral vessel wall (red, by α-smooth muscle actin staining). Nuclei are stained blue.

After several days, a rebound reaction was initiated leading to a several fold increase in blood monocyte concentration (this rebound was similar in mice and rabbits). If the femoral artery of both mice or rabbits was occluded during the monocyte rebound, a significant increase in collateral blood vessel growth was observed. In contrast, if the femoral artery of mice was occluded during the monocyte depletion phase, arteriogenesis was dramatically reduced. However, when a monocyte rescue was performed by injection of isolated monocytes from donor mice, the reduction of collateral artery growth was more than compensated[13].

An additional confirmation of these results was obtained when only blood monocytes were depleted by intravenous injection of liposomes containing cytotoxic bisphosphonates[14]. Bisphosphonates are only cytotoxic when they enter a cell. Since cells did not take up free bisphosphonates, embedding into liposomes was important for its cytotoxic activity. On the other hand, this procedure limited the bisphosphonate effects to phagocyting cells, mainly monocytes, thus giving a rather specific tool to investigate monocyte effects on arteriogenesis. Rabbits, which had been intravenously injected with bisphosphonate liposomes, showed a complete depletion of blood monocytes as early as twelve hours after injection. Monocyte levels returned to normal values at day three (unpublished results). However, the depletion of monocytes during the very brief time frame of 2-3 days, was sufficient to completely abolish arteriogenesis to a level that was similar to acutely ligated animals[14]. When the femoral artery was ligated at day two or three after injection of the bisphosphonate liposome (after monocyte blood concentrations returned to almost normal levels) no inhibition of collateral artery growth was visible (unpublished result). This demonstrated the tight regulation of monocyte infiltration processes during the initial phases of arteriogenesis. Furthermore, it showed that the blood monocyte-controlled phase of arteriogenesis is very short and limited to the very early steps of the process.

Monocytes/macrophages stimulate collateral artery growth

In experimental arteriogenesis using femoral artery ligation, we could show numerous times that monocytes infiltrated the collateral vessel wall and perivascular tissue[8,13,14]. Typically, monocytes did not settle uniformly along the collateral arteriole, but were found accumulated in clusters. This interesting observation could be explained by the morphology of the arteriolar network: Since preexisting collateral arterioles are not linear tubes but are more or less convoluted and additionally split into subbranches, the extent of blood flow and subsequently of endothelial shear

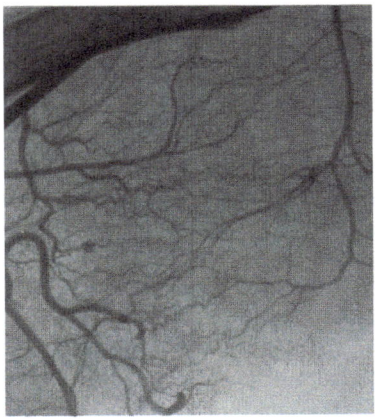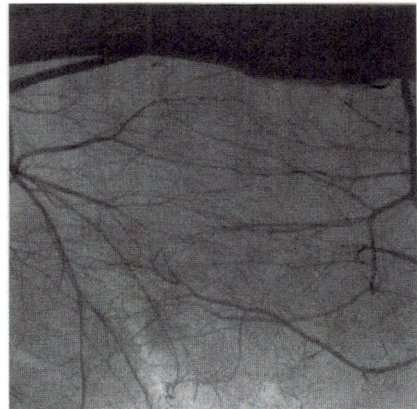

Fig. 5a   *Fig. 5b*

Inhibition of PlGF-stimulated arteriogenesis by injection of bisphosphonate-containing liposomes which induced monocyte depletion from the blood. a: Angiogram of the rabbit thigh seven days after ligation of the right femoral artery and infusion of PlGF. b: Angiogram from a PlGF-treated rabbit with additional monocyte-depletion induced by bisphosphonate-containing liposomes.

stress in collateral vessel network after occlusion of the femoral artery are not consistent. Thus, some areas of the collateral vessel wall are becoming more activated than other areas with less mechanical stress. This in turn may lead to areas with higher density of adhesion molecule expression on the endothelium and higher concentration of chemotactic factors, and conversely. Consequently, monocytes could be more attracted to the more activated areas of the collateral vessel.

Once the monocytes have invaded the vascular wall, they mature into macrophages and become a key stimulator of collateral artery growth. Under these circumstances, monocytes resp. macrophages start to act as "cytokine factories", releasing numerous inflammatory and chemotactic factors (e.g. MCP-1, TNF-α, IL-8, etc.), growth factors (TGF-β, bFGF, PDGF, etc.) and proteinases such as metalloproteinase-2 (MMP-2) (their role in arteriogenesis is described in detail in chapter 6). By immunohistology we previously could show that macrophages, which had accumulated in the perivascular tissue of growing collaterals, express basic fibroblast growth factor (bFGF)[2]. bFGF is one of the few growth factors which have been shown to stimulate collateral artery growth (see chapter 10). In addition, production of tumor necrosis factor-α (TNF-α), a strong inflammatory cytokine with primary effects on endothelial cells,

Cytokines

Cytokines are defined as signaling proteins. They are responsible for cell-to-cell communication and interactions. Cytokines typically act locally as autocrine, paracrine or juxtacrine regulators. In some cases (i.e. IL-1, IL-6, TNF-α) they additionally can act as endocrines. Under these circumstances cytokines can modulate inflammatory reactions within the whole organism.

Cytokine groups of importance for collateral artery growth:
Chemokines are responsible for attraction, migration and activation of leukocytes. Occasionally, chemokines are subdivided into classes describing their target cells. **Monokines** act as monocyte-specific chemokines and **lymphokines** as lymphocyte-specific chemokines.
Growth factors stimulate proliferation of various cell types. Furthermore, they modulate cell activation and migration.
Colony-stimulating factors manage differentiation, proliferation and maturation of hematopoietic stem cells.

was detected in these macrophages[2]. Indeed, *in vivo* studies using a mouse model demonstrated that TNF-α is involved in collateral artery growth[15], probably by activation of endothelial cells (see below). The panel of factors which are released by monocyte-derived macrophages after invading the area of collateral vessels regulate inflammatory processes, proliferation of endothelial cells, vascular smooth muscle cells and fibroblasts and finally create the space for the enlarged collateral artery within the surrounding tissue. Growing collateral arteries have a typical corkscrew like morphology. This is because collateral vessels grow in diamneter as well as in length. Since stem and reentry are fixed, the lengthening collateral vessel folds into corkscrew loops. However, the accumulation of monocytes/macrophages in certain clusters could lead to areas with higher local macrophage-related cytokine levels and subsequently to increased proliferation activity and vessel growth. As a consequence, the corkscrew-like pattern may develop.

Chemokines and chemokine receptors

A major feature of arteriogenesis is that it shares typical mechanisms with other pathophysiological inflammatory processes. Inflammation is based on the successful orchestration of a variety of effector cells which are guided by a heterogenous group of proteins termed cytokines. Cytokines control cell activation, attraction, proliferation and differentiation from progenitor cells. Typically, the cytokine effects on their target cells are exerted by binding to specific cell surface receptors. After ligand binding, the receptors initiate intracellular signaling cascades leading to specific cellular responses.

A subset of cytokines, named chemokines, participate in the activation of leukocytes and the control of their movement during inflammatory processes[16]. Chemokines are small polypeptides with molecular weights between 8 and 12 kDa and share a 20-70% homology in their amino acid sequence. Like all cytokines, chemokines bind to specific cell surface receptors. Four members of the chemokine family are described including CXC- (α-chemokines), CC- (β-chemokines), C- (γ-chemokines) and CX3C- (δ-chemokines). The designation of these subgroups has been conducted on the basis of the relative position of their N-terminal cysteine residues[17,18]. I.e., in CC-chemokines, the first two cysteine residues are adjacent to each other whereas in CXC-chemokines the first two cysteine residues are separated by one amino acid.

While multiple evidence has been gathered that chemokines play an important role in a variety of pathophysiological processes, mainly one group of chemokines, the CC-chemokines, are of certain interest for the understanding of cellular mechanisms in arteriogenesis. The target cells of CC-chemokines are leukocyte subsets which have been related to arteriogenesis, above all monocytes/ macrophages. But CC-chemokines also act on lymphocytes and basophils and all those cells have been associated with arteriogenesis at least by the observation of their morphological appearance in the growing collateral vessel wall. CC-chemokines are dominated by the group of monocyte-chemoattractant-proteins (MCPs) of which five so far have been identified (MCP-1 to MCP-5)[16]. Other members of this group are for example the group of macrophage inflammatory proteines (MIP-1α, MIP-1β, MIP-3α) and RANTES. CC-chemokines are highly specific ligands. Biological activity and cell selectivity are critically controlled by the N-terminal amino acids. The exchange of a single amino acid can reduce activity and specificity by a factor of 100 and more[19].

Chemokine receptors are named after their ligands, i.e., eight CC chemokine receptors are yet identified (CCR1 through CCR8). Chemokine receptors represent a group of G-protein-coupled cell surface receptors and are expressed on different types of leukocytes. Besides the regulation via local expression of the ligands, chemokine signaling is also regulated by the expression pattern of their receptors. While expression of some receptors is restricted to certain types of leukocytes (e.g. CXCR1 is found only on neutrophils) and effects of their ligands are therefore limited to the particular cell types, other chemokine receptors possess a wide expression range. In particular, CCR2 can be found on monocytes, macrophages, T-cells, natural killer cells, dentritic cells and basophils. Never-

6) *Chemokines and chemokine receptors on leukocytes. Chemokines are classified on the basis of the relative position of the cystein residues. In CXC-chemokines (also termed α-chemokines), one amino acid separates the first two cysteins, in CC-chemokines (β-chemokines) the first two amino acids are adjacent to each other. The C-chemokine lymphotactin includes only two cysteins. In CXXXC-chemokines, three variable amino acids separate the first two cystein residues. Abbreviations: MCP: Monocyte chemotattractant protein, MIP: macrophage inflammatory protein, RANTES: regulated upon activation normal T-cell expressed and secreted, GRO: growth-regulated oncogene, SDF: stromal-cell derived factor, R: receptor.*

Chemokine		Receptor	Cell type
CXC	SDF-1	CXCR4	Monocyte 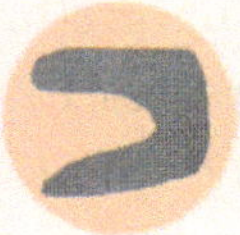
CC	MCP-1, -2, -3, -4, -5	CCR2	
	MCP-3, -4, MIP-1α, RANTES	CCR1	
	MIP-1α, MIP-1β, RANTES	CCR5	
	MCP-1, -2, -3, -4, -5	CCR2	Basophil 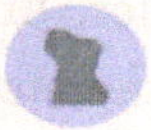
	MCP-3, -4, eotaxin-1,-2, RANTES	CCR3	
	MCP-3, -4, MIP-1α, RANTES	CCR1	Eosinophil 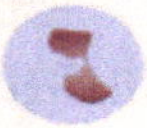
	MCP-3, -4, eotaxin-1,-2, RANTES	CCR3	
CXC	Interleukin-8, GCP-2	CXCR1	Neutrophil 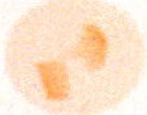
	Interleukin-8, GCP-2, GRO-α, -β, -γ	CXCR2	
C	Lymphotactin	?	Resting T cell 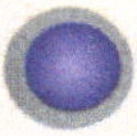
CXXXC	Fractalkine	CX$_3$CR1	
CC	MCP-1, -2, -3, -4, -5	CCR2	
	MCP-3, -4, MIP-1α, RANTES	CCR1	Activated T cell
	TARC	CCR4	
	MIP-1α, MIP-1β, RANTES	CCR5	
	MIP-3β	CCR7	
CC	MCP-1, -2, -3, -4, -5	CCR2	Natural killer cell 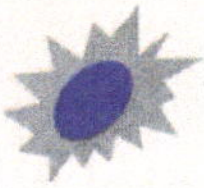
	MIP-1α, MIP-1β, RANTES	CCR5	
CXXXC	Fractalkine	CX$_3$CR1	

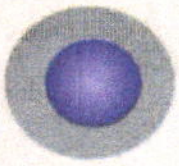

Fig. 6

theless, regulatory mechanisms are also established under these circumstances: Only monocytes and macrophages express CCR2 constitutively on their cell surface. As a negative feedback, expression of the receptor is reduced upon stimulation of the monocytes/ macrophages, e.g. by bacterial lipopolysaccarides. As a consequence, sensitivity of activated cells to the CCR2 ligand MCP-1 is dramatically reduced, but these cells are still sensitive to other CC-chemokines like MIP-1α which binds to CCR1 and CCR5 [20]. In contrast, no basal CCR2 receptor expression is found on other lymphocytes, but expression is induced after stimulation with interleukin-2, therefore making these cells insensitive for MCP-1 signaling in the absence of particular co-stimulating factors [21].

Intracellular signal transduction

Binding of an appropriate chemokine to its receptor induces a complex intracellular signaling cascade leading to a specific cellular response like cell migration or induction of protein biosynthesis. Like other members of the G-protein receptor family, chemokine receptors are functionally

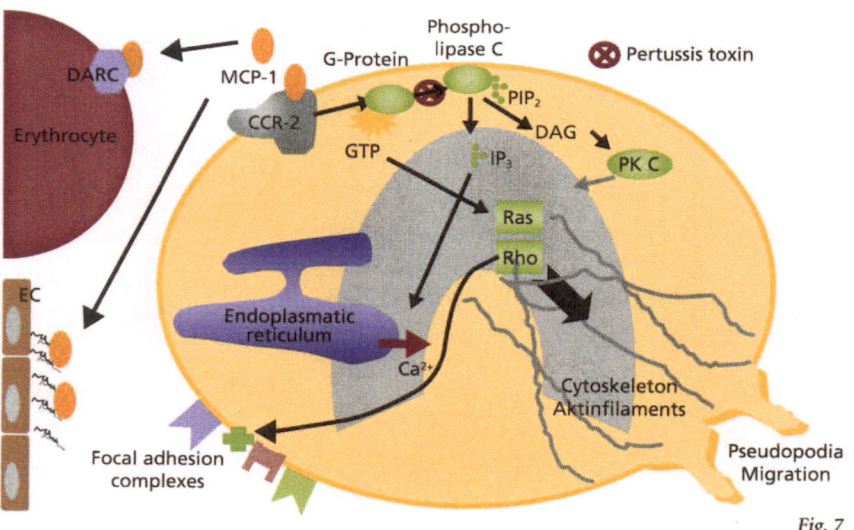

Fig. 7

Chemokine signaling: intracellular signaling pathway. After MCP-1 bound to its receptor on the monocyte surface, an intracellular signal transduction cascade is initiated leading to cell activation, mobility and expression of proteins such as adhesion molecules and cytokines.
Abbreviations: MCP: monocyte chemoattractant protein, CCR chemokine receptor, PKC protein kinase C, IP$_3$: phosphoinositol triphosphate, PIP$_2$: phosphatidylinositol 4,5-diphosphate, GTP: guanosin triphosphate, DARC: duffy-antigen receptor for chemokines, EC: endothelial cell.

linked to phospholipases through G proteins, most of them in particular by G_i-proteins[22-24]. The intracellular signaling cascade comprises generation of inositol triphosphate, release of calcium-ions from their intracellular stores like the endoplasmatic reticulum and activation of protein kinase C^{25}. Subsequently, the signal is transduced to the nucleus where gene expression, e.g. of genes linked to inflammatory processes, is initiated. Moreover, two groups of guanosine triphosphate binding proteins, proteins of the Ras and Rho family are activated[5]. Rho proteins are involved in cell motility because they regulate actin-binding processes along the cytoskeleton: Cell membrane ruffling and pseudopod formation are important steps in the induction of cell migration. Furthermore, so-called focal adhesion complexes comprising a panel of adhesion molecules (mainly integrins and selectins), which are required for interaction procedures with neighboring cells, are formed by contractions and other mechanical modifications of the cytoskeleton. Thus, chemokine receptors activate multiple intracellular signaling pathways guiding the cell to a specific activation and migration route.

The mechanism of action of chemotactic factors is still rather hypothetic. It seems to be more or less obvious, however, that in order to attract cells to a certain area, a concentration gradient of the designed chemotactic factor has to exist. A systemic increase in the concentration may only support cell adhesion and migration by activating effector cells which then in turn increase expression of adhesion molecules. Interestingly, chemokines are basic proteins which can bind to negatively charged heparin and heparan sulfate[26,27]. Therefore, MCP-1 produced and released by endothelial cells of the activated collateral arteriole may bind to the heparan sulfate proteoglycans on the surface of these endothelial cells, thus establishing a gradient with a peak at the area of highest activation[28]. A receptor on erythrocytes termed duffy-antigen receptor for chemokines (DARC) has no signaling function and is assumed to be a sink for plasmatic MCP-1.

Role of chemokines and chemokine receptors in arteriogenesis

In the last twenty years the observation of macrophages in proximity to collateral arteries had been reported several times. As mentioned before, in mice and rabbit studies we were able to correlate the extend of collateral artery growth with the concentration of circulating blood monocytes[13]. These observations inspired us to search for a mechanism which leads to the accumulation of monocytes and -after their maturation- macrophages around growing collateral vessels. The first evidence of a specific attraction process was gathered when MCP-1 was locally infused into the collateral blood vessel network after occlusion of the femoral artery in the rabbit hind limb, thus leading to a dramatic improvement of the growth process[29]. In addition, MCP-1 was tested in a minipig model[30]. Local infusion of MCP-1 enhanced collateral conductance almost twofold compared to controls. Furthermore, investigations in MCP-1 gene deficient mice showed a reduced hind limb perfusion in the knockout group when compared to control animals[31]. This reduction could be rescued by local infusion of MCP-1. Blood flow reduction was associated with decreased rates of monocyte accumulation around the collateral vessel, although monocyte infiltration was completely not abolished. From the results of these studies we hypothesized, that parts of the same mechanism which generates atherosclerosis under different circumstances, may now have beneficial effects in enhancing the growth of collateral arteries. This could be a result of the distinct regulation of the expression pattern of chemokines and their receptors. We were able to collect additional indications for the latter assumption, since in contrast to MCP-1 local application of additional chemokines like MIP-1α, MIP-1β, RANTES and lymphotactin did not improve arteriogenesis (unpublished results) in our rabbit model. The CC-chemokine receptor-2 is the major receptor for MCP-1 in humans and the exclusive MCP-1-receptor in mice. Therefore, we focused on the investigation of the role of the MCP-1-CCR2 signaling pathway during arteriogenesis. Fortunately, a CCR2 gene-deficient mouse strain was established previously[32]. Using this mouse strain we were able to obtain important information on the mechanisms by which monocytes participate in arteriogenesis. Our hypothesis that the CCR2 is responsible for monocyte attraction during the initial phases of collateral artery growth was impressively confirmed. Data obtained from CCR2 knockout (CCR2$^{-/-}$) mice showed a dramatically reduced recovery of blood perfusion distal to the ligation side, which is a strong indication for reduced collateral artery growth[33]. This correlated with other physiological parameters like the reduction in hemoglobin oxygen saturation in the foot from the ligated side but was also reflected by functional parameters: Due to the reduced blood supply distally to the ligation side the knock-out mice showed signs of an impaired active movement of their operated leg. Histological morphometry of the collateral vessel size demonstrated that indeed the mentioned observations were caused by the reduced collateral artery growth rate in the CCR2-deficient mice[34].

By using a specific monoclonal antibody we could illustrate and quantify the accumulation of monocytes and their mature form, macrophages, in the perivascular space around the growing collateral vessel. Interestingly, in CCR2[-/-] mice the monocytes were not completely abolished. A moderate number of cells was concentrated in the collateral adventitia. In contrast, when we investigated the distribution of monocytes and macrophages in corresponding tissue of wildtype animals, we not only found a markedly higher number of accumulating monocytes but also a larger monocyte infiltration area. Parts of the skeletal muscle in close proximity to the collateral vessels showed a strong aggregation of leukocytes. Leukocyte infiltration into tissue is a typical sign for an inflammatory process. Since we can exclude that femoral artery occlusion leads to major ischemia in the adductor muscles of the upper limb, where collateral arteries mainly grow (depending on the mouse strain, ischemia may appear in other parts of the thigh), the mechanism which induces inflammation may not be induced by the lack of oxygen in these areas. Other initiating processes may be operative: Mechanical forces leading to an activation of the preexisting collateral arteriole are the major candidates for a potential trigger of the inflammatory cascade.

Arteriogenic potency of factors can be secondary to monocytes

In addition to chemokines and their receptors other classes of cytokines such as growth factors, colony stimulating factors and proteases can contribute to collateral artery growth. By analyzing the mechanisms of their contribution, it became obvious that many of the processes are secondary to monocyte or macrophage actions.

Vascular endothelial growth factor and Placenta growth factor

Vascular endothelial growth factor (VEGF) is the major inducer of angiogenesis[35]. Because VEGF stimulates capillary growth in response to hypoxia its expression describes a response to the increased need of nutrients and oxygen of growing tissues. Furthermore, VEGF was associated with *de novo* growth of blood vessels in adult organism which is generally termed neovasculogenesis[36], and we could show that VEGF promotes experimental arteriogenesis[14]. Although our own results clearly show that endogenous VEGF does not contribute to arteriogenesis under 'normal' conditions (see Chapter 4 Deindl), we and others found that VEGF applied exogenously has the capacity to promote arteriogenesis, at least to a minor extent.

Some of the VEGF-effects on endothelial cells and vascular system like increase of vascular permeability or induction of tissue factor, a major trigger of blood coagulation[37], may interfere with processes involved in collateral vessel growth. In order to unravel the mechanisms controlling VEGF-activities in arteriogenesis, we performed studies focusing on the role of the two VEGF-receptors, VEGFR-1 (also named flt-1) and VEGFR-2 (also named flk-1/kdr). Endothelial cells express both receptors but VEGFR-2 seems to play a dominant role in mediating activity in those cells[38]. In contrast, monocytes only express VEGFR-1. We therefore hypothesized that VEGF signaling in arteriogenesis could in contrast to angiogenesis be mediated via the VEGFR-1 on monocytes. Our approach to this question was to apply receptor specific ligands of the VEGF-family in our rabbit model. Placenta growth factor (PlGF) was previously identified as a specific ligand for VEGFR-1[39]. Seven days after femoral artery occlusion we found PlGF in the number of visible collateral

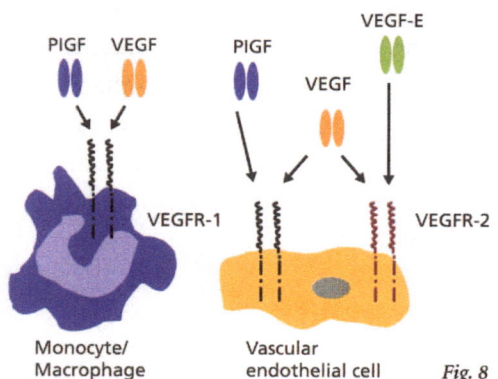

Vascular endothelial growth factor (VEGF) and receptors. VEGF binds to VEGF receptor (VEGFR) -1 and -2. In contrast, the VEGF-homologue placenta growth factor (PlGF) binds specifically to VEGFR-1 only and the orf-virus derived VEGF-E to VEGFR-2.

Fig. 8

arteries and collateral blood conductance superior to both VEGF and the VEGFR-2 specific ligand VEGF-E. In an additional experiment we deleted the monocytes from the blood of PlGF-treated animals which totally abolished collateral artery growth. These findings strongly suggested that the VEGFR-1 is the important VEGF receptor for arteriogenesis. Furthermore, it suggests that the signaling events evoked by VEGFR-1 contribute more to collateral formation than VEGFR-2 mediated signaling. The fact that PlGF was superior to VEGF could have two reasons: First, VEGF could have been immobilized by endothelial cells via their VEGFR-2 which could have made it inaccessible for circulating monocytes. Second, the side effects of VEGF could have been counterproductive to arteriogenesis.

In conclusion, the study shows that VEGF-induced enhancement of arteriogenesis is most probably mediated via the VEGFR-1 and is secondary to monocyte recruitment.

Transforming growth factor-β_1

Transforming growth factor-β_1 (TGF-β_1) was reported to be chemoattractive for monocytes[40] and increase gene expression in a variety of cells including monocytes[40,41]. Furthermore, collateral vessel growth was detected in nonischemic regions[40]. We therefore investigated whether treatment with TGF-ß$_1$ could enhance arteriogenesis[42]. TGF-β_1 that was found to be activated was detected immunohistochemically within and around growing collateral arteries of controls and of TGF-β_1-treated rabbits three days after femoral artery ligation. However, in rabbits with additional infusion of TGF-β_1 immunolabeling was strongly increased. Furthermore, we could demonstrate by flow cytometry that TGF-β_1 increased integrin expression on isolated monocytes and increased their adhesion on endothelial cells. This data, showing that TGF-β_1 has multiple effects on monocytes and macrophages were reflected by our *in vivo* findings: Seven days after ligation of the femoral artery and local infusion of TGF-β_1 collateral conductance was increased when compared to buffer-treated animals. Our data show that –similar to other arteriogenic cytokines- the TGF-β_1 effect is at least partly secondary to monocytes which are activated and attracted by TGF-β_1.

Urokinase-plasminogen activator

Two plasminogen activators, urokinase-plasminogen activator (u-PA) and tissue-plasminogen activator (t-PA) belong to the fibrinolytic system. Both factors can potentially convert the zymogen plasminogen into its active form plasmin[43]. u-PA has been implicated in pericellular prote-

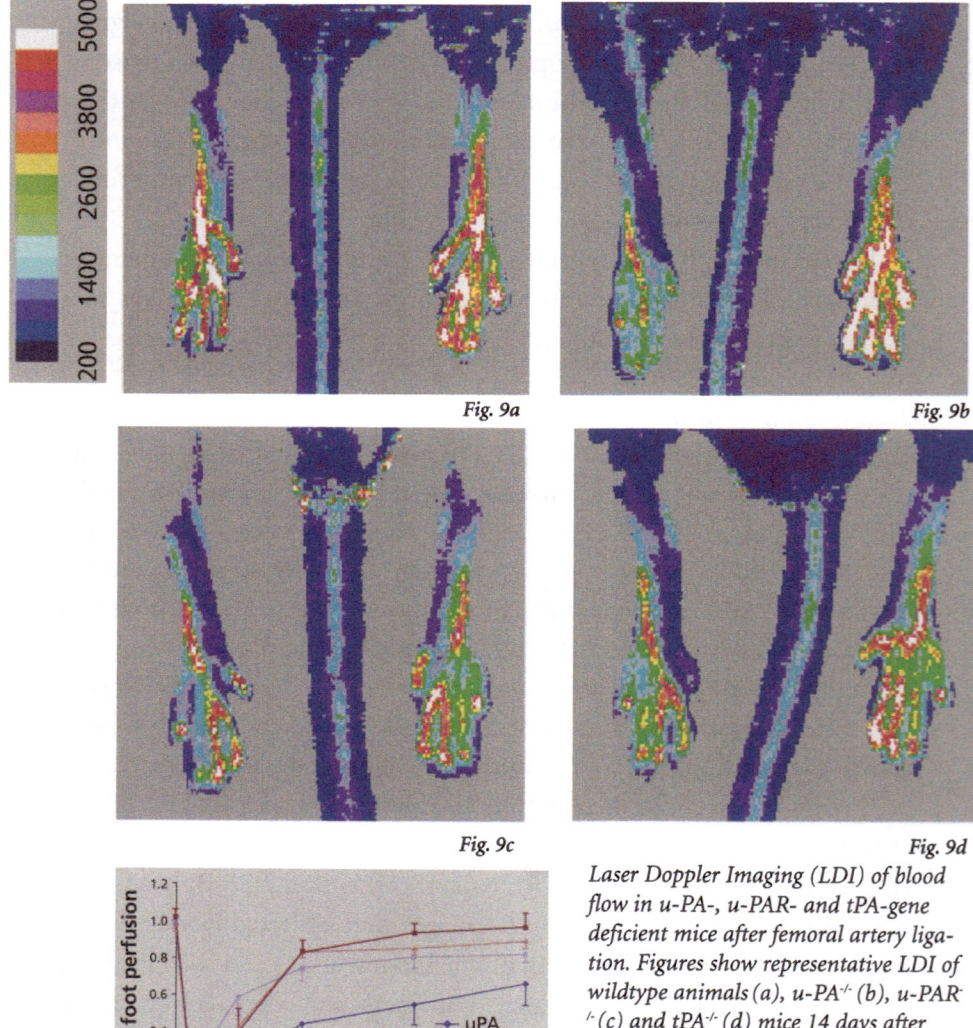

Fig. 9a

Fig. 9b

Fig. 9c

Fig. 9d

Laser Doppler Imaging (LDI) of blood flow in u-PA-, u-PAR- and tPA-gene deficient mice after femoral artery ligation. Figures show representative LDI of wildtype animals (a), u-PA[-/-] (b), u-PAR[-/-] (c) and tPA[-/-] (d) mice 14 days after femoral artery ligation. e: Quantification of hind limb blood perfusion over three weeks using LDI.

Fig. 9e

olysis during cell migration or tissue remodeling. Furthermore, the plasminogen system is known to be involved in angiogenesis and vascular remodeling by modulating adhesion and migration of monocytes and other leukocytes. Consequently, in the rabbit femoral artery occlusion model we found an upregulation of u-PA mRNA in the quadriceps muscle during early phases of arteriogenesis which correlated with increased u-PA activity[44]. In contrast, in accordance with the literature[45], our data did not show any increase in t-PA mRNA expression and activity during arteriogenesis. In order to unravel the role of different factors of the fibrinolytic system in more detail, a second panel of experiments was performed in the mouse model using gene-deficient mice. In addition to the confirmation of our rabbit data, the mice experiments demonstrated that only u-PA[-/-] mice showed a pronounced reduction in blood flow recovery after femoral artery ligation. In contrast, when the u-PA receptor (u-PAR) gene was disrupted, blood flow recovery was not altered from the control group indicating a u-PAR independent role for u-PA in arteriogenesis. Furthermore, t-PA[-/-] mice did not show an effect, either.

Since u-PA was demonstrated to stimulate monocyte invasion[46], at least a part of the u-PA effect could be secondary to monocytes. We therefore analyzed the accumulation of leukocytes in the quadriceps muscle three days after femoral artery occlusion. While numbers of activated macrophages and granulocytes were reduced in u-PA[-/-] mice, no difference to control animals was determined in u-PAR[-/-] and t-PA[-/-] mice, confirming previous data that u-PA promotes monocyte migration independently from the u-PAR[47]. In addition to the stimulation of monocyte migration, u-PA might increase gene expression by monocytes and may stimulate release of matrix metalloproteinases, TNF-α and others[48-50].

Besides its monocyte-specific role in arteriogenesis, u-PA also seems to promote arteriogenesis by an alternative pathway: u-PA has been described to play a role in smooth muscle cell migration, a process where the u-PAR is involved but is not necessarily required[51]. The mechanism most likely is based on the fact, that the serinprotease u-PA converts the zymogen plasminogen to the active protease plasmin. Plasmin in turn degrades the extrecellular matrix and interstitial tissue in the microenvironment of the growing collateral vessel thereby creating pathways for migrating smooth muscle cells. However, there also may be a contribu-

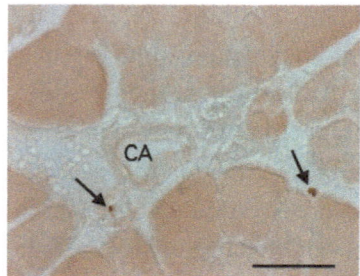

Fig. 10a

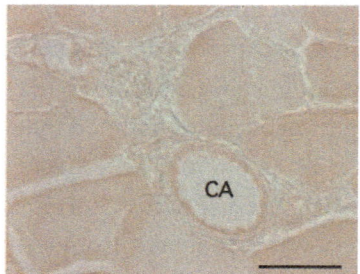

Fig. 10b

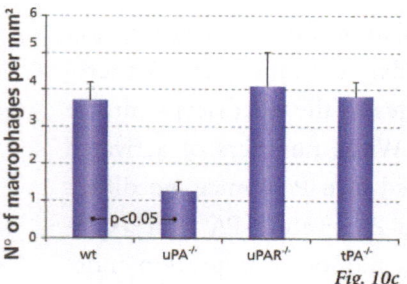

Fig. 10c

Leukocyte distribution in u-PA-, u-PAR and tPA-gene deficient mice after femoral artery ligation. Macrophages were detected three days after ligation around collateral arteries by endogenous biotin. Figure shows section from a wildtype mouse after ligation (a) or sham operation (b). c: Quantification of macrophage accumulation around collateral arteries in wildtype, u-PA$^{-/-}$, u-PAR$^{-/-}$ and tPA$^{-/-}$ animals. CA: collateral artery

tion of macrophages to this process in addition to their own production of tissue-degrading enzymes: u-PA may bind to u-PAR on the macrophage surface, thus accumulating additional lytic activity in the perivascular space of the collateral vessel.

Finally, u-PA may contribute to the production of proteins by smooth muscle cells, since u-PA expression has been correlated to the proliferative phase of vascular smooth muscle cells[52]. Furthermore, it has been shown that u-PA can act as a smooth muscle cell mitogen[47].

Granulocyte monocyte-colony stimulating factor
Colony stimulating factors (CSF) influence the development of blood cells and their release from the bone marrow. Granulocyte-macrophage colony stimulating factor (GM-CSF) in particular is involved in stem cell proliferation, differentiation and survival. Therefore, treatment with GM-CSF stimulates mobilization of monocytes and their progenitors from bone marrow into peripheral blood. However, in our study we decided to apply GM-CSF locally over a period of seven days into the collateral system[53]. Thus, systemic concentrations of GM-CSF remained very low. Consequently, monocyte concentration in the peripheral blood stream did not increase significantly. Nevertheless, we could observe a distinct increase in collateral conductance in GM-CSF-treated rabbits when compared to buffer-treated controls.

By FACS-analysis we could show that GM-CSF strongly reduced apoptosis of blood monocytes. Furthermore, a reduced number of apoptotic macrophages along the collateral network was observed using the TUN-

NEL-assay. In conclusion, we were able to show that in experimental arteriogenesis GM-CSF promoted collateral vessel growth by prolonging the life cycle of both, blood monocytes and tissue macrophages. Subsequently, these cells have a longer time frame to produce and secrete arteriogenic factors. Additionally, a group of rabbits was treated with two factors, thus combining two strategies: Local infusion of MCP-1 was used to increase monocyte attraction and GM-CSF was used to increase their life span. Not surprisingly, this treatment caused a synerigistic effect: Collateral artery growth was strongly enhanced and collateral conductance after seven days was almost 50% of the physiological perfusion values[53].

GM-CSF was the first cytokine which had been successfully tested in coronary artery disease (CAD)-patients[54]: Coronary collateral flow in these patients was significantly increased -compared to a placebo-treated control group- when GM-CSF was applied in a combination of intracoronar (bolus) and subcutaneous (over two weeks) injection. In the GM-CSF-treated group, blood monocyte concentration after treatment was more than twice of the concentration before treatment. Most likely, this is based on two effects, the prolongation of monocyte survival and increased mobilization of monocytes from bone marrow.

Tumor necrosis factor-α

The role of tumor necrosis factor-α (TNF-α) in arteriogenesis has been discussed controversially. Based on unpublished experiments on gene-deficient mice in our group from the nineties which indicated a role for TNF-α in arteriogenesis, immunohistological studies in rabbits revealed that monocytes which had accumulated around the collateral vessel showed TNF-α expression[2]. Also in this study, a group of animals received bacterial endotoxin, which is the strongest inducer of TNF-α in monocytes. However, no enhancement of collateral conductance was achieved by this treatment. Instead, only angiogenesis in the ischemic lower limb was enhanced. Later on, a study was performed using TNF-α and TNF-α-receptor knockout mice[15]. The results from this investigation suggested that arteriogenesis was reduced in either of those gene-deficient mouse strains implicating an involvement of TNF-α in collateral artery growth. However, when this study was repeated with knockout mice and littermates which had been backcrossed into the CS7BL/6 strain, these differences disappeared[55].

This discrepant outcome of the two cited studies suggests that TNF-α does not neccessarily play a crucial role in arteriogenesis. One can hypothesize that the most prominent function of TNF-α in the process would be its ability to potentially stimulate endothelial cell activation. However, it is unclear if such an activation is really needed during collateral artery growth because the main trigger of activation of the collateral endothelial is mechanical stress (shear stress) induced by blood flow (see chapter 3). This is most likely the important step to induce monocyte attraction, activation, adhesion and invasion. A stimulation of collateral endothelial cells by TNF-α (which probably would be monocyte-derived) could only help to maintain the activity potency of the collateral endothelium in a second phase. If such a modulation is required for arteriogenesis is doubtfull, since our studies on monocyte kinetics suggest that monocyte invasion might be important only in the very early phases of arteriogenesis.

Conclusion

Monocytes play a crucial role, since they act as ubiquitous "cytokine factories", responsible for activation, proliferation and migration of other cells types like endothelial cells and smooth muscle cells. Although our studies made it quite obvious that monocytes play the key role in arteriogenesis, optimal collateral vessel growth can only appear if each factor of the chain is available for the system.

Second, monocytes are a possible target for a therapeutic approach to enhance arteriogenesis in patients. This therapy could either be based on a treatment increasing monocyte numbers in the blood, it could increase their ability to invade the collateral vessel wall by increasing expression of adhesion molecules on the monocyte surface or it could stimulate cytokine production. Increased production of arteriogenic factor would then enhance the process as an alternative of a single factors treatment. Finally, a third route is conceivable: Monocytes could act as vectors to deliver arteriogenic factors to the collateral system.

A summary of the findings described is presented in figure 11.

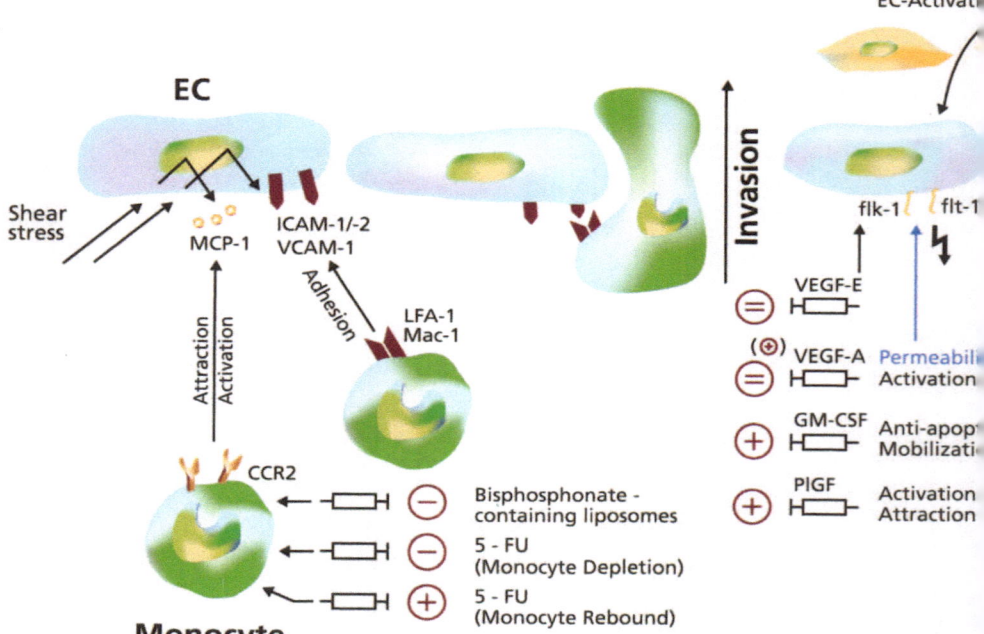

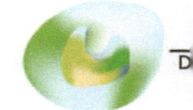

Cellular mechanisms of arteriogenesis.

The initial trigger of arteriogenesis is shear stress which leads to the activation of endothelial cells (EC) in the collateral vessel wall. This EC activation induces surface expression of adhesion molecules like intercellular adhesion molecule-1 and -2 (ICAM-1/-2) and vascular cell adhesion molecule-1 (VCAM-1). The adhesion molecules mediate attachment of leukocytes, namely monocytes, which are attracted by cytokines such as monocyte chemoattractant protein-1 (MCP-1) produced by the collateral endothelium. MCP-1 binds to its receptor, the chemokine receptor-2 (CCR2), on circulating blood monocytes. Monocytes in turn, after being activated by MCP-1, pronouncedly increase surface expression of integrins. Two integrin receptors, Mac-1 and LFA-1, have been identified to be mainly involved in the attachment of monocytes to the collateral endothelium and their subsequent invasion of the collateral vessel wall.

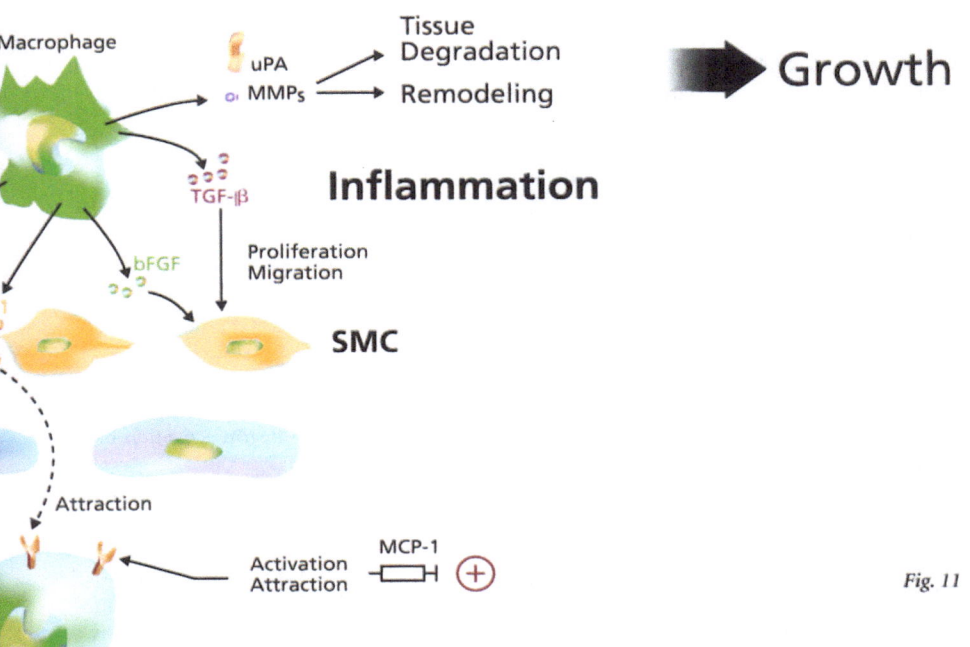

Fig. 11

After entering the collateral vessel wall, monocytes differentiate into macrophages and show increased cytokine synthesis: Tumor necrosis factor-α (TNF-α) modulates the activation status of the collateral endothelium. MCP-1 is transferred to the luminal side of the collateral vessel wall and enhances attraction of more circulating monocytes. Basic fibroblast growth factor (bFGF) and transforming growth factor-β (TGF-β) activate vascular smooth muscle cells (SMC). Proliferation and migration of SMC is induced, thus increasing the blood vessel wall size. The required space for the enlarging collateral artery is created by tissue degradating proteases like uronary plasminogen activator (u-PA) and matrix metalloproteinases (MMPs).
In various experimental setting we could unravel factors, cells and mechanisms leading to the growth of collateral arteries: By either depleting circulating monocytes from the blood using bisphosphonate-containing liposomes or the cytostatic agent 5-fluorouracil (5FU) or increasing the number of blood monocytes via a 5FU induced monocyte rebound we could demonstrate that monocytes play a critical role for arteriogenesis. MCP-1 is one of the most potent stimulators of arteriogenesis when injected locally via an osmotic minipump. Granulocyte-monocyte-colony-stimulating factor (GM-CSF) enhances arteriogenesis most likely via preventing monocytes from entering the apoptotic cell death and mobilizing monocytes from the bone marrow. A number of polypeptides from the vascular endothelial growth factor (VEGF) family was used to show that arteriogenic action of VEGF, if at all, is secondary to monocyte recruitment mediated by the VEGF-receptor-1 (flt-1). Placenta growth factor (PlGF) was shown to pronouncedly enhance arteriogenesis by this mechanism, whereas the VEGFR-2 (flk-1) specific VEGF-E did not stimulate arteriogenesis. VEGF-A only moderately stimulates arteriogenesis at high concentrations, most likely because negative side effects which are induced via flk-1 may partially neutralize flt-1 mediated effects. (-) inhibition of arteriogenesis; (=) no effect on arteriogesis; (+) enhancement of arteriogenesis

References

1. SCHAPER J, KONIG R, FRANZ D, SCHAPER W. The endothelial surface of growing coronary collateral arteries. Intimal margination and diapedesis of monocytes. A combined SEM and TEM study. *Virchows Arch A Pathol Anat Histol.* 1976;370:193-205.
2. ARRAS M, ITO WD, SCHOLZ D, WINKLER B, SCHAPER J, SCHAPER W. Monocyte activation in angiogenesis and collateral growth in the rabbit hind limb. *J Clin Invest.* 1998;101:40-50.
3. TAKAGI J, SPRINGER TA. Integrin activation and structural rearrangement. *Immunol Rev.* 2002;186:141-63.
4. HOGG N, HENDERSON R, LEITINGER B, MCDOWALL A, PORTER J, STANLEY P. Mechanisms contributing to the activity of integrins on leukocytes. *Immunol Rev.* 2002;186:164-71.
5. LAUDANNA C, CAMPBELL JJ, BUTCHER EC. Role of Rho in chemoattractant-activated leukocyte adhesion through integrins. *Science.* 1996;271:981-3.
6. THIAGARAJAN R, WINN R, HARLAN J. The role of leukocyte and endothelial adhesion molecules in ischemia-reperfusion injury. *Thromb Haemost.* 1997;78:310-314.
7. LAUDANNA C, KIM JY, CONSTANTIN G, BUTCHER E. Rapid leukocyte integrin activation by chemokines. *Immunol Rev.* 2002;186:37-46.
8. SCHOLZ D, ITO W, FLEMING I, DEINDL E, SAUER A, WIESNET M, BUSSE R, SCHAPER J, SCHAPER W. Ultrastructure and molecular histology of rabbit hind limb collateral artery growth (arteriogenesis). *Virchows Arch.* 2000;436:257-70.
9. SCHOLZ D, ZIEGELHOEFFER T, HELISCH A, WAGNER S, FRIEDRICH C, PODZUWEIT T, SCHAPER W. Contribution of arteriogenesis and angiogenesis to postocclusive hind limb perfusion in mice. *J Mol Cell Cardiol.* 2002;34:775-87.
10. HEIL M, CLAUSS M, SUZUKI K, BUSCHMANN IR, WILLUWEIT A, FISCHER S, SCHAPER W. Vascular endothelial growth factor (VEGF) stimulates monocyte migration through endothelial monolayers via increased integrin expression. *Eur J Cell Biol.* 2000;79:850-7.
11. BUSCHMANN I, HOEFER I, HEIL M, SCHAPER W. Anti-adhesion monoclonal antibodies against ICAM inhibit arteriogenesis. *J Am Coll Cardiol.* 1999;33:318A.
12. CARLOS TM, HARLAN JM. Leukocyte-endothelial adhesion molecules. *Blood.* 1994;84:2068-101.
13. HEIL M, ZIEGELHOEFFER T, PIPP F, KOSTIN S, MARTIN S, CLAUSS M, SCHAPER W. Blood monocyte concentration is critical for enhancement of collateral artery growth. *Am J Physiol Heart Circ Physiol.* 2002;283:H2411-9.
14. PIPP F, HEIL M, ISSBRUCKER K, ZIEGELHOEFFER T, MARTIN S, VAN DEN HEUVEL J, WEICH H, FERNÁNDEZ B, GOLOMB G, CARMELIET P, SCHAPER W, CLAUSS M. VEGFR-1-selective VEGF homologue PlGF is arteriogenic: evidence for a monocyte-mediated mechanism. *Circ Res.* 2003;92:378-85.
15. HOEFER IE, VAN ROYEN N, RECTENWALD JE, BRAY EJ, ABOUHAMZE Z, MOLDAWER LL, VOSKUIL M, PIEK JJ, BUSCHMANN IR, OZAKI CK. Direct evidence for tumor necrosis factor-alpha signaling in arteriogenesis. *Circulation.* 2002;105:1639-41.
16. LUSTER AD. Chemokines—chemotactic cytokines that mediate inflammation. *N Engl J Med.* 1998;338:436-45.
17. BAGGIOLINI M, MOSER B, CLARK-LEWIS I. Interleukin-8 and related chemotactic cytokines. *The Giles Filley Lecture. Chest.* 1994;105:95S-98S.
18. BAGGIOLINI M, DEWALD B, MOSER B. Human chemokines: an update. *Annu Rev Immunol.*

1997;15:675-705.

19. GONG JH, CLARK-LEWIS I. Antagonists of monocyte chemoattractant protein 1 identified by modification of functionally critical NH2-terminal residues. *J Exp Med.* 1995;181:631-40.

20. SICA A, SACCANI A, BORSATTI A, POWER CA, WELLS TN, LUINI W, POLENTARUTTI N, SOZZANI S, MANTOVANI A. Bacterial lipopolysaccharide rapidly inhibits expression of C-C chemokine receptors in human monocytes. *J Exp Med.* 1997;185:969-74.

21. LOETSCHER P, SEITZ M, BAGGIOLINI M, MOSER B. Interleukin-2 regulates CC chemokine receptor expression and chemotactic responsiveness in T-lymphocytes. *J Exp Med.* 1996;184:569-77.

22. PREMACK BA, SCHALL TJ. Chemokine receptors: gateways to inflammation and infection. *Nat Med.* 1996;2:1174-8.

23. MURPHY PM. The molecular biology of leukocyte chemoattractant receptors. *Annu Rev Immunol.* 1994;12:593-633.

24. BOKOCH GM. Chemoattractant signaling and leukocyte activation. *Blood.* 1995;86:1649-60.

25. LODI PJ, GARRETT DS, KUSZEWSKI J, TSANG ML, WEATHERBEE JA, LEONARD WJ, GRONENBORN AM, CLORE GM. High-resolution solution structure of the beta chemokine hMIP-1 beta by multidimensional NMR. *Science.* 1994;263:1762-7.

26. ROT A. Endothelial cell binding of NAP-1/IL-8: role in neutrophil emigration. *Immunol Today.* 1992;13:291-4.

27. LUSTER AD, GREENBERG SM, LEDER P. The IP-10 chemokine binds to a specific cell surface heparan sulfate site shared with platelet factor 4 and inhibits endothelial cell proliferation. *J Exp Med.* 1995;182:219-31.

28. TANAKA Y, ADAMS DH, HUBSCHER S, HIRANO H, SIEBENLIST U, SHAW S. T-cell adhesion induced by proteoglycan-immobilized cytokine MIP-1 beta. *Nature.* 1993;361:79-82.

29. ITO WD, ARRAS M, WINKLER B, SCHOLZ D, SCHAPER J, SCHAPER W. Monocyte chemotactic protein-1 increases collateral and peripheral conductance after femoral artery occlusion. *Circ Res.* 1997;80:829-37.

30. VOSKUIL M, VAN ROYEN N, HOEFER IE, SEIDLER R, GUTH BD, BODE C, SCHAPER W, PIEK JJ, BUSCHMANN IR. Modulation of collateral artery growth in a porcine hind limb ligation model using MCP-1. *Am J Physiol Heart Circ Physiol.* 2003;284:H1422-8.

31. VOSKUIL M. Abnormal monocyte recruitment and collateral artery formation in monocyte chemoattractant protein-1 deficient mice. In: *Experimental and clinical studies on collateral and epicardial flow in obstructive arterial disease (Thesis).* Amsterdam: Universiteit van Amsterdam; 2003:25-35.

32. KUZIEL WA, MORGAN SJ, DAWSON TC, GRIFFIN S, SMITHIES O, LEY K, MAEDA N. Severe reduction in leukocyte adhesion and monocyte extravasation in mice deficient in CC chemokine receptor 2. *Proc Natl Acad Sci U S A.* 1997;94:12053-8.

33. HEIL M, ZIEGELHOEFFER T, WAGNER S, FERNÁNDEZ B, HELISCH A, MARTIN S, TRIBULOVA S, KUZIEL WA, BACHMANN G, SCHAPER W. Collateral artery growth (arteriogenesis) after experimental arterial occlusion is impaired in mice lacking CC-chemokine-receptor-2. *Circ Res.* 2004;94:671-677.

34. HEIL M, ZIEGELHOEFFER T, PIPP F, MARTIN S, WAGNER S, HELISCH A, SCHAPER W. Functional proof for the pivotal role of blood monocytes in arteriogenesis (Collateral Artery Growth). *FASEB J.* 2003;17:341.23.

35. RISAU W. Mechanisms of angiogenesis. *Nature.* 1997;386:671-4.

36. ASAHARA T, TAKAHASHI T, MASUDA H, KALKA C, CHEN D, IWAGURO H, INAI Y, SILVER M, ISNER JM. VEGF contributes to postnatal neovascularization by mobilizing bone marrow-derived endothelial progenitor cells. *EMBO J.* 1999;18:3964-72.

37. NEMERSON Y. Tissue factor and hemostasis. *Blood.* 1988;71:1-8.

38. SHEN H, CLAUSS M, RYAN J, SCHMIDT AM, TIJBURG P, BORDEN L, CONNOLLY D, STERN D, KAO J. Characterization of vascular permeability factor/vascular endothelial growth factor receptors on mononuclear phagocytes. *Blood.* 1993;81:2767-73.

39. BARLEON B, SOZZANI S, ZHOU D, WEICH HA, MANTOVANI A, MARME D. Migration of human monocytes in response to vascular endothelial growth factor (VEGF) is mediated via the VEGF receptor flt-1. *Blood.* 1996;87:3336-43.

40. WISEMAN DM, POLVERINI PJ, KAMP DW, LEIBOVICH SJ. Transforming growth factor-beta (TGF beta) is chemotactic for human monocytes and induces their expression of angiogenic activity. *Biochem Biophys Res Commun.* 1988;157:793-800.

41. CHANTRY D, TURNER M, ABNEY E, FELDMANN M. Modulation of cytokine production by transforming growth factor-beta. *J Immunol.* 1989;142:4295-300.

42. VAN ROYEN N, PIEK JJ, BUSCHMANN I, HOEFER I, VOSKUIL M, SCHAPER W. Stimulation of arteriogenesis; a new concept for the treatment of arterial occlusive disease. *Cardiovasc Res.* 2001;49:543-53.

43. COLLEN D, LIJNEN HR. Basic and clinical aspects of fibrinolysis and thrombolysis. *Blood.* 1991;78:3114-24.

44. DEINDL E, ZIEGELHOFFER T, KANSE SM, FERNÁNDEZ B, NEUBAUER E, CARMELIET P, PREISSNER KT, SCHAPER W. Receptor-independent role of the urokinase-type plasminogen activator during arteriogenesis. *FASEB J.* 2003;17:1174-6.

45. LOSKUTOFF DJ, VAN AKEN BE, SEIFFERT D. Abnormalities in the fibrinolytic system of the vascular wall associated with atherosclerosis. *Ann N Y Acad Sci.* 1995;748:177-83; discussion 183-4.

46. KIRCHHEIMER JC, REMOLD HG. Endogenous receptor-bound urokinase mediates tissue invasion of human monocytes. *J Immunol.* 1989;143:2634-9.

47. CARMELIET P, MOONS L, HERBERT JM, CRAWLEY J, LUPU F, LIJNEN R, COLLEN D. Urokinase but not tissue plasminogen activator mediates arterial neointima formation in mice. *Circ Res.* 1997;81:829-39.

48. RAO NK, SHI GP, CHAPMAN HA. Urokinase receptor is a multifunctional protein: influence of receptor occupancy on macrophage gene expression. *J Clin Invest.* 1995;96:465-74.

49. SITRIN RG, SHOLLENBERGER SB, STRIETER RM, GYETKO MR. Endogenously produced urokinase amplifies tumor necrosis factor-alpha secretion by THP-1 mononuclear phagocytes. *J Leukoc Biol.* 1996;59:302-11.

50. SYROVETS T, TIPPLER B, RIEKS M, SIMMET T. Plasmin is a potent and specific chemoattractant for human peripheral monocytes acting via a cyclic guanosine monophosphate-dependent pathway. *Blood.* 1997;89:4574-83.

51. CARMELIET P, MOONS L, DEWERCHIN M, ROSENBERG S, HERBERT JM, LUPU F, COLLEN D. Receptor-independent role of urokinase-type plasminogen activator in pericellular plasmin and matrix metalloproteinase proteolysis during vascular wound healing in mice. *J Cell Biol.* 1998;140:233-45.

52. WYSOCKI SJ, ZHENG MH, FAN Y, LAMAWANSA MD, HOUSE AK, NORMAN PE. Expression of transforming growth factor-beta1 (TGF-beta1) and urokinase-type plasminogen activator (u-PA) genes during arterial repair in the pig. *Cardiovasc Res.* 1996;31:28-36.

53. BUSCHMANN IR, HOEFER IE, VAN ROYEN N, KATZER E, BRAUN-DULLEAUS R, HEIL M, KOSTIN S, BODE C, SCHAPER W. GM-CSF: a strong arteriogenic factor acting by amplification of monocyte function. *Atherosclerosis.* 2001;159:343-56.
54. SEILER C, POHL T, WUSTMANN K, HUTTER D, NICOLET PA, WINDECKER S, EBERLI FR, MEIER B. Promotion of collateral growth by granulocyte-macrophage colony-stimulating factor in patients with coronary artery disease: a randomized, double-blind, placebo-controlled study. *Circulation.* 2001;104:2012-7.
55. HELISCH A, WAGNER S, WILLUWEIT A, ITO W, CLAUSS M, SCHAPER W. Tumor Necrosis Factor signaling not important for arteriogenesis but for angiogenesis. *J Am Coll Cardiol.* 2003;41:308A.

Chapter 8

Bone Marrow-Derived Cells

Tibor Ziegelhoeffer, Sawa Kostin, Borja Fernández,
Matthias Heil and Wolfgang Schaper

During embryonic life the vascular system arises from mesodermal precursor cells called angioblasts that invade the different embryonic organ primordia and assemble in situ to form the primary capillary plexus. This process has been termed *vasculogenesis*. It is followed by sprouting and non-sprouting *angiogenesis* of the primary capillary plexus, and further differentiation, maturation and remodeling processes which finally result in the mature vascular system[1,2].

Recently, the concept that *vasculogenesis* is restricted to embryonic life has been questioned. Bone marrow-derived stem or endothelial progenitor cells have been proposed to circulate in adult organisms, to be recruited to, and to incorporate into sites of physiological and pathological neovascularization[3,4]. Furthermore, transplantation of these cells appears to augment recovery of perfusion and function in models of myocardial and peripheral ischemia[5-9]. To differentiate circulating endothelial progenitor or bone marrow-derived cells from native endothelial cells *in vivo* fluorescent carbocyanine DiI-labeled cells, as well as sex-mismatched and reporter gene-labeled cells isolated from bone marrow or from circulating blood have been transplanted into recipient animals[4,7,10,11]. The reported relative contribution of transplanted cells to the endothelium of growing vessels varies widely, from almost no incorporation to more than 50%[7,12]. Moreover, the results of some recent studies using laser scanning confocal microscopy have suggested that the transdifferentiation of bone marrow-derived cells into organ specific cells may occur less frequently than anticipated. Wagers et al.[13] employed a GFP-marked hematopoietic stem cell transplantation model as well as parabiosis model to investigate a tissue chimerism of recipient and parabiotic animals. After cell transplantation they were able to detect only 1 GFP-positive non-hematopoietic cell in the brain and 7 positive cells in the liver of recipient animals, whereas no positive cells were found in the kidney, gut, skeletal muscle, cardiac muscle and lung. In their parabiosis model no partner-derived GFP-positive non-hematopoietic cells were detected in recipient animals. Similarly, Hillebrands et al.[14] reported only a marginal endothelial contribution (1-3%) of bone marrow-derived cells in a model of transplant arteriosclerosis in rats (LEW$_{BM}$ → BN and BN$_{BM}$ → LEW strain combinations). Castro et al.[15] reported the failure of LacZ-positive bone marrow cells from Rosa26 mice to transdifferentiate into neural cells in recipient animals. On the other hand, there are numerous studies describing a positive effects of endothelial progenitor or bone marrow-derived cells on blood flow recovery in various models of ischemic tissue revascularization[4,7,10,11]. The described positive effects on blood flow recovery were interpreted to be related to the incorporation of these cells into growing capillaries. However, there is much evidence to suggest, that after occlusion of a major artery the growth of true "bypass" arteries, *arteriogenesis*, is the most effective and therefore necessary process to restore bulk blood flow to the affected limb[16-18]. Therefore, the crucial question in explaining the positive effect of circulating bone marrow-derived cells on blood flow recovery is whether these cells participate in collateral artery growth. In a recent study, we addressed this question in our mouse model of hind limb ischemia, which allows us to spatially separate angiogenesis (occurring in the distal ischemic bed) and arteriogenesis (occurring in the upper leg). Additionally, we implanted BFS-1 fibrosarcoma cells[19] subcutaneously on the back of the mice and 3 weeks later we studied whether bone marrow-derived cells had incorporated into the vessel walls during the end-stage tumor growth. In order to track and distinguish the cells of bone marrow origin from the tissue-resident ones, we transplanted lethally irradiated C57BL/6J mice with bone marrow from their eGFP-transgenic littermates. Using flow cytometry and histological analysis we confirmed that all of the cells of transgenic animals, with exception of hair cells and erythrocytes, constitutively express GFP (cac/eGFP) as previously reported[20]. Six weeks after transplantation

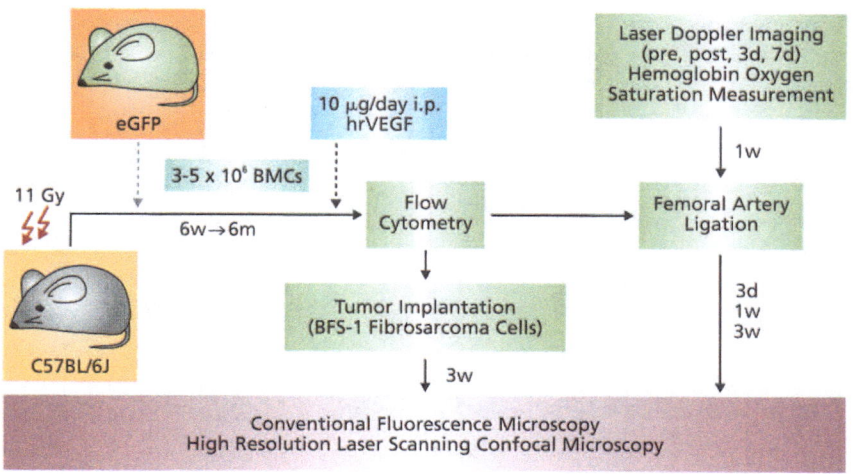

Study design   *Fig. 1*

79-86%, and up to 93% after six months, of nucleated cells in peripheral blood expressed GFP, thus confirming the successful bone marrow engraftment and hematopoietic reconstitution. Moreover, data obtained by colony-forming assays, endothelial progenitor cell assays and flow cytometry analysis indicate that all transplanted animals had an appropriate pool of stem/progenitor cells at the time of surgery.

We performed a rigorous analysis of proximal hind limb tissue with growing collateral arteries, gastrocnemius muscles with ischemic and normoxic tissue, end-stage tumors, spleen, liver, heart, lung, kidney and intestine using conventional fluorescence and high power laser scanning microscopy in order to verify whether bone marrow-derived cells transform into vascular cells under different conditions (Fig. 1). Endothelial and smooth muscle cell markers were used to confirm incorporation of these cells into growing or quiescent vasculature. We never found co-localization of GFP-signals with endothelial or smooth muscle cell markers. GFP-positive cells were frequently found in the perivascular space and interstitium (Fig. 2). These cells were identified as leukocytes, mono-cytes/macrophages, T-lymphocytes, fibroblasts and pericytes by shape and distribution in the tissue as well as by co-localization with specific markers (CD45, F4/80, CD3, vimentin, Figs. 3 and 4). In some cases conventional fluorescence microscopy and confocal microscopy using thick sections of vascular structures showed co-localization of endothelial

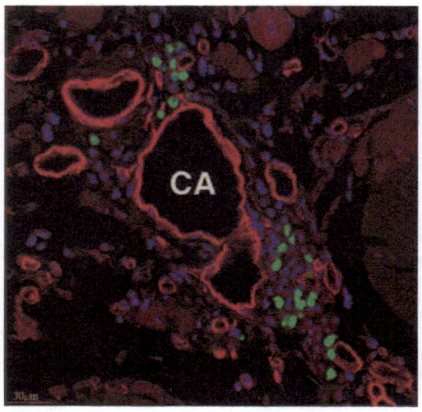 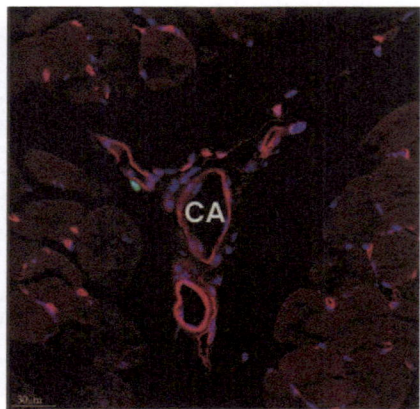

Fig. 2a   *Fig. 2b*

Accumulation of bone marrow-derived cells around growing collateral arteries 3 weeks after femoral artery occlusion. Red = BS-1 lectin; blue = nuclei. a: Numerous GFP-positive cells are clustered around growing collateral artery (CA), however, not co-localizing with endothelial cell marker BS-1 lectin. b: Only a few GFP-positive cells are found around quiescent collateral arteries (CA).

marker BS-1 lectin or smooth muscle cell markers with GFP-signals. However, using high resolution confocal microscopy, we revealed that overlapping of signals was due to the convolution of perivascular cells around vessels and therefore clearly identify these signals as belonging to separate cells.

Thus, in our experimental models of hind limb ischemia and tumor growth, we have not found any evidence of postnatal *vasculogenesis* or an integration of bone-marrow-derived or circulating cells into the endothelium or *tunica media* of vessels. In order to test whether the irradiation or bone marrow transplantation itself had influenced the incorporation of bone marrow-derived cells into the vessel wall and thereby decelerate blood flow recovery we performed relative blood flow and hemoglobin oxygen saturation measurements in the mouse feet before, -immediately

3) *Co-localization of GFP with CD45 (red), F4/80 (red) and CD3 (red) around growing collateral arteries 1 week after femoral artery occlusion. a and b: Clusters of GFP-positive cells around a collateral artery (CA) were mostly composed of CD45-positive cells demonstrating the leukocytic identity of bone marrow cells accumulating specifically around growing collateral arteries. Note that some (approximately 10%) of the CD45-positive cells are GFP-negative (arrows) supporting the results obtained by flow cytometry. c and d: Immunofluorescent signals for F4/80. Most perivascular GFP-positive cells are monocyte/macrophages. e and f: Some of the GFP-positive perivascular cells co-localize with the T lymphocyte-specific CD3 marker.*

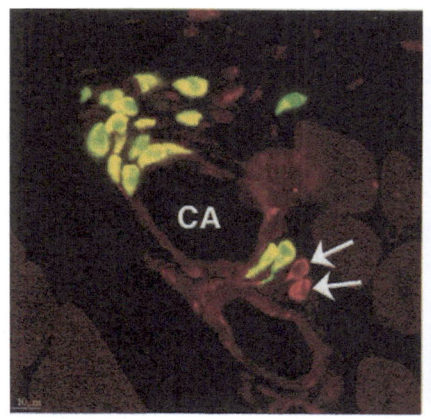

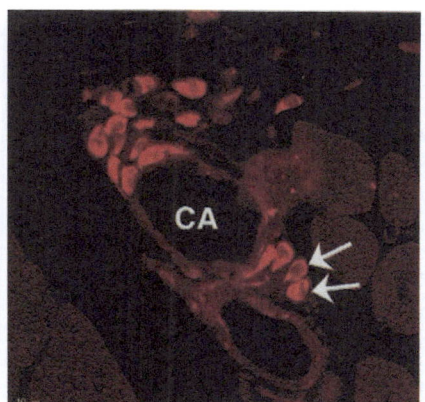

Fig. 3a

Fig. 3b

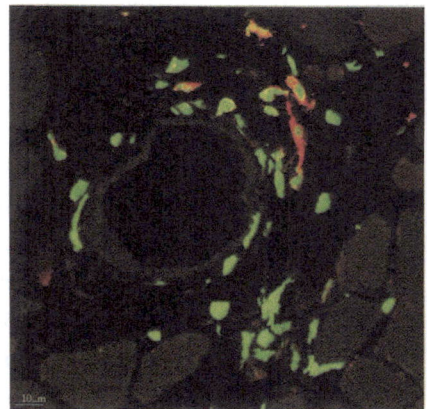

Fig. 3c

Fig. 3d

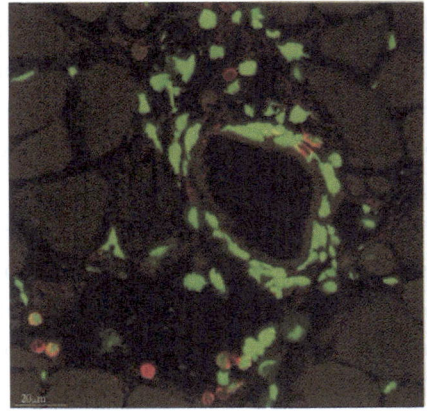

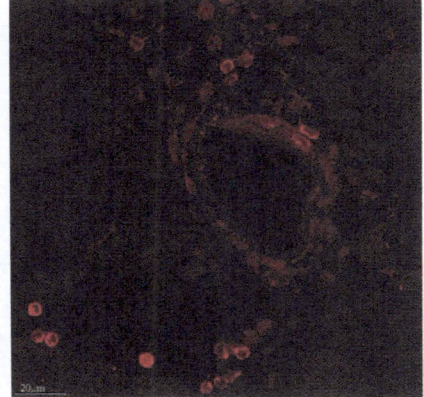

Fig. 3e

Fig. 3f

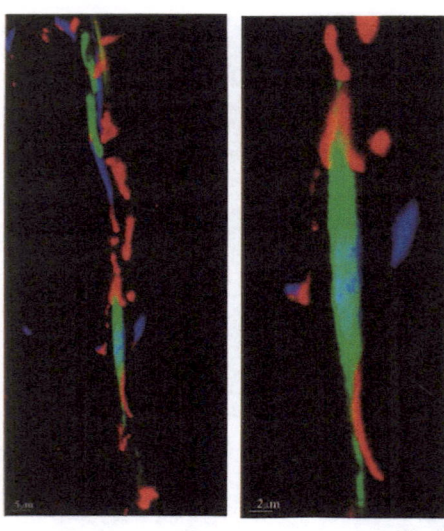

Fig. 4a   *Fig. 4b*

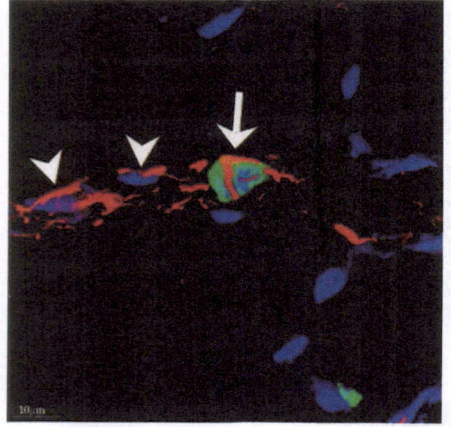

Fig. 4c

Co-localization of GFP with vimentin (red) in the gastrocnemius muscle. Blue = nuclei. a and b: Typical elongated fibroblasts in the fascia of the gastrocnemius muscle show red vimentin filaments together with GFP signals. c: Bone marrow-derived interstitial fibroblast (arrow) shows vimentin filaments (red) surrounding GFP signals into the cytoplasm. Adjacent vimentin-positive fibroblasts are GFP-negative (arrowheads).

after, on day 3 and on day 7 after the femoral artery ligation. We did not observe any differences between transplanted and non-transplanted animals at any timepoint (Fig. 5). Thus, we provide functional data that the incorporation of bone marrow-derived cells into the vessel wall of growing collateral arteries is not required for successful blood flow recovery after femoral artery ligation. Moreover, intraperitoneal administration of rhVEGF, which has been reported to promote mobilization of bone marrow-derived stem cells [21,22], did not lead to any demonstrable incorporation of GFP cells in the vasculature of these mice. These data are conflicting with other studies evaluating the role of endothelial progenitor or bone marrow-derived cells in blood flow recovery using similar or related models of ischemic tissue revascularization [4,7,10,11] reporting various numbers of these cells incorporated into the growing capillaries. However, findings of such incorporation were based on the use of conventional light or fluorescence microscopy with substantial variations between magnifications used.

Our results suggest that conventional microscopy techniques may not be sufficient to rule out "pseudo double-labeling", i.e., immunostaining from two cells in close proximity to each other appearing to originate from a single cell. Moreover, some studies, in which vascular incorporation of progenitor cells was found, used isolated cells of human origin without immunosuppression, which makes the interpretation of these results difficult[4,7]. The use of so called "endothelial progenitor cells" in these studies is also controversial. Endothelial progenitor cells have been isolated from peripheral blood and suggested to enhance *angiogenesis* after infusion into host animals [7,23,24]. The isolation procedure consisted of density gradient centrifugation of peripheral blood and subsequent culturing of the isolated

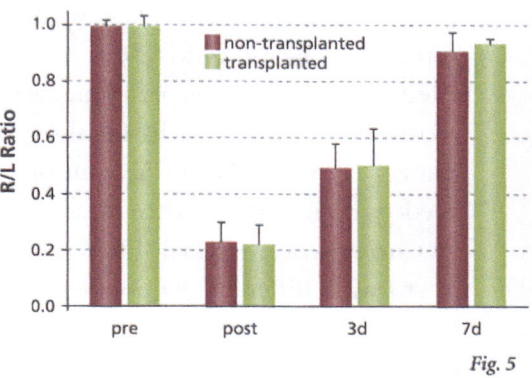

Fig. 5

Serial measurements of Laser-Doppler perfusion in the hind limbs of transplanted and non-transplanted, non-irradiated mice until day 7 after surgery showing that neither irradiation nor subsequent bone marrow transplantation did affect blood flow recovery at the time of histological evaluation.

peripheral blood mononuclear cells on fibronectin. These cells were originally characterized by uptake of acetylated LDL and binding of Ulex-lectin[7,24] and therefore considered to be consistent with endothelial cell lineage. However, such a characterization turns out to be insufficient due to a wide heterogeneity of the isolated cell population and thereby confuses the interpretation of cellular contribution to vessel growth. Although the original cell population referred to as EPCs shared certain characteristics with endothelial cells, such as uptake of acetylated LDL, binding of Ulex-lectin, expression of PECAM (CD31), a marker found on endothelial cells and monocytes, only a minority of them expressed endothelium-specific markers like VE-cadherin or E-selectin (CD62E)[25]. Additionally, only a very small portion of them expressed endothelial and hematopoietic stem or progenitor cells marker CD34 and even less markers for hematopoietic stem or progenitor cells like AC 133 and c-kit (CD117)[25-27].

Moreover, a vast majority of them expressed monocyte/macrophage markers, such as CD11c, CD11b (Mac-1) or CD14, and nearly all of them, more than 99%, expressed the panleukocyte marker CD45 suggesting that they were derived from monocytes/macrophages[25]. Finally, as recently reported, these "EPCs" failed to proliferate in cell culture but were able to secrete some angiogenic factors like vascular endothelial growth factor (VEGF), hepatocyte growth factor (HGF), granulocyte colony-stimulating factor (G-CSF) and granulocyte-macrophage colony-stimulating factor (GM-CSF). This implies that their proangiogenic effect may be due to the paracrine secretion of growth factors rather than providing endothelial cells for the growing capillaries[25]. Thus, a better characterization and purification of single homogenous populations is needed in order to compare these studies and draw a final conclusion.

Currently, the original "EPC" population is suggested to be composed of at least 3 different cell population: the "true" EPCs originating from bone marrow, circulating EPCs originating from bone marrow or from EPCs embedded in different organs and the systemic vasculature, and myelomonocytic cells (for review see[28]). Nevertheless, in the light of our current findings and the relatively high internal proliferative activity in the growing preexisting collateral arteries it is not very likely that bone marrow-derived "true" EPCs would contribute substantially to the enlargement of the endothelial layer of these vessels as a natural response to injury. However, this does not necessarily imply that exogenous application of stem- or progenitor cells will not have a boosting and therapeutically useful effect. First, it is possible that the isolation and subsequent culture of progenitor cells under special conditions change the properties incorporating capacity of these cells. Second, the amount of naturally present bone marrow-derived progenitors in the peripheral blood is very low representing much less than 1% of the cells in the circulation. Although the relatively moderate mobilization of bone marrow-derived cells by application of VEGF did not lead to any incorporation of these cells into the vessel wall of growing arteries in our model, the amount of exogenous cells administered i.v., i.a., or i.p. will exceed this number in magnitude and therefore may lead to their incorporation. Third, the results of some recent studies have suggested differences in bone marrow and stem cell recruitment due to different organ lesions[29].

Therefore, it is possible that these cells will behave differently depending on the conditions and organ investigated. Nevertheless, we did

6) Co-localization of GFP with FGF-2 (a, b), VEGF (c, d), and MCP-1 (e, f) in growing collateral arteries 7 days after femoral artery occlusion. b, d and f show growth factor- or cytokine-specific staining. a, c and e show co-localization with GFP. FGF-2 and VEGF were both mainly found in GFP-positive perivascular leukocytes. MCP-1 was specifically localized in the endothelium and perivascular leukocytes of growing collateral arteries.

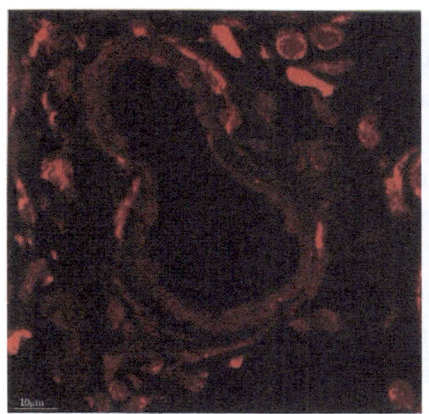
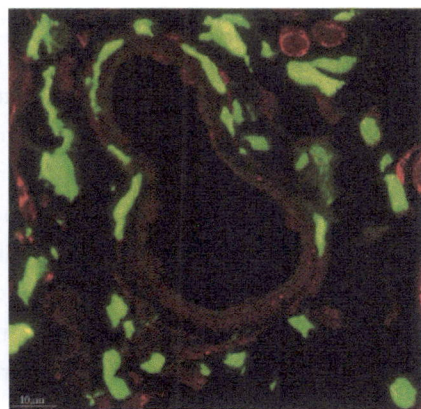

Fig. 6a   *Fig. 6b*

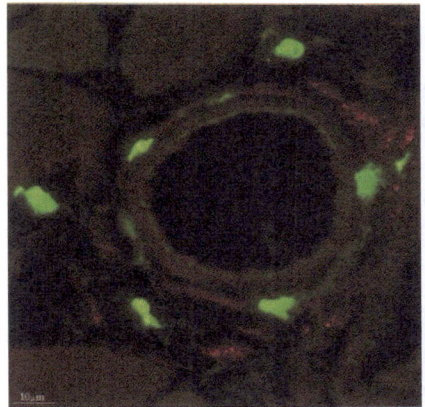

Fig. 6c   *Fig. 6d*

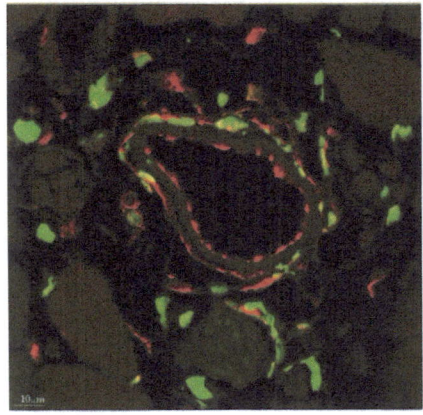
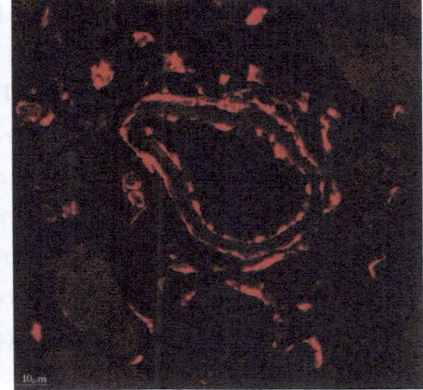

Fig. 6e   *Fig. 6f*

observe an accumulation of GFP-positive cells in regions of collateral artery growth in the proximal thigh and also in the ischemic distal hind limb. Staining for the monocyte/macrophage marker F4/80, T-lymphocytes marker CD3 and the panleukocytic marker CD45, together with morphologic criteria, suggested that these cells were mainly monocytes/macrophages and other leukocytes. They may act as supporting cells providing a variety of growth factors and chemokines. Indeed, monocytes/macrophages have previously been shown to play a critical role in arteriogenesis [18,30-33] by releasing activating cytokines, growth factors and metalloproteinases and thereby creating an inflammatory environment necessary for the enhancement of collateral artery growth [16,17,34-36] (see also chapter 8). Our current data support this hypothesis, since bone marrow-derived GFP-positive cells clustered around growing collateral vessels stained positive for fibroblast growth factor-2 (FGF-2), vascular endothelial growth factor (VEGF) and monocyte chemoattractant protein-1 (MCP-1)(Fig. 6). In the light of these findings it is likely that the reported restoration of limb function in patients suffering from peripheral arterial disease and receiving infusion of autologous whole bone marrow mononuclear cells into the ischemic gastrocnemius muscle [37] is at least partially due to the introduction of myeolomonocytic cells and not to EPCs. More studies and a consensus on markers characterizing the distinct stem and progenitor cell populations and rigorous histological analysis is needed in order to answer these questions. Much progress has been achieved in functional and phenotypic characterization of stem and progenitor cells (for review see [28]), but the analysis of the incorporated cells may also be complicated by cell fusion between donor and recipient cells as recently described [38,39].

One must also consider the possible adverse effects of cell therapy. In particular, tumor formation [40], atheromas [41,42], and arrhythmias [43] represent processes, where such negative effects could be manifested. Therefore, understanding of the mechanisms for recruitment and selective tissue homing of progenitor and bone marrow-derived stem cells is necessary for efficiency and safety of these therapies.

In conclusion, although incorporation of progenitor and bone marrow-derived stem cells into the vessel wall does not seem to contribute naturally to the process of collateral artery growth, these cells may rather support the arteriogenic process by paracrine mechanisms. Nevertheless, the identification of cellular mediators and tissue specific chemokines responsible for bone marrow-derived cell mobilization and selective tissue homing, together with *in vitro* engineering of precursor cells, may open a new possibilities for functional incorporation of these cells into growing arteries and thus raise new horizons in revascularization therapies.

References

1. CARMELIET P. Mechanisms of angiogenesis and arteriogenesis. *Nat Med.* 2000;6:389-395.
2. RISAU W. Mechanisms of angiogenesis. *Nature.* 1997;386:671-674.
3. SHI Q, RAFII S, WU MH, WIJELATH ES, YU C, ISHIDA A, FUJITA Y, KOTHARI S, MOHLE R, SAUVAGE LR, MOORE MA, STORB RF, HAMMOND WP. Evidence for circulating bone marrow-derived endothelial cells. *Blood.* 1998;92:362-367.
4. ASAHARA T, MUROHARA T, SULLIVAN A, SILVER M, VAN DER ZEE R, LI T, WITZENBICHLER B, SCHATTEMAN G, ISNER JM. Isolation of putative progenitor endothelial cells for angiogenesis. *Science.* 1997;275:964-967.
5. FUCHS S, BAFFOUR R, ZHOU YF, SHOU M, PIERRE A, TIO FO, WEISSMAN NJ, LEON MB, EPSTEIN SE, KORNOWSKI R. Transendocardial delivery of autologous bone marrow enhances collateral perfusion and regional function in pigs with chronic experimental myocardial ischemia. *J Am Coll Cardiol.* 2001;37:1726-1732.
6. ORLIC D, KAJSTURA J, CHIMENTI S, BODINE DM, LERI A, ANVERSA P. Transplanted adult bone marrow cells repair myocardial infarcts in mice. *Ann N Y Acad Sci.* 2001;938:221-229.
7. KALKA C, MASUDA H, TAAKAHASHI T, KALKA-MOLL WM, SILVER M, KEARNEY M, LI T, ISNER JM, ASAHARA T. Transplantation of ex vivo expanded endothelial progenitor cells for therapeutic neovascularization. *Proc Natl Acad Sci USA.* 2000;97:3422-3427.
8. KOCHER AA, SCHUSTER MD, SZABOLCS MJ, TAKUMA S, BURKHOFF D, WANG J, HOMMA S, EDWARDS NM, ITESCU S. Neovascularization of ischemic myocardium by human bone-marrow-derived angioblasts prevents cardiomyocyte apoptosis, reduces remodeling and improves cardiac function. *Nat Med.* 2001;7:430-436.
9. SHINTANI S, MUROHARA T, IKEDA H, UENO T, SASAKI K, DUAN J, IMAIZUMI T. Augmentation of postnatal neovascularization with autologous bone marrow transplantation. *Circulation.* 2001;103:897-903.
10. ASAHARA T, MASUDA H, TAKAHASHI T, KALKA C, PASTORE C, SILVER M, KEARNE M, MAGNER M, ISNER JM. Bone marrow origin of endothelial progenitor cells responsible for postnatal vasculogenesis in physiological and pathological neovascularization. *Circ Res.* 1999;85:221-228.
11. TAKAHASHI T, KALKA C, MASUDA H, CHEN D, SILVER M, KEARNEY M, MAGNER M, ISNER JM, ASAHARA T. Ischemia- and cytokine-induced mobilization of bone marrow-derived endothelial progenitor cells for neovascularization. *Nat Med.* 1999;5:434-438.
12. BECK H, VOSWINCKEL R, WAGNER S, ZIEGELHOEFFER T, HEIL M, HELISCH A, SCHAPER W, ACKER T, HATZOPOULOS A, PLATE K. Participation of bone marrow-derived cells in long term repair processes following experimental stroke. *J Cereb Blood Flow Metab.* 2003;23:709-717.

13. WAGERS AJ, SHERWOOD RI, CHRISTENSEN JL, WEISSMAN IL. Little evidence for developmental plasticity of adult hematopoietic stem cells. *Science.* 2002;297:2256-2259.

14. HILLEBRANDS JL, KLATTER FA, VAN DIJK WD, ROZING J. Bone marrow does not contribute substantially to endothelial-cell replacement in transplant arteriosclerosis. *Nat Med.* 2002;8:194-195.

15. CASTRO RF, JACKSON KA, GOODELL MA, ROBERTSON CS, LIU H, SHINE HD. Failure of bone marrow cells to transdifferentiate into neural cells *in vivo. Science.* 2002;297:1299.

16. SCHOLZ D, ZIEGELHOEFFER T, HELISCH A, WAGNER S, FRIEDRICH C, PODZUWEIT T, SCHAPER W. Contribution of arteriogenesis and angiogenesis to postocclusive hind limb perfusion in mice. *J Mol Cell Cardiol.* 2002;34:775-787.

17. HELISCH A, SCHAPER W. Arteriogenesis - the development and growth of collateral arteries. *Microcirculation.* 2003;10:83-97.

18. HEIL M, ZIEGELHOEFFER T, PIPP F, KOSTIN S, MARTIN S, CLAUSS M, SCHAPER W. Blood monocyte concentration is critical for enhancement of collateral artery growth. *Am J Physiol Heart Circ Physiol.* 2002;283:H2411-H2419.

19. HAFNER M, OROSZ P, KRUGER A, MANNEL DN. TNF promotes metastasis by impairing natural killer cell activity. *Int J Cancer.* 1996;66:388-392.

20. OKABE M, IKAWA M, KOMINAMI K, NAKANISHI T, NISHIMUNE Y. "Green mice" as a source of ubiquitous green cells. *FEBS Lett.* 1997;407:313-319.

21. ASAHARA T, TAKAHASHI T, MASUDA H, KALKA C, CHEN D, IWAGURO H, INAI Y, SILVER M, ISNER JM. VEGF contributes to postnatal neovascularization by mobilizing bone marrow-derived endothelial progenitor cells. *EMBO J.* 1999;18:3964-3972.

22. GABRILOVICH D, ISHIDA T, OYAMA T, RAN S, KRATSOV V, NADAF S, CAROBE DP. Vascular endothelial growth factor inhibits the development of dendritic cells and dramatically affects the differentiation of multiple hematopoietic lineages *in vivo. Blood.* 1998;92:4150-4166.

23. KAWAMOTO A, GWON HC, IWAGURO H, YAMAGUCHI JI, UCHIDA S, MASUDA H, SILVER M, MA H, KEARNEY M, ISNER JM, ASAHARA T. Therapeutic potential of ex vivo expanded endothelial progenitor cells for myocardial ischemia. *Circulation.* 2001;103:634-637.

24. VASA M, FICHTLSCHERER S, AICHER A, ADLER K, URBICH C, MARTIN H, ZEIHER AM, DIMMELER S. Number and migratory activity of circulating endothelial progenitor cells inversely correlate with risk factors for coronary artery disease. *Circ Res.* 2001;89:E1-E7.

25. REHMAN J, LI J, ORSCHELL CM, MARCH KL. Peripheral blood "endothelial progenitor cells" are derived from monocyte/macrophages and secrete angiogenic growth factors. *Circulation.* 2003;107:1164-1169.

26. RAFII S. Circulating endothelial precursors: mystery, reality, and promise. *J Clin Invest.* 2000;105:17-19.

27. PEICHEV M, NAIYER AJ, PEREIRA D, ZHU Z, LANE WJ, WILLIAMS M, OZ MC, HICKLIN DJ, WITTE L, MOORE MA, RAFII S. Expression of VEGFR-2 and AC133 by circulating human CD34(+) cells identifies a population of functional endothelial precursors. *Blood.* 2000;95:952-958.

28. RAFII S, LYDEN D. Therapeutic stem and progenitor cell transplantation for organ revascularization and regeneration. *Nat Med.* 2003;9:702-712.

29. FORBES S, VIG P, POULSOM R, THOMAS H, ALISON M. Hepatic stem cells. *J Pathol.* 2002;197:510-518.

30. ARRAS M, ITO WD, SCHOLZ D, WINKLER B, SCHAPER J, SCHAPER W. Monocyte activation in angiogenesis and collateral growth in the rabbit hind limb. *J Clin Invest.* 1998;101:41-50.

31. DEINDL E, ZIEGELHOEFFER T, KANSE SM, FERNÁNDEZ B, NEUBAUER E, CARMELIET P, PREISSNER K, SCHAPER W. Receptor-independent role of the urokinase-type plasminogen activator during arteriogenesis. *FASEB J.* 2003; published online 08.04.2003:

32. SCHOLZ D, ITO W, FLEMING I, DEINDL E, SAUER A, WIESNET M, BUSSE R, SCHAPER J, SCHAPER W. Ultrastructure and molecular histology of rabbit hind limb collateral artery growth (arteriogenesis). *Virchows Arch.* 2000;436:257-270.

33. SCHAPER J, KOENIG R, FRANZ D, SCHAPER W. The endothelial surface of growing coronary collateral arteries. Intimal margination and diapedesis of monocytes. A combined SEM and TEM study. *Virchows Arch A (Pathol Anat).* 1976;370:193-205.

34. PIPP F, HEIL M, ISSBRUECKER K, ZIEGELHOEFFER T, MARTIN S, VAN DEN HEUVEL J, WEICH H, FERNÁNDEZ B, CARMELIET P, SCHAPER W, CLAUSS M. The VEGFR-1 selective VEGF-homologue PlGF is arteriogenec: evidence for a monocyte-mediated mechanism. *Circ Res.* 2003;92:378-385.

35. WOLF C, CAI WJ, VOSSCHULTE R, KOLTAI S, MOUSAVIPOUR D, SCHOLZ D, AFSAH-HEDJRI A, SCHAPER W, SCHAPER J. Vascular remodeling and altered protein expression during growth of coronary collateral arteries. *J Mol Cell Cardiol.* 1998;30:2291-2305.

36. MALIK N, GREENFIELD BW, WAHL AF, KIENER PA. Activation of human monocytes through CD40 induces matrix metalloproteinases. *J Immunol.* 1996;156:3952-60.

37. Tateishi-Yuyama E, Matsubara H, Murohara T, Ikeda U, Shintani S, Masaki H, Amano K, KISHIMOTO Y, YOSHIMOTO K, AKASHI H, SHIMADA K, IWASAKA T, IMAIZUMI T. Therapeutic Angiogenesis using Cell Transplantation (TACT) Study Investigators. Therapeutic angiogenesis for patients with limb ischaemia by autologous transplantation of bone-marrow cells: a pilot study and a randomised controlled trial. *Lancet.* 2002;360:427-435.

38. TERADA N, HAMAZAKI T, OKA M, HOK IM, MASTALERZ DM, NAKANO Y, MEYER EM, MOREL L, PETERSEN BE, SCOTT EW. Bone marrow cells adopt the phenotype of other cells by spontaneous cell fusion. *Nature.* 2002;416:542-545.

39. WURMSER AE, GAGE FH. Stem cells: cell fusion causes confusion. *Nature.* 2002;416:485-487.

40. DAVIDOFF AM, NG CY, BROWN P, LEARY MA, SPURBECK WW, ZHOU J, HORWITZ E, VANIN EF, NIENHUIS AW. Bone marrow-derived cells contribute to tumor neovasculature and, when modified to express an angiogenesis inhibitor, can restrict tumor growth in mice. *Clin Cancer Res.* 2001;7:2870-2879.

41. SATA M, SAIURA A, KUNISATO A, TOJO A, OKADA S, TOKUHISA T, HIRAI H, MAKUUCHI M, HIRATA Y, NAGAI R. Hematopoietic stem cells differentiate into vascular cells that participate in the pathogenesis of atherosclerosis. *Nat Med.* 2002;8:403-409.

42. CAPLICE N, BUNCH T, STALBOERGER P, WANG S, SIMPER D, MILLER D, RUSSELL S, LITZOW M, EDWARDS W. Smooth muscle cells in human coronary atherosclerosis can originate from cells administered at marrow transplantation. *Proc Natl Acad Sci USA.* 2003;100:4754-4759.

43. ZHANG Y, HARTZELL C, NARLOW M, DUDLEY SJ. Stem cell-derived cardiomyocytes demonstrate arrhythmic potential. *Circulation.* 2002;106:1294-1299.

Cell-Cell and Cell-Matrix Interactions

Borja Fernández and Kerstin Broich

Normal organs in physiological conditions maintain tissue homeostasis due to continuous interactions between the cells and the extracellular matrix. These interactions are responsible for sensing changes in the environment and transmitting information into the cell, mediating specific cellular responses to different environmental cues. Normally, the response of the tissue is not restricted to individual cells, and the environmental signal, or the mediated effect, is transmitted to adjacent cells through cell-cell interactions. Thus, the molecular apparatus governing cell-cell and cell-matrix communications is normally linked to the molecular pathways that regulate specific cellular functions (i.e. proliferation, migration, cell death, differentiation).

As discussed above, the arteriogenic process is initiated in collateral arteries by a sudden increase in shear stress. Shear stress is sensed on the surface of endothelial cells by mechano-transducers that link the extracellular space with the intracellular skeleton. The endothelial cells then become activated and express cell surface proteins that mediate leukocyte attachment and recruitment. Communication between vascular and perivascular cells initiates a tissue response that affects the whole artery. Interactions of SMCs with the surrounding matrix determine their phenotypical status (synthetic vs. contractile). Synthetic SMCs migrate to form an intimal layer. Cell migration is controlled by refined interactions between proteins of the matrix and the cytoskeleton through specific membrane receptors. Mechano-sensing, cell attachment and recruitment, cell-cell communication, and migration: all rely on cell-to-cell and cell-to-matrix interactions.

Integrins

Cellular effects of the extracellular matrix are primarily mediated by integrins. Virtually all molecules of the matrix are able to communicate with cells by binding to integrins [1,2]. They form a family of heterodimeric cell surface glycoprotein receptors composed of one α- and one β-subunit non-covalently bound [2]. Currently, there are 18 different α- and 8 different β-subunits known in man, which form at least 24 different integrins [3]. Sixteen of these are expressed by blood as well as vascular cells including leukocytes, platelets, endothelial and SMCs [4,5].

Integrin $\alpha_v\beta_3$ is used by endothelial and SMCs to migrate and form the neointima that characterizes proliferative vascular diseases such as restenosis and atherosclerosis [8-12]. In addition, $\alpha_v\beta_3$ integrin is involved in angiogenesis [6] as well as macrophage adhesion and migration [7]. The process of arteriogenesis shares several cellular mechanisms with proliferative vascular diseases, like leukocyte recruitment, proliferation, and formation of a neointimal layer. Therefore, we decided to investigate the possible involvement of this integrin in collateral artery growth by means of quantitative immunohistochemistry using the rabbit model of femoral artery occlusion.

Figure 1a shows the localization of $\alpha_v\beta_3$ integrin protein in quiescent arteries. It is expressed in endothelial and SMCs of the vascular wall at very low concentrations. Three days after femoral artery occlusion, the $\alpha_v\beta_3$ integrin localization pattern and amount has changed substantially. Most growing collateral arteries show an increased protein content in the subendothelium (Fig 1b), or in the subendothelium and the media. However, we did not find any artery with increased expression of integrin in the media only. These results already indicate that: 1) $\alpha_v\beta_3$ integrin is selectively increased in the wall of growing collateral arteries during the first 3 days after femoral artery occlusion. 2) Integrin upregulation first occurs in endothelial cells and later spreads to the SMCs of the media. The specific localization of $\alpha_v\beta_3$ integrin signals in the abluminal surface of the endothelium is an interesting finding. The same observation was obtained *in vitro*, when $\alpha_v\beta_3$ integrin expression or activation was increased in endothelial layers subjected to elevated shear stress [13]. As shear stress is considered the main initiator of arteriogenesis, it is tempting to speculate that the abluminal pattern of $\alpha_v\beta_3$ integrin expression in the endothelium is a specific result of elevated shear stress. However, it is currently not known whether this restriction in $\alpha_v\beta_3$ integrin localization is a general feature of endothelial cell behavior, or a specific consequence of shear stress signaling. The former hypothesis is also reasonable since active integrins in the endothelial luminal surface might be highly thrombogenic.

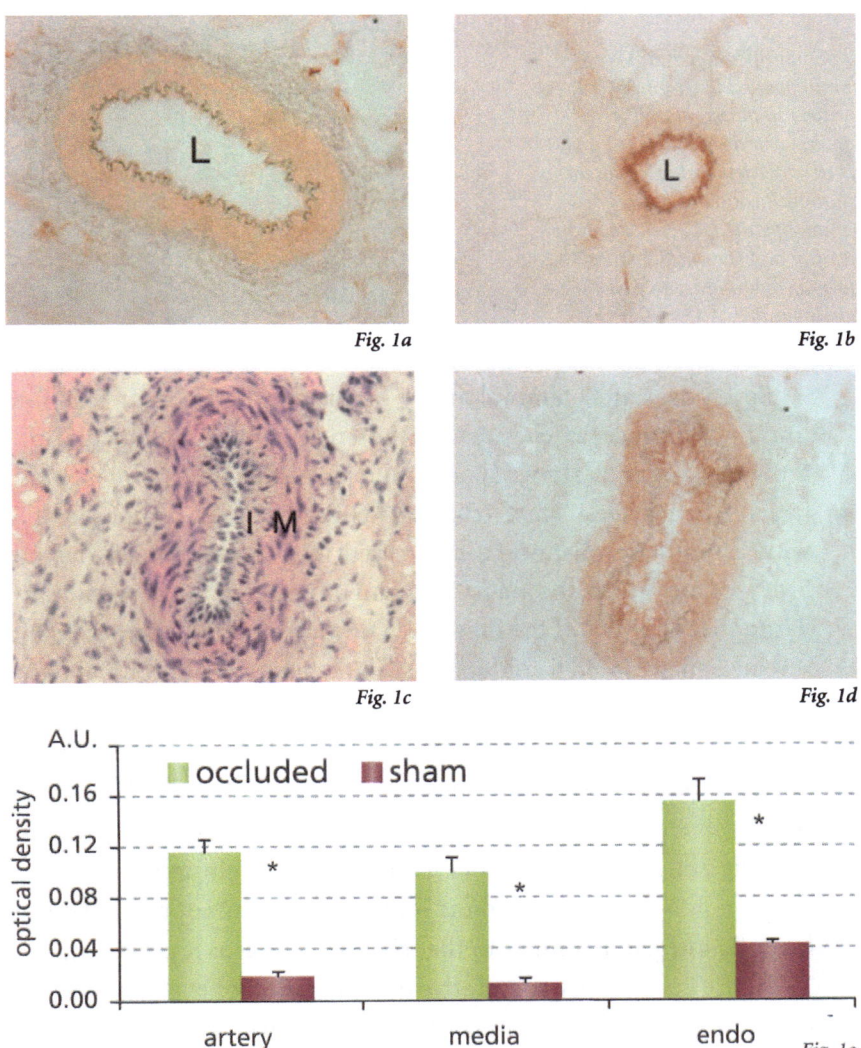

Fig. 1a

Fig. 1b

Fig. 1c

Fig. 1d

Fig. 1e

*Hematoxylin-Eosin (c) and $\alpha_v\beta_3$ integrin immunoperoxidase stainings (a, b, d) in quiescent (a), and growing (b-d) collateral arteries. a: in a quiescent collateral artery, $\alpha_v\beta_3$ signals are just above the detection level. b: three days after femoral artery occlusion, most growing arteries show intense staining in the subendothelium. c and d: seven days after occlusion, increased expression of $\alpha_v\beta_3$ integrin is evident in the neointima (I) and the media (M). e: quantification of the immunoperoxidase signals seven days after occlusion. L = Lumen. optical density in A.U. = arbitrary units. *p < 0.001*

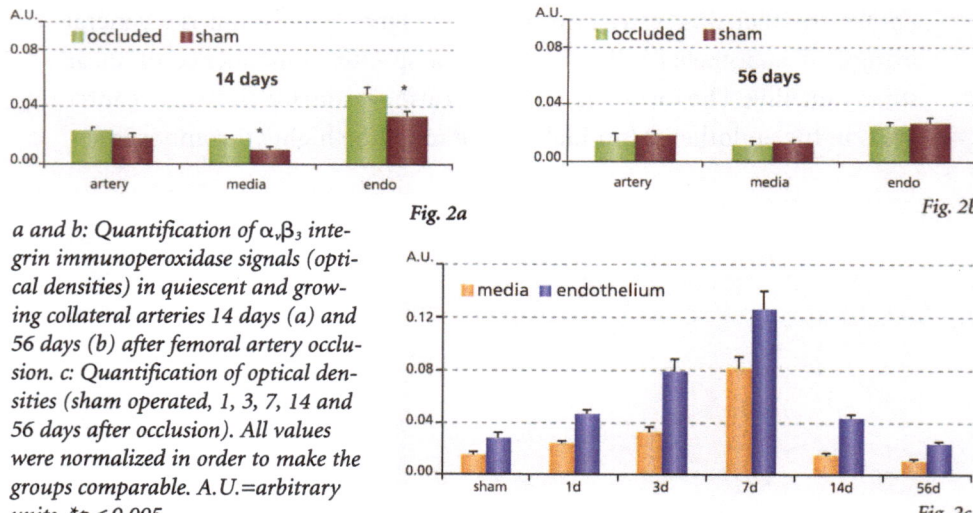

Fig. 2a

Fig. 2b

Fig. 2c

a and b: Quantification of $\alpha_v\beta_3$ *integrin immunoperoxidase signals (optical densities) in quiescent and growing collateral arteries 14 days (a) and 56 days (b) after femoral artery occlusion. c: Quantification of optical densities (sham operated, 1, 3, 7, 14 and 56 days after occlusion). All values were normalized in order to make the groups comparable. A.U.=arbitrary units.* *$p < 0.005$

Seven days after femoral artery occlusion, the levels of $\alpha_v\beta_3$ integrin immunostaining are elevated in the endothelium and media of most growing collateral arteries (Figs 1c and d). At this time point, some growing collateral arteries start to form a neointimal layer, composed of SMCs with a synthetic phenotype embedded in a loose extracellular matrix. SMCs of the intima show a pattern and intensity of integrin staining similar to that of SMCs of the media. Quantification of the immunostainings revealed an averaged 6-fold increase in the amount of protein in growing collateral vessel walls compared to quiescent ones (Fig. 1e).

After 14 days of occlusion, some collateral arteries still show an increased integrin content in the endothelium, intima, and media. However, most collaterals show an intensity of staining similar to that of quiescent vessels (Fig 2a). Fifty-six days after femoral artery occlusion, collateral arteries are notably enlarged, and the intensity of immunoperoxidase staining for $\alpha_v\beta_3$ integrin is similar to that of quiescent arteries (Fig 2b).

Figure 2c shows a comparative quantification of $\alpha_v\beta_3$ integrin protein levels in the five time points analyzed. Integrin protein levels steadily increase in the endothelium and media of growing collateral arteries during the first week from the onset of arteriogenesis, returning to basal levels during the second week. These results clearly indicate that $\alpha_v\beta_3$ integrin plays a role in arteriogenesis. One important function of $\alpha_v\beta_3$ integrin in vessel remodeling events is the promotion of SMC migration to form the neointima[8-12]. Vitronectin, the main $\alpha_v\beta_3$ integrin ligand, has been shown to promote cell adhesion, spreading, and migration in vascular cells by $\alpha_v\beta_3$ binding[14,15]. Thus, to further explore the precise function of $\alpha_v\beta_3$ integrin during arteriogenesis we analyzed the localization and amount of vitronectin in growing collateral arteries. Seven and fourteen days after femoral artery occlusion were the selected time points, together with sham operation, coinciding with maximal levels of $\alpha_v\beta_3$ integrin content in growing collaterals (7 days), and its return to basal levels (14 days).

Figure 3 shows the localization and quantification of vitronectin in the wall of collateral arteries. In control vessels, vitronectin signals are strong in the endothelium, whereas the media shows a light staining. Seven days after femoral artery occlusion, the amount of vitronectin has substantially decreased in the endothelium of growing collateral arteries. Fourteen days after occlusion, the pattern of vitronectin immunostaining is similar to that of quiescent vessels. Quantification of the immunoperoxidase signals confirmed the downregulation of vitronectin in the endothelium after 7 days of occlusion and its return to basal levels after 14 days.

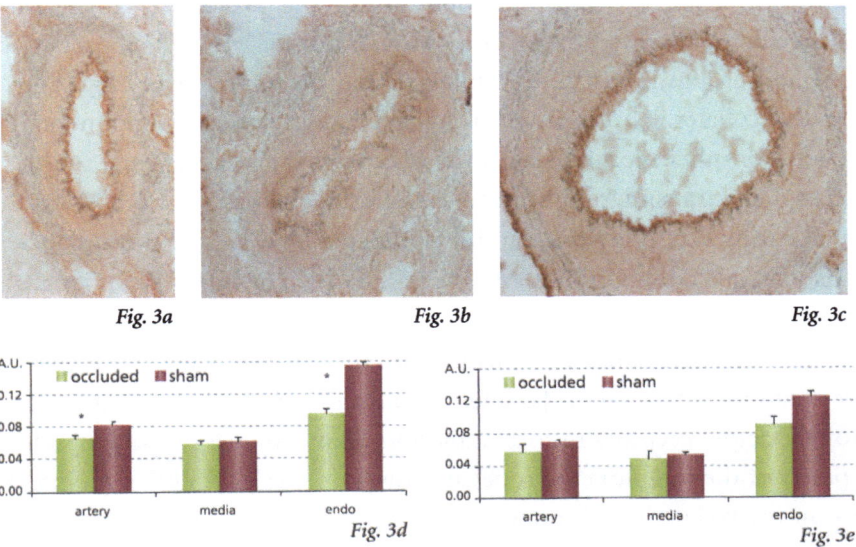

Fig. 3a   Fig. 3b   Fig. 3c

Fig. 3d   Fig. 3e

Immunoperoxidase staining of quiescent (a), 7 day-occluded (b), and 14 day-occluded (c) collateral arteries stained for vitronectin. Quantification of immunoperoxidase signals was also performed after 7 days (d) and 14 days (e) of occlusion. *p<0.005

These results clearly indicate that vitronectin is not the main $\alpha_v\beta_3$ integrin ligand in arteriogenesis. Moreover, the strong down-regulation of vitronectin after one week of surgery, when integrin levels peak, suggests that a specific signaling mechanism is preventing $\alpha_v\beta_3$-vitronectin binding. Thus, it seems that the cellular functions stimulated by $\alpha_v\beta_3$-vitronectin binding are not necessary during arteriogenesis, and ligand downregulation may be the way to avoid them. As indicated above, $\alpha_v\beta_3$-vitronectin binding has been demonstrated to mediate SMC migration during neointima formation in atherosclerotic and restenotic arteries[8,9], whereas in arteriogenesis vitronectin is downregulated. Neointima formation in collateral arteries is a highly coordinated process of growth. Atherosclerotic and restenotic vessels develop a neointimal layer in response to an aggressive stimulus, in order to protect the vessel wall from an altered environment. Thus, it is a protective mechanism more than a mechanism of growth. Blocking $\alpha_v\beta_3$-vitronectin binding might serve as therapy to change the fate of the pathological neointima in atherosclerotic and restenotic vessels. Although vitronectin is the main ligand for $\alpha_v\beta_3$ integrin, this integrin receptor can bind to other proteins of the extracellular matrix with adhesive and locomotive properties (osteopontin[16]; fibrinogen[17]; thrombin, fibronectin and proteolysed forms of collagen and laminin[18,19]). Additional studies must clarify, which particular ligand, if any, binds to $\alpha_v\beta_3$ integrin and promotes SMC migration into the collateral neointima. In addition, integrin upregulation may account for other mechanisms of the arteriogenic process at early stages. Macrophage transmigration through the collateral vessel wall, a critical event during arteriogenesis, can be modulated by $\alpha_v\beta_3$ integrin interactions with cell adhesion molecules like PECAM[20], or ICAM[21], which are known to be upregulated early in arteriogenesis. The gradient of integrin upregulation, first in the endothelium and then in the media, is a suggestive result in this regard. $\alpha_v\beta_3$ integrin can also physically associate with growth factor receptors in focal adhesion points, thereby regulating the capacity of the receptors to propagate downstream signaling[22]. $\alpha_v\beta_3$ integrin in the collateral wall might also serve as an anti-apoptotic signal[23], and as a mechanosensor[24]. Currently, we are conducting *in vivo* experiments with specific $\alpha_v\beta_3$ integrin blockers in order to elucidate the specific cellular function/s of this integrin during arteriogenesis. These

experiments are of special relevance because current anti-restenotic therapies, applied for example after balloon angioplasty, use different non-
specific integrin blockers to inhibit post-surgical clotting[25,26]. These treatments may interfere with proper arteriogenesis, the natural mechanism
of the body to fight against arterial stenosis that angioplasty is expected
to cure. Unraveling the functions of integrins during arteriogenesis is an
important challenge for the near future given that integrins may well
serve as one class of "master regulators" of cell function[27].

Jagged/Notch

The Jagged/Notch system is an evolutionary conserved intercellular signaling mechanism that regulates cell fate decisions and differentiation in
a broad spectrum of precursor cells throughout embryonic development[27].
Both, Notch (receptor) and Jagged (ligand) are membrane bound proteins,
mediating signals between cells in contact. Upon activation, the Notch
intracellular domain is proteolyzed and translocated to the nucleus, where
it co-regulates transcription of target genes including transcription factors[28]. Jagged ligands can also activate transcription, consistent with a
model of bi-directional signaling. The general net effect of Jagged/Notch
activation is that cells become refractory to differentiation signals,
remaining competent to adopt different fates[28,29]. In vertebrates, 4 different Notch and 5 different Jagged members have been described[27,30]. The

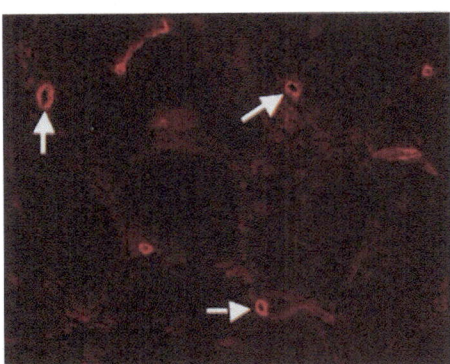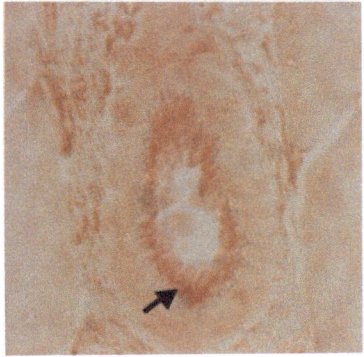

Fig. 4

Jagged1 immunofluorescent (left) and immunoperoxidase (right) staining of rabbit quad-
riceps muscles. Jagged1 is restricted to endothelial cells of the microvasculature (arrows
left), arteries (arrow right), and veins (not shown). Note that in arteries, staining is con-
centrated in the subendothelium.

specific ligand receptor interactions have yet to be fully elucidated, but appear to be variable depending on the tissue studied[31].

Expression and phenotypic analyses have demonstrated the importance of Jagged1 and Notch3 in the vascular system. Mice homozygote for a null mutation of the Jagged1 gene die *in utero* due to failure of remodeling of the primary vascular plexus[32]. In addition, Jagged1 has been dem-

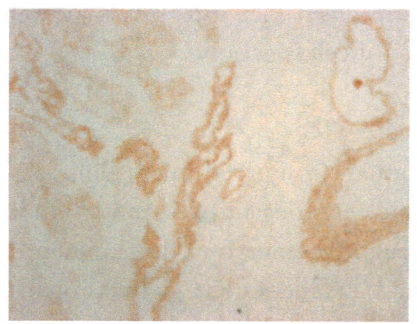 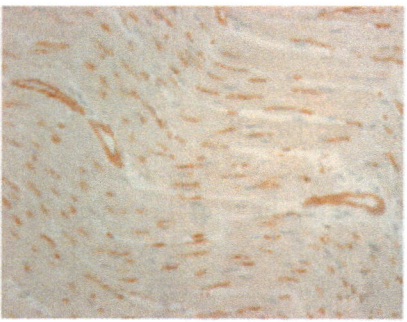

Fig. 5a   *Fig. 5b*

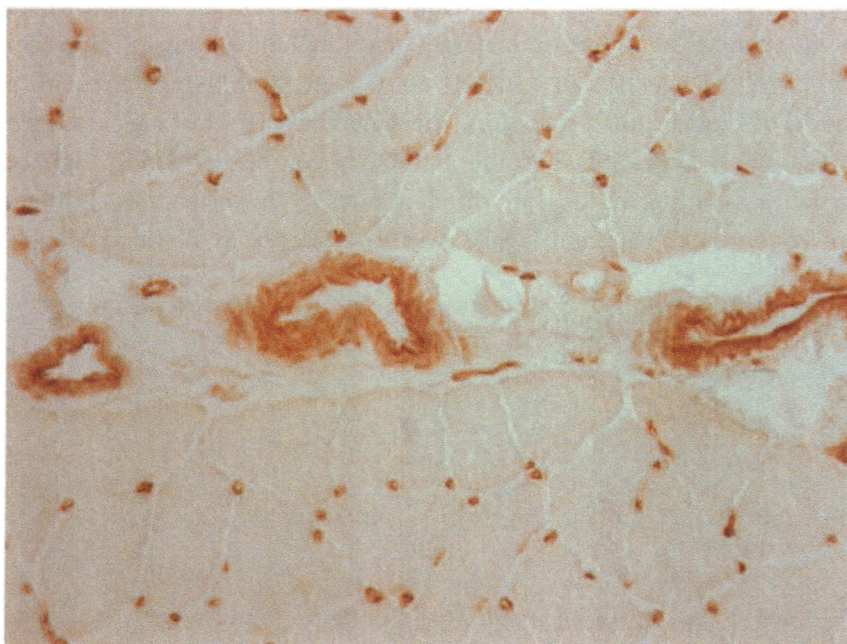

Fig. 5c

Notch3 immunoperoxidase staining of human (a) and rabbit (b) hearts, and rabbit adductor muscle (c). SMCs of the coronary arteries are the only positive structure in the human heart. In the rabbit, arteries and capillary vessels show a strong and specific staining. The same results were obtained with two different Notch3 polyclonal and monoclonal antibodies.

onstrated to regulate human endothelial cell differentiation *in vitro*[33,34]. Moreover, spontaneous mutations in the human Jagged1 gene cause the autosomal dominant disorder Algille syndrome that includes congenital heart defects[35,36]. Mutations in the Notch3 gene cause cerebral autosomal dominant arteriopathy with subcortical infarcts and leukoencephalopathy (CADASIL), an inherited vascular dementia syndrome[37-39].

We have studied the localization of Jagged1 and Notch3 proteins by immunohistochemistry in quiescent and growing collateral arteries of the rabbit hind limb and other organs in order to inspect the possible involvement of this signaling system in arteriogenesis. As previously described for mouse and man, rabbit Jagged1 is normally localized in the endothelium of capillaries and bigger vessels, but it is absent from SMCs (Fig 4). In arteries, the protein is clearly restricted to the abluminal surface of the endothelium. The expression of Notch3 receptor, one putative ligand for Jagged1, has been shown to be restricted to the SMCs of the human vasculature in adult life[37]. Our immunohistochemical analyses revealed however a more general distribution of the protein in the vascular system of the rabbit, where endothelial cells show a clear and specific staining as well (Fig. 5).

Thus, in the rabbit vasculature, endothelial cells express Jagged1 ligand, whereas both endothelial and SMCs express the Notch3 receptor. The relevance of Notch3 function in the arterial system was discovered in 1996 by Joutel and collaborators[38]. They found that mutations in the Notch3 gene were responsible for the human syndrome CADASIL, characterized by alterations of vascular SMCs in small cerebral and dermal arteries. Some years later[37], the same group reported the restricted expression of Notch3 protein in SMCs of arteries of the whole body, suggesting that it may be involved in the phenotypic modulation of these cells by inducing the differentiated contractile phenotype in adult tissues. Our results support this hypothesis. Cell – cell contacts between Jagged1[+ positive] endothelial cells and Notch3[+ positive] SMCs in the arterial wall may activate a differentiation pathway in SMCs that keeps the cells in a quiescent, contractile phenotype. Likewise, a differentiation pathway might also be activated in endothelial cells due to the known transcriptional capacity of Jagged1 ligand[40]. Moreover, it has been shown in Drosophila embryos that individual cells often express both, Notch receptor and Jagged ligand[41,42], and studies in cultured cells indicate that Notch and Jagged can interact *in cis*[42]. Thus, the co-expression of both Jagged1 and Notch3 in the endothelial cells of the rabbit microvasculature may result in cell-autonomous activation of Notch3 receptor, controlling differentiation and quiescent status of adult microvessels.

In our experiments in rabbits, we found that soon after femoral occlusion, Jagged1 is markedly downregulated in the endothelium of growing

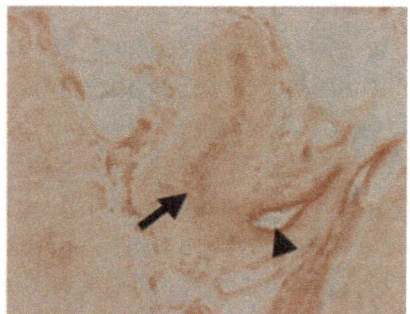

Fig. 6a

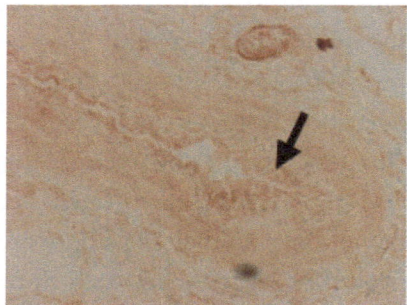

Fig. 6b

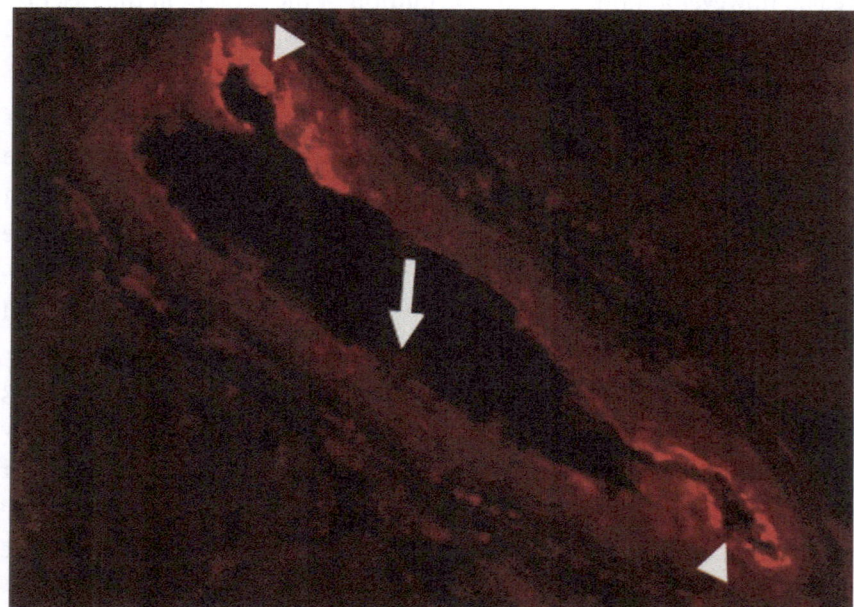

Fig. 6c

J1 Immunoperoxidase (a and b) and immunofluorescent (c) stainings of growing collateral arteries 3 days after femoral artery occlusion. J1 has almost disappeared from the endothelium of growing collateral arteries (arrows; compare with Fig. 4). Note that the branches of the collateral arteries (arrowheads) show basal high levels of J1.

collateral arteries (Fig 6). This downregulation was consistent, occurring progressively during the first days after femoral artery occlusion. In addition, Jagged1 downregulation was very finely restricted to the wall of the collateral vessels and did not affect the collateral branches (Figs 6a and c). When we analyzed the localization of Notch3 receptor, we found a strong downregulation of the protein in the SMCs of the media during the first days of growth. The amount of protein gradually decreased until it almost disappeared from the collateral media 1 week after surgery (Fig 7). The process of arteriogenesis is based on the remodeling of preexisting collateral arteries into larger arterial conduits. This remodeling requires a phenotypic shift of the SMCs of the arterial media, which in mice and rabbits takes place during the first week after femoral artery occlusion. The observed downregulation of Jagged1 and Notch3 may block the differentiation signaling pathway normally active in mature SMCs and perhaps also in endothelial cells, resulting in the acquisition of a dedifferentiated phenotype.

The acquisition of a synthetic phenotype by SMCs of the collateral media is followed by, or occurs concomitantly with, their migration to the subendothelial space to form a neointimal layer. The

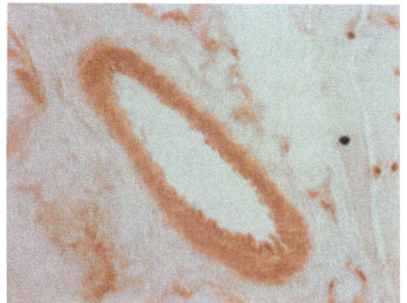

Fig. 7a

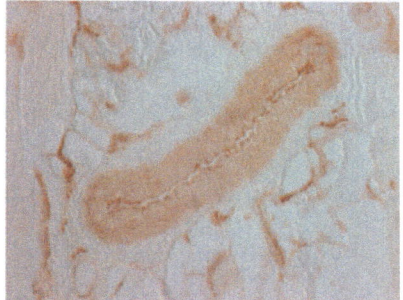

Fig. 7b

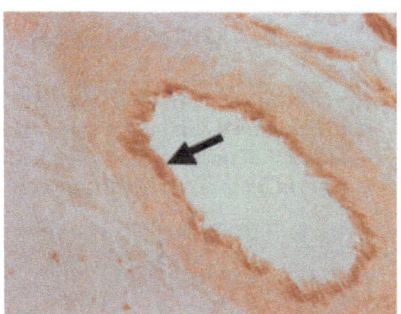

Fig. 7c

Notch3 immunoperoxidase staining of rabbit collateral arteries after sham operation (a), 3 days (b), and 7 days (c) of femoral occlusion. The strong staining of the media is gradually reduced during arteriogenesis. Note that the intensity of Notch staining does not change in the endothelium (arrow in c).

neointimal layer, common to most proliferative events in arteries, serves as the backbone of the regenerating collateral vessel. Proliferating neointimal cells are the source of new cellular material in the growing artery.

These cells must finally re-differentiate into mature SMCs, stabilizing the wall of the thicker and wider collateral artery (Fig 8).

Figure 9 shows the distribution of Jagged1 protein in the neointima of a growing collateral artery. Jagged1 is expressed by neointimal SMCs, whereas it is still downregulated in the endothelium. Upregulation of Jagged1 occurs very early during neointima formation. Notch3 immunostainings revealed, however, no signs of upregulation in the neointima of collateral arteries (Fig 10). The intensity of staining seems even lower than in the media. The immunostaining shown in figure 10 was performed with monoclonal antibodies that specifically recognize the extracellular domain of Notch3. When we used polyclonal antibodies against

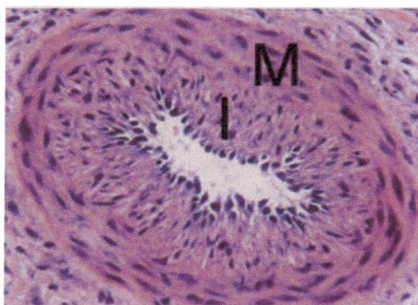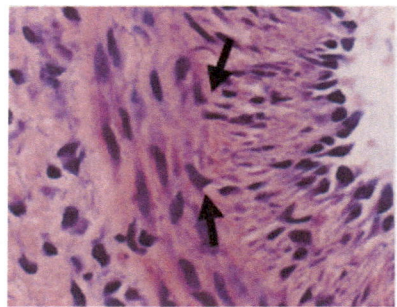

Fig. 8

Hematoxylin-Eosin staining of a rabbit collateral artery 10 days after femoral artery occlusion. Neointimal cells appear loosely packed in the subendothelium and occupy half of the collateral wall thickness (I = intima; M = media). Note that SMCs of the media seem to migrate into the neointima (arrows).

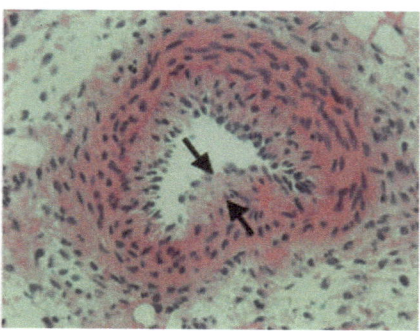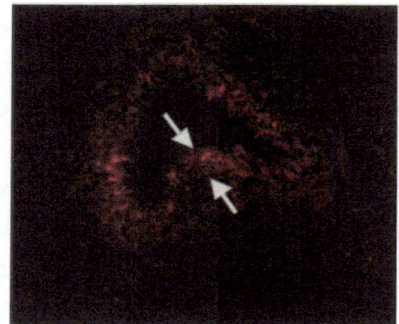

Fig. 9

Hematoxylin-Eosin staining (left) and Jagged1 immunofluorescence (right) of a rabbit collateral artery 10 days after femoral artery occlusion. The neointimal layer (between arrows) can be distinguished by its pale appearance compared to the media. Jagged1 staining is evident in the neointimal layer (red, right).

the intracellular part of the molecule the picture changed substantially (Fig 11). In many SMCs of the neointima, the intracellular domain of the Notch3 protein has been cleavaged and translocated to the nucleus, where it presumably regulates the transcription of specific genes. This observation is surprising, as Jagged/Notch studies have shown that minimal amounts of the Notch3 intracellular domain are enough to activate transcription *in vivo*, and it is usually not detectable by immunohistochemical methods[43]. Therefore, we interpret our results as a strong activation of the Jagged/Notch dependent pathway in neointimal cells, which may result in progressive redifferentiation of SMCs.

In summary, our results indicate that the embryonic Jagged/Notch signaling system plays a role in arteriogenesis. The downregulation of Jagged1 in the endothelium and Notch3 in the media of growing collateral arteries correlates well with the loss of the mature phenotype of these cells during arteriogenesis. Moreover, the re-expression of Jagged1 and activation of the Notch3 nuclear pathway in neointimal cells suggests that

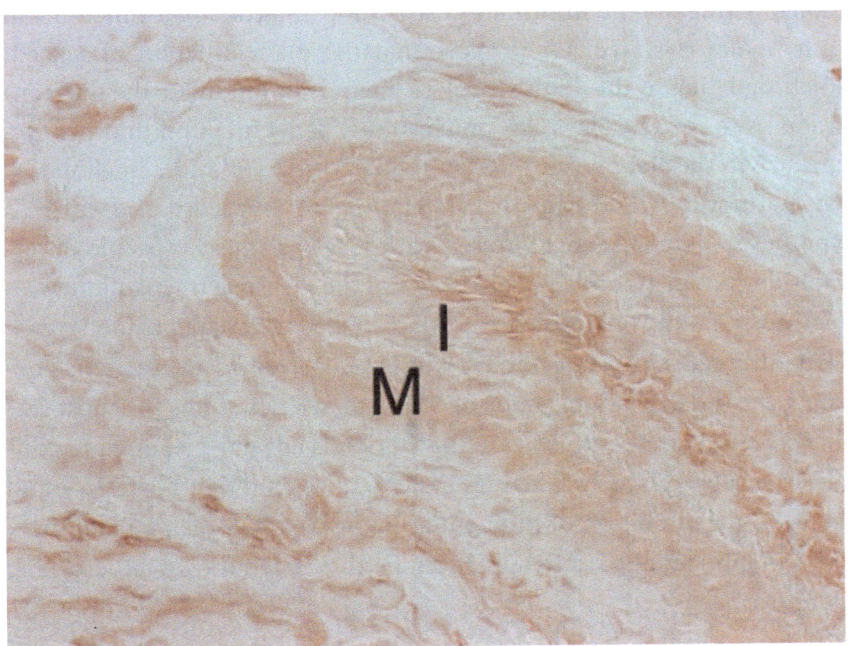

Fig. 10

Notch3 immunoperoxidase staining of a rabbit collateral artery 7 days after femoral artery occlusion. Small amounts of Notch3 are found in the media (M) at this stage, and even less in the neointima (I). (Compare to Fig. 7a)

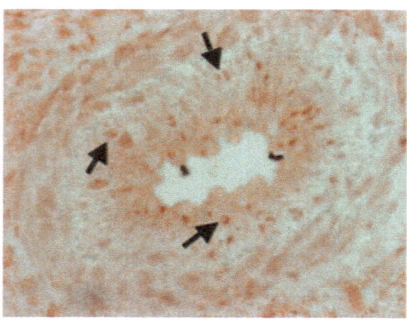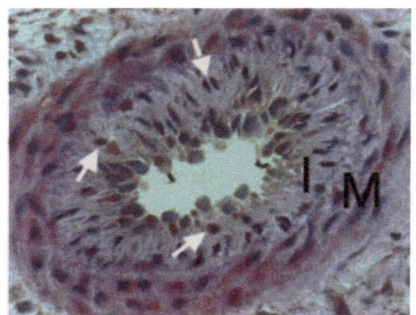

Fig. 11

Notch3 (intracellular domain) immunoperoxidase (left) and Hematoxylin-Eosin staining of a rabbit collateral artery 7 days after femoral artery occlusion. Nuclear localization of the intracellular domain of Notch3 (arrows) is prevalent in intimal cells (I) but not in the media (M).

both dedifferentiation and redifferentiation of the collateral wall components are regulated by this very conserved signaling system.

The Jagged/Notch system during embryonic life has been extensively studied. However, the information regarding Jagged/Notch functions in adult tissues is scarce. We propose that the main function of Jagged/Notch signaling in the adult vascular system is to modulate the differentiation status of vascular cells, much similar to its function in other systems like in skeletal muscle[44] and in retinal[45] differentiation, in chondrocyte maturation[46], and in feather development[47]. In accordance with this hypothesis, Notch3 is co-expressed with HeyL (a muscle specific differentiation transcription factor) in SMCs of the digestive tract and the vasculature, so far the only Notch pathway detected in vascular smooth muscles[48]. Although simplistic, the view of Jagged1-Notch3 interactions governing the differentiation status of SMCs of arteries seems the most feasible current hypothesis. At least, this notion is attractive enough to consider the Jagged/Notch signaling system as a good candidate to build strategies for inhibition of differentiation in the arteriogenic neointima, and for induction of differentiation in the restenotic or atherogenic neointima.

References

1. HYNES RO, BADER BL, HODIVALA-DILKE K. Integrins in vascular development. *Braz J Med Biol Res.* 1999;32:501-10
2. HYNES RO. Integrins: versatility, modulation, and signaling in cell adhesion. *Cell.* 1992; 69:11-25
3. VAN DER FLIER A, SONNENBERG A. Function and interactions of integrins. *Cell Tissue Res.* 2001; 305:285-98
4. CLEMETSON KJ, CLEMETSON JM. Integrins and cardiovascular disease. *Cell Mol Life Sci.* 1998; 54:502-13
5. RUPP PA, LITTLE CD. Integrins in vascular development. *Circ Res.* 2001;89:566-72
6   FRIEDLANDER M, BROOKS PC, SHAFFER RW, KINCAID CM, VARNER JA, CHERESH DA. Definition of two angiogenic pathways by distinct alpha v integrins. *Science.* 1995;270:1500-2
7. WEERASINGHE D, MCHUGH KP, ROSS FP, BROWN EJ, GISLER RH, IMHOF BA. A role for the alphavbeta3 integrin in the transmigration of monocytes. *J Cell Biol.* 1998;142:595-607
8. NAITO M, HAYASHI T, FUNAKI C, KUZUYA M, ASAI K, YAMADA K, KUZUYA F. Vitronectin-induced haptotaxis of vascular smooth muscle cells *in vitro.* *Exp Cell Res.* 1991;194:154-6
9. DUFOURCQ P, COUFFINHAL T, ALZIEU P, DARET D, MOREAU C, DUPLAA C, BONNET J. Vitronectin is up-regulated after vascular injury and vitronectin blockade prevents neointima formation. *Cardiovasc Res.* 2002;53:952-62
10. HOSHIGA M, ALPERS CE, SMITH LL, GIACHELLI CM, SCHWARTZ SM. Alpha-v beta-3 integrin expression in normal and atherosclerotic artery. *Circ Res.* 1995;77:1129-35
11. KAPPERT K, BLASCHKE F, MEEHAN WP, KAWANO H, GRILL M, FLECK E, HSUEH WA, LAW RE, GRAF K. Integrins alphavbeta3 and alphavbeta5 mediate VSMC migration and are elevated during neointima formation in the rat aorta. *Basic Res Cardiol.* 2001;96:42-9
12. CORJAY MH, DIAMOND SM, SCHLINGMANN KL, GIBBS SK, STOLTENBORG JK, RACANELLI AL. alphavbeta3, alphavbeta5, and osteopontin are coordinately upregulated at early time points in a rabbit model of neointima formation. *J Cell Biochem.* 1999;75:492-504
13. TZIMA E, DEL POZO MA, SHATTI SJ, CHIEN S, SCHWARTZ MA. Activation of integrins in endothelial cells by fluid shear stress mediates Rho-dependent cytoskeletal alignment. *EMBO J* 2001; 20(17):4839-4847
14. HESS S, KANSE SM, KOST C, PREISSNER KT. The versatility of adhesion receptor ligands in haemostasis: morpho-regulatory functions of vitronectin. *Thromb Haemost.* 1995;74:258-65
15. BROWN SL, LUNDGREN CH, NORDT T, FUJII S. Stimulation of migration of human aortic smooth muscle cells by vitronectin: implications for atherosclerosis. *Cardiovasc Res.* 1994; 28:1815-20
16. LIAW L, ALMEIDA M, HART CE, SCHWARTZ SM, GIACHELLI CM. Osteopontin promotes vascular cell adhesion and spreading and is chemotactic for smooth muscle cells *in vitro.* *Circ Res.* 1994;74:214-24
17. HYNES RO, BADER BL, HODIVALA-DILKE K. Integrins in vascular development. *Braz J Med Biol Res.* 1999;32:501-10
18. CLYMAN RI, MAURAY F, KRAMER RH. Beta 1 and beta 3 integrins have different roles in the adhesion and migration of vascular smooth muscle cells on extracellular matrix. *Exp Cell Res.* 1992;200:272-84
19. HOOD JD, CHERESH DA. Role of integrins in cell invasion and migration. *Nature Rev Cancer.* 2002;2:91-100
20. PIALI L, HAMMEL P, UHEREK C, BACHMANN F, GISLER RH, DUNON D, IMHOF BA. CD31/PECAM-1 is a ligand for alpha v beta 3 integrin involved in adhesion of leukocytes to endothelium. *J Cell Biol.* 1995;130:451-60

21. WEERASINGHE D, MCHUGH KP, ROSS FP, BROWN EJ, GISLER RH, IMHOF BA. A role for the alphavbeta3 integrin in the transmigration of monocytes. *J Cell Biol.* 1998;142:595-607

22. ELICEIRI BP. Integrin and growth factor receptor crosstalk *Circ Res.* 2001;89:1104-1110

23. COLEMAN KR, BRADEN GA, WILLINGHAM MC, SANE DC. Vitaxin, a humanized monoclonal antibody to the vitronectin receptor (alphavbeta3), reduces neointimal hyperplasia and total vessel area after balloon injury in hypercholesterolemic rabbits. *Circ Res.* 1999;84:1268-76

24. JALALI S, DEL POZO MA, CHEN K-D, MIAO H, LI YS, SCHWARTZ MA, SHYY JY, CHIEN S. Integrin-mediated mechanotransduction requires its dynamic interaction with specific extracellular matrix (ECM) ligands. *Proc Natl Acad Sci USA.* 2001;98(3):1042–1046

25. PROIMOS G. Platelet aggregation inhibition with glycoprotein IIb—IIIa inhibitors. *J Thromb Thrombolysis.* 2001;11:99-110

26. TOPOL EJ, LINCOFF AM, KEREIAKES DJ, KLEIMAN NS, COHEN EA, FERGUSON JJ, TCHENG JE, SAPP S, CALIFF RM. Multi-year follow-up of abciximab therapy in three randomized, place-bo-controlled trials of percutaneous coronary revascularization. *Am J Med.* 2002;113:1-6

27. ARTAVANIS-TSAKONAS S, RAND MD, LAKE RJ. Notch signaling: cell fate control and signal integration in development. SCIENCE 1999;284:770–776

28. ARTAVANIS-TSAKONAS S, MATSUNO K, FORTINI ME. Notch1 signaling. *Science* 1995; 268: 225–232

29. GREENWALD I, RUBIN GM. Making a difference: the role of cell-cell interactions in establishing separate identities for equivalent cells. *Cell* 1992; 68:271–281

30. SHIMIZU K, CHIBA S, KUMANO K, HOSOYA N, TAKAHASHI T, KANDA Y, HAMADA Y, YAZAKI Y, HIRAI H. Mouse Jagged1 physically interacts with notch2 and other notch receptors. Assessment by quantitative methods. *J Biol Chem.* 19992; 74:32961–32969

31. LOOMES KM, TAICHMAN DB. GLOVER CL, WILLIAMS PT, MARKOWITZ JE, PICCOLI DA, BALDWIN HS, OAKEY RJ. Characterization of Notch receptor expression in the developing mammalian heart and liver. *Am J Med Genet.* 2002; 112:181–189.

32. XUE Y, GAO X, LINDSELL CE, NORTON CR, CHANG B, HICKS C, GENDRON- MAGUIRE M, RAND EB, WEINMASTER G, GRIDLEY T. Embryonic lethality and vascular defects in mice lacking the Notch ligand Jagged1. *Hum Mol Genet.* 1999; 8:723–730

33. ZIMRIN AB, PEPPER MS, MCMAHON GA, NGUYEN F, MONTESANO R, MACIAG T. An antisense oligonucleotide to the Notch ligand Jagged enhances fibroblast growth factor-induced angiogenesis *in vitro. J Biol Chem.* 1996; 271(51):32499–32502.

34. WONG MKK, PRUDOVSKY I, VARY C, BOOTH C, LIAW L, MOUSA S, SMALL D, MACIAG T. A Non-Transmembrane Form of Jagged 1 Regulates the Formation of Matrix-Dependent Chord-like Structures. *Biochem Biophys Res Commun.* 2000; 268:853–859

35. LI L, KRANTZ ID, DENG Y, GENIN A, BANTA AB, COLLINS CC, QI M, TRASK BJ, KUO WL, COCHRAN J, COSTA T, PIERPONT ME, RAND EB, PICCOLI DA, HOOD L, SPINNER NB. Alagille syndrome is caused by mutations in human Jagged1, which encodes a ligand for Notch1. *Nat Genet.* 1997; 16:243–251

36. ODA T, ELKAHLOUN AG, PIKE BL, OKAJIMA K, KRANTZ ID, GENIN A, PICCOLI DA, MELTZER PS, SPINNER NB, COLLINS FS, CHANDRASEKHARAPPA SC. Mutations in the human 01 gene are responsible for Alagille syndrome. *Nat Genet.* 1997; 16:235–242

37. JOUTEL A, ANDREUX F, GAULIS S, DOMENGA V, CECILLON M, BATTAIL N, PIGA N, CHAPON F, GODFRAIN C, TOURNIER-LASSERVE E. The ectodomain of the Notch3 receptor accumulates within the cerebrovasculature of CADASIL patients. *Clin Invest* 2000; 105:597–605

38. JOUTEL A, CORPECHOT C, DUCROS A, VAHEDI K, CHABRIAT H, MOUTON P, ALAMOWITCH S, DOMENGA V, CECILLION M, MARECHAL E, MACIAZEK J, VAYSSIERE C, CRUAUD C, CABANIS EA, RUCHOUX MM, WEISSENBACH J, BACH JF, BOUSSER MG, TOURNIER-LASSERVE E. Notch3 mutations in CADASIL, an hereditary adultonset condition causing stroke and dementia. *Nature* 1996; 383:707–710

39. JOUTEL A, VAHEDI K, CORPECHOT C, TROESCH A, CHABRIAT H, VAYSSIERE C, CRUAUD C, MACIAZEK J, WEISSENBACH J, BOUSSER MG, BACH JF, TOURNIER-LASSERVE E. Strong clustering and stereotyped nature of Notch3 mutations in CADASIL patients. *Lancet* 1997; 350:1511–1515

40. BLAND CE, KIMBERLY P, RAND MD. Notch-induced proteolysis and nuclear localization of the Delta ligand. *J Biol Chem.* 2003;278(16):13607-13610

41. HEITZLER P, SIMPSON P. Altered epidermal growth factor-like sequences provide evidence for a role of Notch as a receptor in cell fate decisions. *Development* 1993;117(3):1113-23

42. FEHON RG, JOHANSEN K, REBAY I, ARTAVANIS-TSAKONAS S. Complex cellular and subcellular regulation of notch expression during embryonic and imaginal development of Drosophila: implications for notch function. *J Cell Biol.* 1991;113(3):657-669

43. SCHROETER EH, KISSLINGER JA, KOPAN R. Notch-1 signaling requires ligand-induced proteolytic release of intracellular domain. *Nature* 1998;28:393(6683):382-386

44. DELFINI M-C, HIRSINGER E, POURQUIÉ O, DUPREZ D. Delta 1-activated Notch inhibits muscle differentiation without affecting Myf5 and Pax3 expression in chick limb myogenesis. *Development* 2000; 127:5213-5224

45. HENRIQUE D, HIRSINGER E, ADAM J, LE ROUX I, POURQIUÉ O, ISH-HOROWICZ D, LEWIS J. Maintenance of neuroepithelial progenitor cells by Delta-Notch signaling in the embryonic chick retina. *Curr Biol.* 1997; 7:661-670

46. CROWE R, ZIKHERMAN J, NISWANDER L. Delta1 negatively regulates the transition from pre-hypertrophic to hypertrophic chondrocytes during cartilage formation. *Development* 1999; 126:987-998

47. MARTINE VIALLET JP, PRIN F, OLIVERA Z I, HIRSINGER E, POURQUIE O, DHOUAILLY D. Chick Delta1 gene expression and the formation of the feather primordia. *Mech Dev.* 1998; 72:159-168

48. LEIMEISTER C, SCHUMACHER N, STEIDL C, GESSLER M. Analysis of HeyL expression in wild-type and Notch pathway mutant mouse embryos. *Mech Dev.* 2000; 98:175-178

Chapter 10

Fibroblast Growth Factors

René Zimmermann, Borja Fernández, Alexandra Buehler, Alessandra Martire, Sawa Kostin, Claudia Strohm, Swen Wolfram and Elisabeth Deindl

The fibroblast growth factor (FGF) family consists of at least 23 structurally related polypeptides[1] with new ones added at a regular basis. FGFs bind heparin and heparansulfat and their important activities in numerous aspects of embryogenesis, angiogenesis, growth and cell survival (for review: see[2,3]) are mediated through four structurally related membrane associated tyrosine kinase receptors that derive from separate genes.[4,5] The prototype and best-known members of the FGF family are acidic FGF (FGF-1)[6-8] and basic FGF (FGF-2) (reviewed in[9,10]). It is beyond the scope of this review to discuss the role of FGF-1 and -2 in angiogenesis. Instead, we aim to provide evidence for a role of FGF-1 and some of the other FGFs in collateral vessel growth/arteriogenesis. Furthermore, some recent findings from the literature will be discussed in view of the role of FGFs other than FGF-1 and -2 in vessel growth as such.

FGF-1 and FGF-2

During embryonic development FGF-1 is involved in the differentiation of mesoderm derived tissues including the heart. The proliferation and growth of the myocardium and the coronary vasculature correlates well with the expression of FGF-1 and its receptors FGFR1-4 on endothelial and smooth muscle cells as well as on cardiomyocytes.[11-15]

In 1989 our group reported the isolation of FGF-1 and FGF-2 from bovine, canine and porcine myocardial tissue.[16] The presence of potent growth factors in a normal heart where proliferation of cells is absent indicates that these factors must have functions other than being a mitogen, e.g acting as trophic factors for terminally differentiated cells like cardiomyocytes.[17] In addition, we and others showed that in the adult heart, FGF-1 and its receptors are upregulated during ischemia in several animal models.[17-19] Collateral flow and left ventricular function can be significantly improved by either local or systemic administration of FGF-1 or FGF-2 protein during myocardial ischemia. This process is characterized by the formation of new vessels and hyperplasia of smooth muscle cells, mainly in arteriolar vessels.[20-22] Further evidence for a vessel-promoting role of FGF-1 came from clinical studies on patients with coronary heart disease. Local intramyocardial injection of the growth factor resulted in a 3-fold increase in capillary density, followed by the improvement of myocardial perfusion as well as a reduction of symptoms and an increase in working capacity.[23] From all of these studies it became obvious that FGF-1 (and FGF-2; see below) is somehow involved in vascular growth associated with ischemia and in cardiomyocyte protection.

Since the only FGF-1 transgenic mouse available showed lens-specific FGF-1 overexpression due to fusion of the human FGF-1 to α A-crystallin promoter[24] it was not an appropriate model to study the effect of FGF-1 in the heart and on coronary vessel development in more detail. Therefore, we generated transgenic mice with heart-specific overexpression of FGF-1 driven by the MLC2v promoter. Three transgenic lines, two with and one without the CMV enhancer, were studied. All 3 lines showed similar results except that in the line without enhancer the effects were weaker.[25]

In general, animals appeared normal despite a 1.9-fold overexpression of FGF-1 mRNA and protein. Although increased in transgenic animals, FGF-1 expression patterns were similiar in wildtype and transgenic animals. The protein localized in cardiomyocytes and the extracellular matrix with a clear epicardial to endocardial gradient. No difference was found in gross anatomy and histomorphology between wildtype and transgenic animals. Atria, ventricles, septae, valves and chambers were anatomically and histologically intact. In addition, there were no ultrastructural alterations in FGF-1 overexpressing cardiomyocytes and the surrounding tissue.

Capillary density was unchanged between wildtype and transgenic animals, indicating that angiogenesis is not pertubed in these lines. However, to our suprise the density of arteries and arterioles in transgenic mice was significantly different (1.3-1.45 fold increase) in transgenic mice, mostly due to an increase in the number of small arterioles (Fig 1). In addition, the number of branches of the coronary arteries was significantly elevated (1.4-1.5 fold) in all transgenic lines compared to non-transgenic littermates. The differences in the anatomic pattern between transgenic and wildtype animals were established between the second and the sixth week of postnatal life and were still detectable with 36 weeks of age. Furthermore, *ex vivo* hemodynamic experiments in isolated hearts showed that the coronary flow was enhanced 1.2 -1.3 fold in the transgenic hearts which was not due to the vasodilatation capacity of FGF-1.[25]

These findings so far indicate FGF-1 as a key regulatory molecule of the differentiation of the arterial system. It also sheds new light on the cardioprotective effect of FGF-1 seen in pigs following intramyocardial infusion of the protein[22] that may be due to its known growth promoting effects for blood vessels or mediated by a non-vascular mechanism. The first possibility would result in a higher coronary bloodflow, thereby reducing maximal infarct size, while the latter one may be due to the stimulation of ERKs in ischemic myocardium.[26]

To test for both possibilities infarct development was studied in transgenic mice after coronary occlusion for 15 to 75 min[27]. Results clearly showed unaltered final infarct size (about 60 % of the risk area) between transgenic and wildtype animals, suggesting a non-vascular

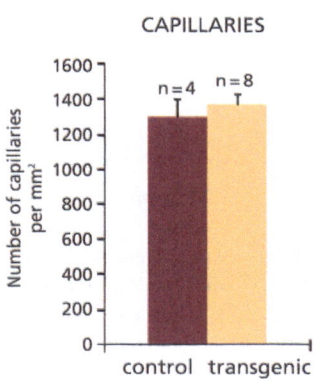

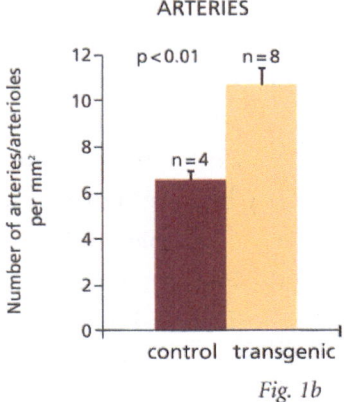

Fig. 1b

Capillary density per mm² (a) versus arteriolar density per mm² (b) Capillary density is not changed in FGF-1 transgenic mice but arteriolar density is significantly increased.

mode of cardioprotection. However, infarct development in transgenic animals was significantly delayed when compared to non-transgenic littermates. The maximal or final infarct size was reached after 45 min of ischemia in wildtype animals, but at 75 min in the transgenics (Fig 2). This delay of infarct development for 30 min is similar to the one seen in pigs following intramyocardial infusion of FGF-1 protein.[22] Most proba-

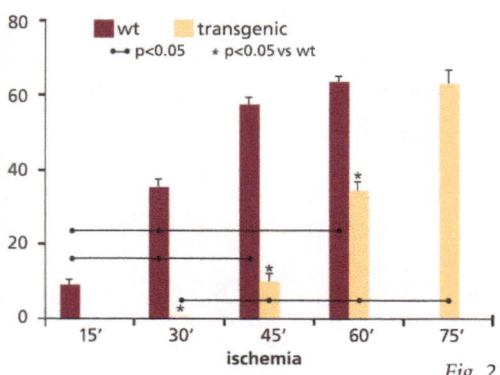

Delay of infarct development in FGF-1 transgenic mice. Transgenic mice with cardiac-specific over-expression of FGF-1 show a delay in infarct development of about 30 min (reprinted with permission from[25]).

bly, binding of the ligand FGF-1 to its receptors FGFR-1 and -2 induces a signaling cascade, characterized by receptor dimerization and phosphorylation, followed downstream by signaling via the mitogen-activated protein kinases (MAPK). Further analysis of this effect revealed that transgenic FGF-1 mice are characterized by a constitutive higher expression of the extracellular signal-regulated kinases ERK-1 and ERK-2 in the myocardium. Following injection of UO126, an ERK-1/2 inhibitor, a decreased cardioprotective effect of FGF-1 was observed.

In summary, these studies of the FGF-1 transgenic mouse showed a dual effect of FGF-1 in the heart. On one side, FGF-1 is involved in the differentiation and growth of the coronary artery system. On the other side, FGF-1 is cardioprotective by delaying infarct size development. However, the cardioprotective effect of FGF-1 is not due to increased arteriolar density because maximal infarct size was not reduced in FGF-1 transgenic mice. Further studies will clarify the role of other molecules involved in the FGF-1 mediated cardioprotection and arterial vessel growth (Fig 3).

Heparin-binding FGF-2, like FGF-1, is a prototype member of the FGF family. Originally, it was identified as a 18k Da protein of 146 amino acids, mitogenic for mesoderm and neuroectoderm derived cells.[12] In addition to the 18 kDa isoform, several higher molecular weight isoforms (22, 22.5, 24 and 34 kDa) have been identified which arise from the use of CUG start codons upstream of the traditional AUG codon. While the 18kDa isoform is mainly localized to the cytoplasm, the higher molecular weight forms of FGF-2 are found in the nucleus due to a nuclear localization signal.[10] Another interesting feature of FGF-2 is the presence of an antisense RNA transcribed from its 3' end.[28,29]

Although FGF-2, like FGF-1, lacks a signal sequence for secretion it acts as a multifunctional growth factor with pleiotropic functions in a large number of cells. The protein is mitogenic, induces tissue remodeling and regeneration, is neurotrophic for neural cells, a potent angiogenic stimulatory agent for vascular cells such as endothelial and smooth muscle cells and is involved in the pathogenesis of atherosclerosis.[9,10,30-32] Its actions are mediated by binding to four different receptors (FGFR1-4)[9,33,34] and are potentiated by heparansulfate sidechains of proteoglycans like syndecan-2 and -4[35-38] and perlecan.[39] This is not only true for the setting of angiogenesis, but also in arteriogenesis/collateral growth. In the quail chorioallantoic membrane FGF-2 directly increases arterial density and stimulates the growth of small but not large vessels via FGFR1-4.[40]

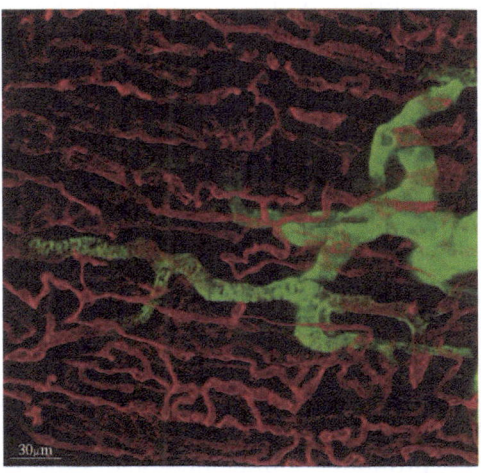

Fig. 3

Three-dimensional immunoconfocal image of a 100 µm thick section from a FGF-1 transgenic mouse heart double labeled for smooth muscle α-actin (green) and Bandeiraea simplicifolia lectin (red). Shown is a single arteriolar tree (green) surrounded by the capillary network (red). (reprinted by permission from[25])

However, the unstimulated temporal and spatial expression of FGF-2 as well as FGF-1 and their high and low affinity receptors during adaptive arteriogenesis has never been elucidated *in vivo*. To address this question, we performed studies in our rabbit model of arteriogenesis. Results of Northern blot analysis for FGF-2 (and FGF-1) showed that neither of these growth factors is differentially expressed. In contrast to these results, the expression of the FGFRs and their isoforms (which have unique ligand binding properties) is tempospatially restricted throughout the body during development and disease, delineating that the mode of action of the FGFs is not only regulated by the expression of the ligands but also by the availability of their receptors. Our results displayed a rapid and pronounced induction of FGFR-1 on

RNA and protein level as well as an increased tyrosine kinase activity of FGFR-1 in the early phase of arteriogenesis. Immunohistochemical studies showed a specific localization of FGFR-1 in SMCs of arteries in the m. quadriceps (Fig 4). Fibroblasts and pericytes were also stained, but not ECs of capillaries, arteries and veins, or skeletal muscle. The time relationship between the FGFR-1 expression and arteriogenesis, the strong expression of FGFR-1 in collateral arteries, the specific immunoreactivity in vascular SMCs, as well as the fact that the FGFR-1 mRNA (which is, like FGF-1 and FGF-2, already expressed in vascular SMCs under normal conditions[41,42]) is the major form of the four known FGFRs expressed by proliferating human arterial SMCs[43] strongly suggest an important role of FGFR-1 for signal-transduction in the arterial wall during the early phase of collateral artery growth.[44]

As mentioned before, ligand induced dimerization of the high-affinity receptor (FGFR) mediated by low-affinity receptors (heparan sulfate proteoglycans, HSPGs) is a key event in transmembrane signaling. Attention is focused on the syndecans, a group of transmembrane HSPGs.[35-38] Analyzing the expression of distinct syndecans in our model, we found a pronounced upregulation of syndecan-4 in the m. quadriceps at the early phase of arteriogenesis. Syndecan-4 has been described as a primary response gene induced by FGF-2 in vascular SMCs *in vivo.*[36] Furthermore, overexpression of syndecan-4 resulted in a significant increase in cell growth and migration in response to FGF-2.[45] In addition, syndecan-4 has been implicated in various processes like regulation of focal adhesion assembly and protein kinase C activation.[46] However, which functional properties might be assigned to syndecan-4 during arteriogenesis remains to be clarified.

Most probably, FGFR ligands, similar to TNF, are supplied by monocytes/macrophages during arteriogenesis.[47] Monocytes are known to play an important role in adaptive and cytokine induced collateral artery growth (see chapter 7). These mononuclear cells that have the capacity to transmigrate the EC-layer have been shown to deliver growth factors like FGF-2 to the vessel during arteriogenesis[48] and accumulate in the perivascular space already at 12h of femoral artery ligation.[49] Our *in vitro* results showed that stimulation of monocytes with LPS leads to an increased level of FGF-2 in these types of cells[44]. Furthermore, flow

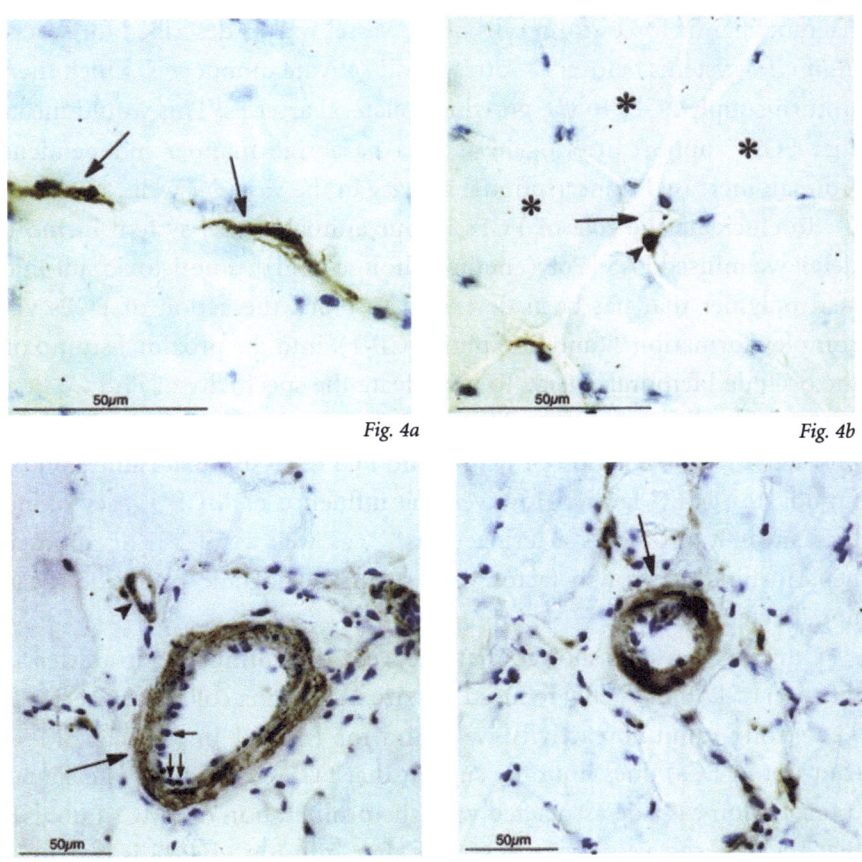

Fig. 4a

Fig. 4b

Fig. 4c

Fig. 4d

Immunohistochemical analysis of FGFR-1 in m. quadriceps after femoral artery occlusion. a: Fibroblasts were the main cells showing strong immunoreactivity after 3 days. b: Capillary ECs (arrow) and skeletal muscle cells (asteriks) were negative at 12 h and all other time points studied. Some pericytes were also labeled (arrowhead). c: SMCs of arteries (arrow) and arterioles (arrowhead) were immunoreactive at 1d as well as at later time points. No staining was found in ECs (small arrows). d: A growing collateral artery is shown 3 d after femoral artery occlusion (arrow). (reprinted by permission from[44])

cytometry results revealed that monocytes treated with FGF-2 show an increased expression of integrins that are part of the MAC-1 (α_M/β_2) or LFA-1 (α_L/β_2) heterodimer. These two heterodimeres are receptors that are responsible for monocyte interaction with the endothelium (see chapter 7). Our adhesion assays revealed that FGF-2 as well as FGF-1 have the ability to stimulate monocyte adhesion to EC-layers and that FGF-1 is an even more potent factor than MCP-1. These data strongly suggest that during adaptive arteriogenesis FGFs – which might be released by

haemodynamic forces from cells of the vessel wall as described for several *in vitro* systems before[50,51] – attract and activate monocytes, which then
in turn supply FGFs to the growing collateral arteries. This would mean
that FGFs support arteriogenesis in a paracrine manner independent
from an increased transcriptional activity in the vascular wall.

To elucidate the role of FGFs in our animal model system in more
detail we infused PAS [Poly(anetholsulfonoc Acid)], a non-toxic sulfonic
acid polymer that has been described to block the action of FGFs via
complex formation[52] (and PAS plus MCP-1), into the proximal stump of
the occluded femoral artery. To investigate the specificity of PAS we first
performed adhesion assays. The results showed that PAS significantly
interfered with the action of FGF-1 and FGF-2 to stimulate adhesion of
monocytes to EC layers. However, the influence of MCP-1, a cytokine
that strongly promotes arteriogenesis[48,53], as well as of VEGF, another
heparin-binding growth factor with strong angiogenic properties, was
not affected by PAS.

Our *in vivo* results showed that one week of continuous intra-arterial
infusion of PAS markedly reduced the size of growing collateral arteries[44].
The strong immunoreactivity we found for FGFR-1 in vascular SMCs
(but not in ECs) does not only suggest that FGFR-1 mediates the signal
transduction cascade associated with the proliferation of SMCs but also
that the reduced vessel size observed after infusion of PAS is due to a
reduced SMC proliferation in growing collateral arteries resulting from
an interference of PAS with the action of FGFs. This assumption is cor-
roborated by results from Ueno et al. who recently showed that FGF-2
induced DNA synthesis and arterial SMC proliferation was abolished by
overexpressing a dominant-negative truncated FGFR-1.[54] Concomitant
application of PAS, owing to its property to pass the EC layer of a vessel
(personal communication with S. Liekens), and MCP-1 showed an even
stronger negative effect on collateral artery growth than the application
of PAS alone, indicating that a significant part of the monocyte-related
arteriogenesis is caused by FGFs. Our *in vitro* results evidenced that PAS
can block the action of both FGF-1 and FGF-2 (and maybe of other
FGFs, too), and that FGF-1 is an even more potent factor than MCP-1 in
terms of stimulation of monocyte adhesion. Despite these findings, we
consider it likely that the observed *in vivo* effect of PAS was particularly

due to an interference with the action of FGF-2, since the FGF-1 function has been associated more with vessel differentiation and branching than with growing proper.[25]

Additional hints for a „positive" role of FGF-1 and -2 in collateral artery growth come from a recently published study which shows that *in vivo* application of FGF-2 in combination with PDGF-BB leads to a significant improvement of collateral flow in a rabbit model of hind limb ischemia[55], similar to the one seen in SHR rats after infusion of FGF-2 alone[56] (see also chapter 10). It is also noteworthy to mention that FGFs released from the cell surface or secreted via a non-classical pathway were described to regulate the expression of osteoglycin/mimecan, a proteoglycan component of the extracellular matrix, which is significantly decreased during collateral growth[57,58] (see also chapter 9).

Doukas and co-workers reported that the application of plasmid and adenoviral vectors encoding either FGF-2 or FGF-6 transgenes produced early angiogenic responses followed by arteriogenesis when these constructs/vectors were delivered directly to excisional wounds.[59] FGF-2 was much more potent than FGF-6, leading to a more than 11-fold increased arteriolar density at day 21. FGF-2 also enhanced muscle repair because gene-treated wounds filled with regenerating myotubes expressing CD56 at an average 20-fold higher level. They also showed that these responses required the transfection of a threshold number of cells only in injured muscles. In their hands, neither delivery of FGF-2 protein nor PDGF-B gene produced similar results.

While numerous *in vitro* and *in vivo* studies indicate that FGF-1 and FGF-2 are involved in angiogenesis and collateral growth, the findings in transgenic and knockout mice do not inevitably confirm these results. Transgenic mice with FGF-2 overexpression under the control of a phosphoglycerate kinase promoter develop chondrodysplasia[60] with absence of any vascular defects, but they show enhanced angiogenesis if an angiogenic substrate is provided.[61] Furthermore, overexpression of FGF-2 in mouse lens using the a A-crystallin promoter does not result in any vascular abnormalities[62] while overexpression in the heart using the Rous sarcoma virus promoter results in a 20% increase in capillary density with unchanged FGFR-1 expression and an up to 45% increase in cardiac myocyte viability after injury.[63]

Ablation of FGF-2 gene expression, in contrast, generally resulted in only mild vascular defects while otherwise the knockout mice were viable, fertile and phenotypically indistinguishable from the wildtype littermates. Dono et al. reported the generation of FGF-2$^{-/-}$ mice in which the first coding exon was replaced by a neomycin resistance gene, resulting in autonomic dysfunctions in adult mice, including impaired cerebral cortex development and dysregulation of blood pressure as a consequence thereof.[64] Similar results with regard to the neural defects were observed in another strain of FGF-2$^{-/-}$ mice in which exon 1 was deleted. In addition, these animals showed a delay in wound healing which, despite the redundancy of the FGF family, cannot be compensated by other family members.[65] The role of FGF-2 in the control of vascular tone was confirmed by Zhou et al. who showed that FGF-2 knockout mice display decreased vascular smooth muscle contractility, low blood pressure and thrombocytosis. Nevertheless, vessels of these animals undergo a normal hyperplastic response following intra-arterial mechanical injury.[66] Closer analysis of the same strain implicated a role of FGF-2 in bone development, because disruption of FGF-2 led to a decrease in bone mass and to a slower bone formation.[67] Furthermore, osteoclast formation was markedly decreased in response to stimulation with parathyroid hormone, a potent bone resorbing agent.[68] Disruption of exon 2 of the FGF-2 gene demonstrated that FGF-2 is not essential for tumor formation of the retinal pigment epithelium, thereby indicating that tumor growth as such is not dependent on the presence of FGF-2.[69] The possibility that missing FGF-2 is compensated by other members of the FGF family cannot be excluded, although FGF-1/FGF-2 double knockout animals do not have other mild phenotypic defects than those observed in FGF-1$^{-/-}$ mice.[70] In general, studies in FGF-2 knockout mice revealed thrombocytosis, neurological defects, defects in bone formation, decreased vascular smooth muscle cell contractility, followed by low blood pressure and impaired wound healing, but no other vascular defects.

Still the question remains if there is a role for FGF-2 in arteriogenesis. All studies using FGF-2 transgenic or knockout animals deal with angiogenesis. None addressed arteriogenesis or collateral growth. Studies are currently undertaken in the FGF-2 transgenic mice described by Coffin et al[60] and in the FGF-2 null mice generated by Foletti and co-workers.[69]

FGF-3 and higher

Studies in the chicken embryo indicated that FGF plays a role in coronary arterialization which then induces Purkinje fiber differentiation.[71] Ablation of the cardiac neural crest resulted in a 70% reduction in the density of intramural coronary arteries and associated Purkinje fibers. However, retrovirus-mediated overexpression of FGF (the authors do not say which one they used) induced hypervascularization, followed by Purkinje fiber differentiation adjacent to this newly induced coronary arteries. This indicates that a developing arterial bed is necessary and sufficient to convert myocytes into Purkinje fibers. Furthermore, the results point to a function of FGF in heart development distinct from its role in establishing coronary blood circulation, similiar to our findings in FGF-1 transgenic animals.[25] Interestingly, based on these results one may ask if there is a direct link between arteriogenesis (or the development of blood vessels as such) and neurogenesis. This hypothesis is supported by the well known fact that in culture embryonic myocytes can differentiate into Purkinje cells if ET-1, a vascular cytokine secreted from arteries in a shear-stress dependent manner, is added.[72]

In 1994 FGF-3 was described as an "oncogenic growth factor produced locally in mouse mammary tumor virus-induced tumorigenesis".[73] It is not expressed during normal mammary development, but shows high expression in tumorous mammary gland tissue. First hints for a possible role of FGF-3 in angiogenesis came from the high degree of cellular proliferation and angiogenesis that accompany the growth of this tissue.

Similar results were presented by Mario and co-workers who showed that the FGF-3 retrovirus infected human epithelial mammary cell line MCF-10A implanted in the chicken chorioallantoic membrane induced a dense capillary network.[74] Conditioned medium from these cells, injected twice daily i.p. over a period of 10 d in rats, induced numerous small blood vessels, originating from the place where the conditioned medium was injected. They concluded that FGF-3/int-2 is associated with the acquisation of the angiogenic phenotype. When normal mouse mammary EF43 cells were transformed by a retroviral vector carrying either FGF-3 or FGF-4 cDNA these cells displayed different tumorigenic potentials when injected in nude mice.[75] Cells transfected with FGF-3 developed slowly growing tumors only in the fat pad while tumors induced by FGF-4 were rapidly growing at all sites of injection. Interestingly, conditioned medium of FGF-4 transformed EF43 induced an angiogenic phenotype in HUVECs while FGF-3 has no effect. In parallel, MMP-1 and ETS-1 mRNA levels were significantly increased in these cells, while TIMP-1 mRNA levels were decreased simultaneously. VEGF mRNA and protein were also expressed at high levels while they were unchanged in FGF-3 transfected cells. The angiogenic phenotype of the HUVECs induced by the conditioned medium of FGF-4 transfected cells could be suppressed by the inhibition of PKC.

These results are somehow in contrast to others cited before, making it difficult to decide if FGF-3 has vessel growth promoting effects or not. This is especially true in view of the fact that studies on FGF-3[-/-] mice had shown that some of these animals are viable (although only at a low number) and without any visible vascular defects in the surviving (and dead) animals. However, FGF-3[-/-] animals show developmental defects in the tail and inner ear[76], indicating that FGF-3 is required for the normal development of these parts of the body.

As already mentioned, the role of FGF-4/hst, a 21 kDa protein mitogenic for endothelial cells, in angiogenesis is discussed controversially. First clues for a positive role in promoting vascularization in tumors came from studies of adrenal cortical carcinoma cells, genetically engineered to express FGF-4. Following exposure to ionizing radiation cells expressing FGF-4 survive at a higher rate or higher doses, probably due to a significant increase in the duration of G2 arrest, suggesting perturbation of a cell cycle checkpoint.[77] In contrast to these results, levels of FGF-4 mRNA expression were significantly lower in both endometrial cancers and normal endometria when compared to those of FGF-1 and –2, indicating no participation of FGF-4 in neovascularization.[78]

Furthermore, cells from a rat bladder carcinoma cell line (NBT-II cells) transfected with FGF-4 and injected into nude mice behave like non-transfected carcinoma cells, which is in contrast to FGF-1 transfected NBT-II cells which, when injected, form rapidly growing, highly vascularized carcinomas. Conditioned medium from FGF-4 transfected cells does not induce vascular structures *in vitro*.[79] In contrast to these results which do not imply FGF-4 as an angiogenic factor is the fact that fusion of its signal petide to other FGF family members which do not have such a secretion signal (e.g. FGF-1; FGF-2) induces or enhances the angiogenic properties of these molecules.[54,80] Furthermore, recent results from Rissanen et al. even suggest a role of FGF-4 in arteriogenesis.[81]

FGF-4 knockout animals which would give anambiguous clues to the role of the molecule in blood vessel growth are not viable due to severely impaired proliferation of the inner cell mass.[82] However, there is evidence that FGF-4 may be required for survival during the early postimplantation period of development.[83]

FGF-5 was first described as an angiogenesis-inducing factor in a pig ameroid model of stress induced ischemia.[84] Injection of a recombinant adenovirus expressing human FGF-5 in the heart resulted in a significant improvement of regional abnormalities in stress-induced function and blood flow. These effects persisted for up to 12 weeks and were associated with evidence of angiogenesis in the myocardial tissue but without increased capillary density.

In addition, Schneeberger and co-workers found immunoreactive FGF-5 present in most cells, including endothelial cells of vascular and avascular epiretinal membranes from patients with proliferative diabetic retinopathy or proliferative vitreoretinopathy where it colocalizes with VEGF. These results seem to question the concept that the presence of a single angiogenic factor determines the vascular status of epiretinal proliferation.[85] FGF-5$^{-/-}$ mice are viable and show no obvious vascular defects.[83] These animals, however, indicate that the normal function of FGF-5 is the regulation of one step in the progression of the hair follicle through its growth cycle, because FGF-5$^{-/-}$ mice have 50% longer hair.

FGF-6 protein displays a strong mitogenic activity on 3T3 cells while there is only a limited response from bovine aortic endothelial cells that is also highly dependent on heparin concentration.[86] However, just recently Doukas et al. reported that plasmid or adenoviral vectors encoding either FGF-2 or FGF-6 and delivered to excisional muscle wounds produced early angiogenic responses that subsequently remodeled into arteriogenesis[59], results, which are in contrast to our own showing that collateral arteries do not grow *de novo* but develop exclusively from preexisting anastomoses.[87] Furthermore, they found significant increases in

EC present at treatment sites as well as enhancement of muscular arteriole density and an increase in regenerating myotubes. These results imply a role of FGF-6 not only in angiogenesis and arteriogenesis or collateral growth but also in myogenesis, thereby confirming previously published results on myotubes as the primary source for FGF-6 expression in both developing embryos and adults[88] and confirming the findings from Floss et al. in FGF-6 $^{-/-}$ mice that „FGF-6 is a critical component of the muscle regeneration machinery, possibly by stimulating or activating satellite cells".[89] In addition, no significant difference in microvessel number was found in these mice. Studies by Fiore et al., however, on FGF-6 $^{-/-}$ mice showed an apparently normal phenotype of these animals, indicating that „FGF-6 is not required for vital functions in the laboratory mouse".[90]

FGF-7, also called keratinocyte growth factor, so far has been linked only indirectly to neovascularization. Coleman-Krnacik & Rosen reported high expression of FGF-7 in mammary preneoplasias, tumors and immortal cell lines, although at levels less than those seen during normal mammary gland growth.[73] These data do not implicate that FGF-7 has a role in angiogenesis. However, when gene expression of the ubiquitous heparan sulfate proteoglycan perlecan, a potent inducer of angiogenesis was obliterated, the growth of colon carcinoma cells was markedly attenuated. These effects correlated well with reduced responsiveness to and affinity for FGF-7, implying a role of FGF-7 in capillary sprouting.[91] Supporting results came from Tilson et al.[92] reporting FGF-7 as one of the most upregulated genes in abdominal aortic aneurysms (besides VEGF and TNF), characterized by extensive angiogenesis in the adventitia.

Wound healing is another process in which angiogenesis is a necessary step. The role of FGF-7 in this process is controversially discussed. Studying wound healing in mice Werner et al. reported a 160-fold overexpression of the growth factor, implying an important role of FGF-7 in this process.[93] Knockout mice, however, do not show any disturbances or delay in wound healing, indicating that KGF/FGF-7 is dispensable.[94] Note added in proof: FGF-7 mRNA was found strongly upregulated in rabbit collaterals under high shear stress.

There is some evidence for an angiogenic potential of FGF-8, a secreted heparin-binding protein which is most homologous to FGF-18 among the FGF family members. It potentially codes for eight protein isoforms (a-h) which differ in their capacity to transform cells. When overexpressed in S115 mouse mammary tumor cells only isoforms 8a and 8b show angiogenic properties. While FGF-8a only slightly increased tumor growth and probably tumor vascularization recombinant FGF-8b protein stimulates proliferation, migration and vessel-like tube formation in immortomouse brain capillary endothelial cells and in CAM assays.[95]

Supporting evidence for a role of FGF-8 in neovascularization comes from data published by West et al.[96] They investigated 67 cases of prostate cancer, previously checked for the expression of FGF-8, for the expression of VEGF which is known to cooperate with the FGF-system to facilitate angiogenesis in a synergistic manner. A significant association was found between tumor VEGF and FGF-8 expression, indicating a tumor and possibly angiogenesis promoting activity of FGF-8.

With the exception of FGF-13 and -18 no data are available supporting a role of FGF-9 to -23, in vessel growth.

FGF-13 was shown to induce cell growth of lung fibroblasts and aortic smooth muscle cells but had no effect on dermal vascular endothelial cells, making it difficult to decide on its angiogenic properties.[97]

FGF-18 was cloned in 1999.[98] It is most homologous to FGF-8 and expressed primarily in the heart, skeletal muscle, and pancreas as well as, at much lower levels, in other tissues and in certain cancer cell lines. When transfected in mammalian cells, FGF-18 is secreted due to its typical secretion sequence. The fact that recombinant protein stimulates proliferation of NIH3T3 cells in a dose-dependent manner suggest that FGF-18 acts as a typical growth factor. Its localization in certain tumor cell lines points to possible role in tumor invasion and metastasis, driven by neovascularization.

Although a lot of data are available on the role of FGFs in general, little is known about the role of individual FGFs in arteriogenesis. Current literature favors a function of FGF-2 in this process. However, our own results showed no reduction in arteriogenesis upon femoral artery ligation in FGF-2$^{-/-}$ mice (T. Ziegelhoeffer, unpublished). Interestingly, these mice showed an activation by increased phosphorylation of the FGFR-1 during the early phase of collateral artery growth, similar to that observed in wt mice upon femoral artery occlusion (M. Barancik, unpublished). From our studies we conclude that arteriogenesis is more dependent on the availability of the FGFR-1 that becomes activated exclusively within a limited time frame than on the presence of specific FGFs. We even hypothesize that individual FGFs might substitute for each other.

Acknowledgement

The authors would like to thank E. Neubauer, C. Ullmann and M. Granz for technical assistance.

References

1. YAMASHITA T, YOSHIOKA M, ITOH N. Identification of a novel fibroblast growth factor, FGF-23, preferentially expressed in the ventrolateral thalamic nucleus of the brain. *Biochem Biophys Res Comm.* 2000;277:494-498.
2. FOLKMAN J, KLAGSBRUN M. Angiogenic factors. *Science.* 1987;235:442-447.
3. KLEIN S, ROGHANI M, RIFKIN DB. Fibroblast growth factors as angiogenesis factors: new insights into their mechanism of action. *Exs.* 1997;79:159-92.
4. FERNIG DG, GALLAGHER JT. Fibroblast growth factors and their receptors: an information network controlling tissue growth, morphogenesis and repair. *Prog Growth Factor Res.* 1994;5:353-377.
5. PARTANEN J, VAINIKKA S, KORHONEN J, ARMSTRONG E, ALITALO K. Diverse receptors for fibroblast growth factors. *Prog Growth Factor Res.* 1992;4:69-83.
6. BURGESS WH, MEHLMAN T, MARSHAK DR, FRASER BA, MACIAG T. Structural evidence that endothelial cell growth factor beta is the precursor of both endothelial cell growth factor alpha and acidic fibroblast growth factor. *Proc Natl Acad Sci USA.* 1986;83:7216-20.
7. JAYE M, HOWK R, BURGESS W, RICCA GA, CHIU IM, RAVERA MW, O'BRIEN SJ, MODI WS, MACIAG T, DROHAN WN. Human endothelial cell growth factor: cloning, nucleotide sequence, and chromosome localization. *Science.* 1986;233:541-5.
8. BURGESS WH, MACIAG T. The heparin binding (Fibroblast growth factor) family proteins. *Ann Rev Biochem.* 1989;58:575-606.
9. NUGENT MA, IOZZO RV. Fibroblast growth factor-2. *Int J Biochem Cell Biol.* 2000;32:115-20.
10. OKADA-BAN M, THIERY JP, JOUANNEAU J. Fibroblast growth factor-2. *Int J Biochem Cell Biol.* 2000;32:263-7.
11. BAIRD A, ESCH F, MORMEDE P, UENO N, LING N, BOHLEN P, YING SY, WEHRENBERG WB, GUILLEMIN R. Molecular characterization of fibroblast growth factor: distribution and biological activities in various tissues. *Recent Prog Horm Res.* 1986;42:143-205.
12. GOSPODAROWICZ D, NEUFELD G, SCHWEIGERER L. Molecular and biological characterization of fibroblast growth factor, an angiogenic factor which also controls the proliferation and differentiation of mesoderm and neuroectoderm derived cells. *Cell Differ.* 1986;19:1-17.
13. CASSCELLS W, SPEIR E, SASSE J, KLAGSBRUN M, ALLEN P, LEE M, CALVO B, CHIBA M, HAGGROTH L, FOLKMAN J, EPSTEIN SE. Isolation, characterization, and localization of heparin-binding growth factors in the heart. *J Clin Invest.* 1990;85:433-441.

14. SPIRITO P, FU Y-M, YU Z-X, EPSTEIN SE, CASSCELLS W. Immunohistochemical localization of basic and acidic fibroblast growth factors in the developing rat heart. *Circulation.* 1991; 84:322-332.
15. MIMA T, UENO H, FISCHMAN DA, WILLIAMS LT, MIKAWA T. Fibroblast growth factor receptor is required for *in vivo* myocyte proliferation at early embryonic stages of heart development. *Proc Natl Acad Sci USA.* 1995;92:467-471.
16. QUINKLER W, MAASBERG M, BERNOTAT-DANIELOWSKI S, LUTHE N, SHARMA HS, SCHAPER W. Isolation of heparin-binding growth factors from bovine, porcine and canine hearts. *Eur J Biochem.* 1989;181:67-73.
17. SCHAPER W. Collateral vessel growth in the human heart - role of fibroblast growth factor-2. *Circulation.* 1996;94:600-601.
18. BERNOTAT-DANIELOWSKI S, SHARMA HS, SCHOTT RJ, SCHAPER W. Generation and localisation of monoclonal antibodies against fibroblast growth factors in ischaemic collateralised porcine myocardium. *Cardiovas Res.* 1993;27:1220-1228.
19. ENGELMANN GL, DIONNE CA, JAYE MC. Acidic fibroblast growth factor and heart development. Role in myocyte proliferation and capillary angiogenesis. *Circ Res.* 1993;72:7-19.
20. HARADA K, GROSSMAN W, FRIEDMAN M, EDELMAN ER, PRASAD PV, KEIGHLEY CS, MANNING WJ, SELLKE FW, SIMONS M. Basic fibroblast growth factor improves myocardial function in chronically ischemic porcine hearts. *J Clin Invest.* 1994;94:623-630.
21. LAZAROUS DF, SCHEINOWITZ M, SHOU M, HODGE E, RAJANAYAGAM MAS, HUNSBERGER S, ROBISON WG, STIBER JA, CORREA R, EPSTEIN SE, UNGER EF. Effects of chronic systemic administration of basic fibroblast growth factor on collateral development in the canine heart. *Circulation.* 1995;91:145-153.
22. HTUN P, ITO WD, HOEFER IE, SCHAPER J, SCHAPER W. Intramyocardial infusion of FGF-1 mimics ischemic preconditioning in pig myocardium. *J Mol Cell Cardiol.* 1998;30:867-877.
23. SCHUMACHER B, PECHER P, VON SPECHT BU, STEGMANN T. Induction of neoangiogenesis in ischemic myocardium by human growth factors: first clinical results of a new treatment of coronary heart disease. *Circulation.* 1998;97:645-650.
24. ROBINSON M, OVERBEEK P, VERRAN D, GRIZZLE W, STOCKARD C, FRIESEL R, MACIAG T, THOMPSON J. Extracellular FGF-1 acts as a lens differentiation factor in transgenic mice. *Development.* 1995;121:505-514.
25. FERNÁNDEZ B, BUEHLER A, WOLFRAM S, KOSTIN S, ESPANION G, FRANZ WM, NIEMANN H, DOEVENDANS PA, SCHAPER W, ZIMMERMANN R. Transgenic myocardial overexpression of fibroblast growth factor-1 increases coronary artery density and branching. *Circ Res.* 2000; 87:207-213.
26. STROHM C, BARANCIK M, VON BRUEHL M-L, KILIAN SAR, SCHAPER W. Inhibition of the ER-kinase cascade by PD98059 and UO126 counteracts ischemic preconditioning in pig myocardium. *J Cardiovasc Pharmacol.* 2000;36:216-229.
27. BUEHLER A, MARTIRE A, STROHM C, WOLFRAM S, FERNÁNDEZ B, PALMEN M, WEHRENS XHT, DOEVENDANS PA, FRANZ WM, SCHAPER W, ZIMMERMANN R. Angiogenesis-independent cardioprotection in FGF-1 transgenic mice. *Cardiovasc Res.* 2002;55:768-777.
28. MURPHY PR, KNEE RS. Identification and characterization of an antisense RNA transcript (gfg) from the human basic fibrobalst growth factor gene. *Mol Endocrinol.* 1994;8:852-859.
29. LI AW, TOO CKL, KNEE R, WILKINSON M, MURPHY PR. FGF-2 antisense RNA encodes a nuclear protein with MutT-like antimutator activity. *Mol Cell Endocrinol.* 1997;133:177-182.
30. LINDNER V. Role of basic fibroblast growth factor and platelet-derived growth factor (B-chain) in neointima formation after arterial injury. *Z Kardiol.* 1995;84:137-144.

31. LECONTE I, FOX JC, BALDWIN HS, BUCK CA, SWAIN JL. Adenoviral-mediated expression of antisense RNA to fibroblast growth factors disrupts murine vascular development. *Dev Dyn.* 1998;213:421-430.

32. SEGHEZZI G, PATEL S, REN CJ, GUALANDRIS A, PINTUCCI G, ROBBINS ES, SHAPIRO RL, GALLOWAY AC, RIFKIN DB, MIGNATTI P. Fibroblast growth factor-2 (FGF-2) induces vascular endothelial growth factor (VEGF) expression in the endothelial cells of forming capillaries: an autocrine mechanism contributing to angiogenesis. *J Cell Biol.* 1998;141:1659-1673.

33. LEE SH, SCHLOSS DJ, SWAIN JL. Maintenance of Vascular Integrity in the Embryo Requires Signaling through the Fibroblast Growth Factor Receptor. *J Biol Chem.* 2000;275:33679-33687.

34. KRANENBURG AR, DE BOER WI, VAN KRIEKEN HJM, MOOI WJ, WALTERS JE, SAXENA PR, STERK PJ, SHARMA HS. Enhanced expression of fibroblast growth factors and receptor FGFR-1 during vascular remodeling in chronic obstructive pulmonary disease. *Am J Respir Cell Mol Biol.* 2002;27:517-525.

35. CLASPER S, VEKEMANS S, FIORE M, PLEBANSKI M, WORDSWORTH P, DAVID G, JACKSON DG. Inducible expression of the cell surface heparan sulfate proteoglycan syndecan-2 (fibroglycan) on human activated macrophages can regulate fibroblast growth factor action. *J Biol Chem.* 1999;274:24113-24123.

36. CIZMECI-SMITH G, LANGAN E, YOUEKY J, SHOWALTER LJ, CAREY DJ. Syndecan-4 is a primary response gene induced by basic fibroblast growth factor and arterial injury in vascular smooth muscle cells. *Arterioscler Thromb Vasc Biol.* 1997;17:172-180.

37. WOODS A, COUCHMAN JR. Syndecans: synergistic activators of cell adhesion. *Trends Cell Biol.* 1998;8:189-192.

38. TUMOVA S, WOODS A, COUCHMAN JR. Heparan sulfate proteoglycans on the cell surface: versatile coordinators of cellular functions. *Int J Biochem Cell Biol.* 2000;32:269-288.

39. KNOX S, MERRY C, STRINGER S, MELROSE J, WHITELOCK J. Not all perlecans are created equal. Interactions with fibroblast growth factor (FGF) 2 and FGF receptors. *J Biol Chem.* 2002; 277:14657-14665.

40. PARSONS-WINGERTER P, ELLIOTT KE, CLARK JI, FARR AG. Fibroblast growth factor-2 selectively stimulates angiogenesis of small vessels in arterial tree. *Arterioscler Thromb Vasc Biol.* 2000;20:1250-1256.

41. BROGI E, WINKLES JA, UNDERWOOD R, CLINTON SK, ALBERTS GF, LIBBY P. Distinct patterns of expression of fibroblast growth factors and their receptors in human atheroma and nonatherosclerotic plaques. *J Clin Invest.* 1993;92:2408-2415.

42. HUGHES SE, CROSSMAN D, HALL PE. Expression of basic and acidic fibroblast growth factors and their receptors in normal and atherosclerotic human arteries. *Cardiovasc Res.* 1993;27:1214-1219.

43. XIN X, JOHNSON AD, SCOTT-BURDEN T, ENGLER D, CASSCELLS W. The predominant form of fibroblast growth factor receptor expressed by proliferating human arterial smooth muscle cells in culture is type I. *Biochem Biophys Res Commun.* 1994;204:557-564.

44. DEINDL E, HOEFER IE, FERNÁNDEZ B, BARANCIK M, HEIL M, STRNISKOVA M, SCHAPER W. Involvement of the fibroblast growth factor system in adaptive and chemokine-induced arteriogenesis. *Circ Res.* 2003;92:561-568.

45. VOLK R, SCHWARTZ JJ, LI J, ROSENBERG RD, SIMONS M. The role of syndecan cytoplasmic domain in basic fibroblast growth factor-dependent signal transduction. *J Biol Chem.* 1999;274:24417-24424.

46. COUCHMAN RC, WOODS A. Syndecan-4 and integrins: combinatorial in cell adhesion. *J Cell Sci.* 1999;112:3415-3420.

47. ARRAS M, STRASSER R, MOHRI M, DOLL R, ECKERT P, SCHAPER W, SCHAPER J. Tumor necrosis factor-alpha is expressed by monocytes/macrophages following coronary microemboliza-tion and is antagonized by cyclosporine. *Basic Res Cardiol.* 1998;93:97-107.

48. ARRAS M, ITO WD, SCHOLZ D, WINKLER B, SCHAPER J, SCHAPER W. Monocyte activation in angiogenesis and collateral growth in the rabbit hind limb. *J Clin Invest.* 1997;101:40-50.

49. SCHOLZ D, ITO W, FLEMING I, E. D, SAUER A, WIESNET M, BUSSE R, SCHAPER J, SCHAPER W. Ultrastructure and molecular histology of rabbit hind limb collateral artery growth (arte-riogenesis). *Virchows Arch.* 2000;436:257-270.

50. RHOADS DN, ESKIN SG, McINTIRE LV. Fluid flow releases fibroblast growth factor-2 from human aortic smooth muscle cells. *Arterioscler Thromb Vasc Biol.* 2000;20:416-421.

51. GLOE T, SOHN HY, MEININGER GA, POHL U. Shear stress-induced release of basic fibroblast growth factor from endothelial cells Is mediated by matrix interaction via integrin alpha Vbeta 3. *J Biol Chem.* 2002;277:23453-23458.

52. LIEKENS S, NEYTS J, DEGRÉVE B, DE CLERCQ E. The sulfonic acid polymers PAMPS [Poly(2-Acrylamido-2-Methyl-1-Propanesulfonoc Acid)] and related analogons are highly potent inhibitors of angiogenesis. *Oncology Res.* 1997;9:173-181.

53. ITO WD, ARRAS M, WINKLER B, SCHOLZ D, SCHAPER J, SCHAPER W. Monocyte chemotactic protein-1 increases collateral and peripheral conductance after femoral artery occlusion. *Circ Res.* 1997;80:829-837.

54. UENO H, LI J-J, MASUDA S, QI Z, YAMAMOTO H, TAKESHITA A. Adenovirus-mediated expres-sion of the secreted form of basic fibroblast growth factor (FGF-2) induces cellular prolif-eration and angiogenesis *in vivo. Arterioscler Thromb Vasc Biol.* 1997;17:2453-2460.

55. CAO R, BRAKENHIELM E, PAWLIUK R, WARIARO D, POST MJ, WAHLBERG E, LEBOULCH P, CAO Y. Angiogenic synergism, vascular stability and improvement of hind limb ischemia by a combination pf PDGF-BB and FGF-2. *Nat Med.* 2003;

56. SRIVASTAVA S, TERJUNG RL, YANG HT. Basic fibroblast growth factor increases collateral blood flow in spontaneously hypertensive rats. *Am J Physiol Heart Circ Physiol.* 2003; 285:H1190-1197.

57. SHANAHAN CM, CARY NRB, OSBOURN JK, WEISSBERG PL. Identification of osteoglycin as a component of the vascukar matrix. Differential expression during neointima formation and in atherosclerotic plaques. *Arterioscler Thromb Vasc Biol.* 1997;17:2437-2447.

58. KAMPMANN A, FERNÁNDEZ B, VON DER AHE D, SCHAPER W, ZIMMERMANN R. Changes in osteoglycin gene expression are linked to arteriogenesis. *J Mol Cell Cardiol.* 2001;33:A55.

59. DOUKAS J, BLEASE K, CRAIG D, MA C, CHANDLER LA, SOSNOWSKI BA, PIERCE GF. Delivery of FGF genes to wound repair cells enhances arteriogenesis and myogenesis in skeletal muscle. *Mol Therapy.* 2002;5:517-527.

60. COFFIN JD, FLORKIEWICZ RZ, NEUMANN J, MORT-HOPKINS T, DORN II GW, LIGHTFOOT P, GERMAN R, HOWLES PN, KIER A, O'TOOLE BA, SASSE J, GONZALEZ AM, BAIRD A, DOETSCHMAN T. Abnormal bone growth and slective translational regulation in basic fibroblast growth factor (FGF-2) transgenic mice. *Mol Biol Cell.* 1995;6:1861-1873.

61. FULGHAM DL, WIDHALM SR, MARTIN S, COFFIN JD. FGF-2 dependent angiogenesis is a latent phenotype in basic fibroblast growth factor transgenic mice. *Endothelium.* 1999;6:189-195.

62. STOLEN C, JACKSON M, GRIEP A. Overexpression of FGF-2 modulates fiber cell differentia-tion and survival in the mouse lens. *Development.* 1997;124:4009-4017.

63. SHEIKH F, SONTAG DP, FANDRICH RR, KARDAMI E, CATTINI PA. Overexpression of FGF-2 increases cardiac myocyte viability after injury in isolated mouse hearts. *Am J Physiol.* 2001;280:H1039-1050.

64. DONO R, TEXIDO G, DUSSEL R, EHMKE H, ZELLER R. Impaired cerebral cortex development and blood pressure regulation in FGF-2-deficient mice. *EMBO J.* 1998;17:4213-4225.

65. ORTEGA S, ITTMANN M, TSANG SH, EHRLICH M, BASILICO C. Neuronal defects and delayed wound healing in mice lacking fibroblast growth factor 2. *Proc Natl Acad Sci USA.* 1998; 95:5672-5677.

66. ZHOU M, SUTLIFF RL, PAUL RJ, LORENZ JN, HOYING JB, HAUDENSCHILD CC, YIN M, COFFIN JD, KONG L, KRANIAS EG, LUO W, BOIVIN GP, DUFFY JJ, PAWLOWSKI SA, DOETSCHMAN T. Fibroblast growth factor 2 control of vascular tone. *Nat Med.* 1998;4:201-207.

67. MONTERO A, OKADA Y, TOMITA M, ITO M, TSURUKAMI H, NAKAMURA T, DOETSCHMAN T, COFFIN JD, HURLEY MM. Disruption of the fibroblast growth factor-2 gene results in decreased bone mass and bone formation. *J Clin Invest.* 2000;105:1085-1093.

68. OKADA Y, MONTERO A, ZHANG X, SOBUE T, LORENZO J, DOETSCHMAN T, COFFIN JD, HURLEY MM. Impaired osteoclast formation in bone marrow cultures of FGF2 null mice in response to parathyroid hormone. *J Biol Chem.* 2003;278:21258-21266.

69. FOLETTI A, ACKERMANN J, SCHMIDT A, HUMMLER E, BEERMANN F. Absence of fibroblast growth factor 2 does not prevent tumor formation originating from the RPE. *Oncogene.* 2002;21:1841-1847.

70. MILLER DL, ORTEGA S, BASHAYAN O, BASCH R, BASILICO C. Compensation by fibroblast growth factor 1 (FGF1) does not account for the mild phenotypic defects observed in FGF2 null mice. *Mol Cell Biol.* 2000;20:2260-2268.

71. HYER J, JOHANSEN M, PRASAD A, WESSELS A, KIRBY ML, GOURDIE RG, MIKAWA T. Induction of Purkinje fiber differentiation by coronary arterialization. *Proc Natl Acad Sci USA.* 1999;96:13214-13218.

72. GOURDIE RG, WEI Y, KIM D, KLATT SC, MIKAWA T. Endothelin-induced conversion of embryonic heart muscle cells into impulse-conducting Purkinje fibers. *Proc Natl Acad Sci USA.* 1998;95:6815-6818.

73. COLEMAN-KRNACIK S, ROSEN J. Differential temporal and spatial gene expression of fibroblast growth factor family members during mouse mammary gland development. *Mol Endocrinol.* 1994;8:218-229.

74. COSTA M, DANESI R, AGEN C, DI PAOLO A, BASOLO F, DEL BIANCHI S, DEL TACCA M. MCF-10A cells infected with the int-2 oncogene induce angiogenesis in the chick chorioallantoic membrane and in the rat mesentery. *Cancer Res.* 1994;54:9-11.

75. DEROANNE C, HAJITOU A, CALBERG-BACQ C, NUSGENS B, LAPIERE C. Angiogenesis by fibroblast growth factor 4 is mediated through an autocrine up-regulation of vascular endothelial growth factor expression. *Cancer Res.* 1997;57:5590-5597.

76. MANSOUR S, GODDARD J, CAPECCHI M. Mice homozygous for a targeted disruption of the proto-oncogene int-2 have developmental defects in the tail and inner ear. *Development.* 1993;117:13-28.

77. JUNG M, KERN F, JORGENSEN T, MCLESKEY S, BLAIR O, DRITSCHILO A. Fibroblast growth factor-4 enhanced G2 arrest and cell survival following ionizing radiation. *Cancer Res.* 1994;54:5194-5197.

78. FUJIMOTO J, HORI M, ICHIGO S, TAMAYA T. Expressions of the fibroblast growth factor family (FGF-1,-2 and -4) mRNA in endometrial cancers. *Tumour Biol.* 1996;17:226-233.

79. JOUANNEAU J, MOENS G, MONTESANO R, THIERRY JP. FGF-1 but not FGF-4 secreted by carcinoma cells promotes *in vitro* and *in vivo* angiogenesis and rapid tumor proliferation. *Growth Factors.* 1995;12:37-47.

80. PARTRIDGE CR, HAWKER JR JR, FOROUGH R. Overexpression of a secretory isoform of FGF-1 promotes MMP-1-mediated endothelial cell migration. *J Cell Biochem.* 2000;78:487-499.

81. RISSANEN TT, MARKKANEN JE, ARVE K, RUTANEN J, KETTUNEN MI, VAJANTO I, JAUHIAINEN S, CASHION L, GRUCHALA M, NARVANEN O, TAIPALE P, KAUPPINEN RA, RUBANYI GM, YLA-HERTTUALA S. Fibroblast growth factor-4 induces vascular permeability, angiogenesis, and arteriogenesis in a rabbit hind limb ischemia model. *FASEB J.* 2002;02-0377fje.

82. FELDMAN B, POUEYMIROU W, PAPAIOANNOU VE, DECHIARA TM, GOLDFARB M. Requirement of FGF-4 for postimplantation mouse development. *Science.* 1995;267:246-249.

83. HÉBERT JM, ROSENQUIST T, GOETZ J, MARTIN GR. FGF5 as a regulator of the hair growth cycle: evidence from targeted and spontaneous mutations. *Cell.* 1994;78:1017-1025.

84. GIORDANO FJ, PING P, MCKIRNAN MD, NOZAKI S, DEMARIA AN, DILLMANN WH, MATHIEU-COSTELLO O, HAMMOND HK. Intracoronary gene transfer of fibroblast growth factor-5 increases blood flow and contractile function in an ischemic region of the heart. *Nat Med.* 1996;2:534-539.

85. SCHNEEBERGER SA, HJELMELAND LM, TUCKER RP, MORSE LS. Vascular endothelial growth factor and fibroblast growth factor 5 are colocalized in vascular and avascular epiretinal membranes. *Am J Ophthalmol.* 1997;124:447-454.

86. PIZETTE S, BATOZ M, PRATS H, BIRNBAUM D, COULIER F. Production and functional characterization of human recombinant FGF-6 protein. *Cell Growth Differ.* 1991;2:561-566.

87. SCHOLZ D, ZIEGELHOEFFER T, HELISCH A, WAGNER S, FRIEDRICH C, PODZUWEIT T, SCHAPER W. Contribution of arteriogenesis and angiogenesis to postocclusive hind limb perfusion in mice. *J Mol Cell Cardiol.* 2002;34:775-787.

88. DELAPEYRIERE O, OLLENDORFF V, PLANCHE J, OTT M, PIZETTE S, COULIER F, BIRNBAUM D. Expression of the FGF6 gene is restricted to developing skeletal muscle in the mouse embryo. *Development.* 1993;118:601-611.

89. FLOSS T, ARNOLD H-H, BRAUN T. A role for FGF-6 in skeletal muscle regeneration. *Genes Dev.* 1997;11:2040-2051.

90. FIORE F, PLANCHE J, GIBIER P, SEBILLE A, DELAPEYRIERE O, BIRNBAUM D. Apparent normal phenotype of FGF6-/- mice. *Int J Dev Biol.* 1997;41:639-642.

91. SHARMA B, HANDLER M, EICHSTETTER I, WHITELOCK JM, NUGENT MA, IOZZO RV. Antisense Targeting of Perlecan Blocks Tumor Growth and Angiogenesis *In Vivo. J Clin Invest.* 1998;102:1599-1608.

92. TILSON MD, FU C, XIA SX, SYN D, YOON Y, MCCAFFREY T. Expression of molecular messages for angiogenesis by fibroblasts from aneurysmal abdominal aorta dermal fibroblasts. *Int J Surg Investig.* 2000;1:453-457.

93. WERNER S, PETERS K, LONGAKER M, FULLER-PACE F, BANDA M, WILLIAMS L. Large Induction of Keratinocyte Growth Factor Expression in the Dermis During Wound Healing. *Proc Natl Acad Sci USA.* 1992;89:6896-6900.

94. GUO L, DEGENSTEIN L, FUCHS E. Keratinocyte growth factor is required for hair development but not for wound healing. *Genes Dev.* 1996;10:165-175.

95. MATTILA MMT, RUOHOLA JK, VALVE EM, TASANEN MJ, SEPPAENEN JA, HAERKOENEN PL. FGF-8b increases angiogenic capacity and tumor growth of androgen-regulated S115 breast cancer cells. *Oncogene.* 2001;20:2791-2804.

96. WEST AF, O'DONNELL M, CHARLTON RG, NEAL DE, LEUNG HY. Correlation of vascular endothelial growth factor expression with fibroblast growth factor-8 expression and clinico-pathologic parameters in human prostate cancer. *Br J Cancer.* 2001;85:576-583.

97. LEUNG KH, PIPALLA V, KREUTTER A, CHANDLER M. Functional effects of FGF-13 on human lung fibroblasts, dermal microvascular endothelial cells, and aortic smooth muscle cells. *Biochem Biphys Res Comm.* 1998;250:137-142.

98. HU MC-T, WANG Y, QIU WR. Human fibroblast growth factor-18 stimulates fibroblast cell proliferation and is mapped to chromosome 14p11. *Oncogene.* 1999;18:2635-2642.

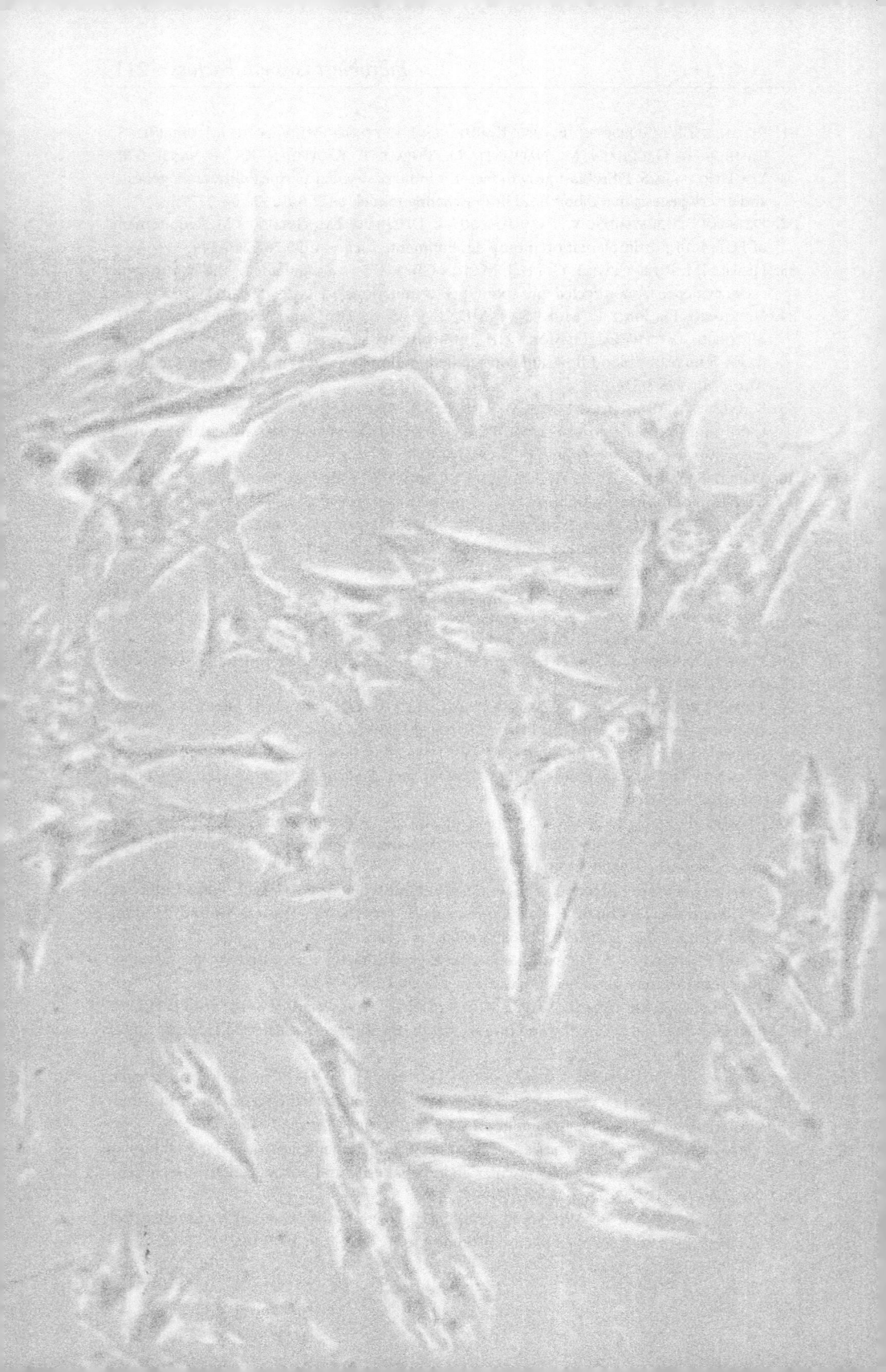

Chapter 11

Signal Transduction Pathways in Smooth Muscle Cells

Sabina Vogel, Thomas Kubin, Miroslav Barancik,
Elisabeth Deindl, Dietmar von der Ahe and
René Zimmermann

Phenotypic modulation of vascular smooth muscle cells

Vascular smooth muscle cells (SMCs) form the backbone of functioning arteries and play an indispensable role in the development of collateral vessels. They possess a high degree of plasticity in terms of their ability to respond to different growth factors. In addition to blood vessel development, various physiological processes including injury response and vascular remodeling all require SMC proliferation. Their role has been extensively studied, particularly in the pathophysiology of vascular diseases associated with excessive and accelerated SMC proliferation and migration. SMCs mediate these versatile cellular responses by inducing autocrine and paracrine growth mechanisms.

SMCs in the arterial vessel wall display morphological, phenotypical and functional heterogeneity. There is substantial evidence that certain medial SMCs are particularly prone to replicate and accumulate within the intima in response to appropriate stimuli.[1-3] It is, however, unclear if this heterogeneity is due to spatio-temporal differences in expression of differentiation markers or to differences in origin, as shown for normal and atherosclerotic aorta.[4]

It has been described that two distinct SMC populations coexist in the rat arterial media: spindle-shaped SMCs (S-SMCs) and epitheloid SMCs, both exhibiting different biological features.[5] Recently, the notion of SMC heterogeneity has been extended to a porcine coronary artery model and, therefore, to a well-accepted model for human atherosclerosis and restenosis.[6] Similar to the porcine arterial media the presence of two populations of SMCs was demonstrated in the normal media of the porcine coronary artery. Spindle-shaped (S-SMCs) display a classic "hill-and-valley" growth pattern at confluence and clearly express the 4 differentiation markers smooth muscle myosin heavy chain (SMMHC), smoothelin, desmin and α-smooth muscle actin. Furthermore, they switch their phenotype to rhomboid SMCs when co-cultured with endothelial cells. In contrast, rhomboid SMCs (R-SMCs) grow rapidly as a monolayer but cease to proliferate at confluence. They display higher migratory activity compared to S-SMCs, which is associated with an increased urokinase-plasminogen activator (u-PA) activity. In contrast to S-SMCs, R-SMCs express no desmin or smoothelin but some α-smooth muscle actin and SMMHC type 2. Upon co-culture with endothelial cells, R-SMCs proliferation increased but no change in phenotype was observed.[6]

When SMCs were isolated from stent-induced intimal thickening instead of normal media, R-SMCs were recovered maximally, indicating that this sub-population predominantly participates in intimal thickening formation *in vivo* [6]. This is in accordance with the finding that R-SMCs display low levels of differentiation markers while showing high proliferative and migratory activity.[6]

There is also some evidence that SMCs do not necessarily require growth factors for proliferation. Cell cycle entry in response to mechanical forces such as cyclic strain, stretch and shear stress has been extensively studied but yielded controversial results as discussed below.

Activation of bovine or rat aortic SMCs by cyclic strain led to an enhanced proliferation[7,8] and this phenomenon was not mediated by PKC or PKA activity[7] but rather by activated p70S6K in bovine[9] and p38 in rat SMCs.[8] On the contrary, cyclic strain decreased the proliferation of porcine aortic SMCs,[10] suggesting that SMC responsiveness to cyclic strain varies significantly depending on the species under study. Oscillatory shear stress, which corresponds to turbulent flow pattern in vessels, augmented DNA-synthesis rate in cultured bovine aortic SMCs,[11] similarly as cyclic stretch, which also increased the number of proliferating SMCs.[12] However, opposing results have been provided by Sterpetti et al., who showed that increasing shear stress hindered SMC proliferation.[13] This is in agreement with findings obtained in the *in vivo* baboon graft model where elevated shear stress induced neointimal regression in the grafts, resulting from decreased SMC proliferation and increased apoptosis.[14]

Collateral growth is associated with profound phenotypic modulation of SMCs, i.e., the change from the contractile to the synthetic phenotype. Changes in morphological appearance include myofilament disassembly and their replacement by a widespread endoplasmic reticulum and abundant Golgi complex.[15,16] The increase in synthetic cellular organelles correlates with an augmented capacity to synthesize proteins and lipids required for cellular proliferation, migration and secretory activity.

Although the mechanisms behind the transition of the SMCs from a contractile to a synthetic phenotype are not completely understood, it has been hypothesized that the process is at least in part a consequence of alterations in the cellular environment, including extracellular matrix, growth factor expression and lipid composition. Hedin et al. postulated that the basement membrane (comprising laminin, collagen type IV, and heparan sulfate proteoglycans), which usually surrounds the SMCs, favours the contractile phenotype.[17] Following its destruction, plasma and fibronectin come into closer contact with SMCs to promote their conversion into the synthetic phenotype. In the neointima of growing collateral vessels that contain numerous SMCs of the synthetic phenotype high amounts of collagen VI and fibronectin have been reported[18], which would confirm Hedin's assumption.

In addition to qualitative changes including the reorganization of contractile and cytoskeletal proteins within the cell, the modulation from contractile to synthetic phenotype is associated with a significant quantitative change in expression of structural proteins. Expression of α-smooth muscle actin, SMMHC, calponin and desmin is present in differentiated SMCs but significantly diminished in the de-differentiated state (reviewed by [19]). This is confirmed by our own study showing the modified SMCs of the neointima of growing arteries are characterized by reduced amounts of α-smooth muscle actin and vinculin, almost no desmin and calponin but abundant vimentin.[18]

Further hallmarks of the transition are the early rise in expression of the transcription factors c-jun, c-fos, and ets-1, as well as a sustained increase in matrix metalloproteinases (MMPs) and osteopontin gene expression. An elevated expression of the PDGF-A chain and PDGFRα was also observed [20]. In growing collaterals, MMP-2 and MMP-9 were highly expressed in addition to being activated.[21] Phenotypic modulation is further supported by kinase activation, whereby ERK1/2 phosphorylation[22] and focal adhesion kinase seem to play a predominant role.[23]

The molecular mechanisms of signal transduction behind phenotypic modulation of SMCs have been investigated to some extent. Hayashi et al. studied the signaling pathways triggered by IGF-I involved in the maintenance of the differentiated phenotype of vascular SMCs in culture, and compared them with those elicited by PDGF-BB, FGF-2 and EGF which trigger SMC dedifferentiation.[24] They demonstrated that PDGF-BB, FGF-2 and EGF activated the MAP kinases ERK1/2 and p38 which play an essential role in dedifferentiation of SMCs. IGF-I, however, failed to activate these two MAP kinases, but triggered the PI3K/Akt pathway, indicating that this pathway is critical in maintaining the differentiated state. Interestingly, PDGF-BB, in addition to stimulating ERK1/2 and p38, also activated the PI3K/Akt cascade, suggesting that changes in the balance between the strength of the PI3K/Akt pathway and the ERK and p38 MAPK pathways are likely to be the determinant of the phenotype of vascular SMCs.

Growth factors of the FGF and PDGF family have been implicated in multiple aspects of vascular development. So far at least 5 isoforms of PDGF have been identified, consisting of disulphide-bound homodimers and heterodimers of A, B, C and D chains. Studies using mice deficient either for PDGF or PDGF receptor genes confirmed the utmost importance of these genes in lung, kidney, blood vessel, and CNS development. In adults, PDGFs stimulate cardiac angiogenesis,[25] regulate the structural integrity of blood vessels by promoting the recruitment of pericytes,[26] and, being potent inducers of SMC proliferation and migration, have a crucial function in vascular pathophysiology (reviewed by [27]).

The family of FGFs comprises at least 23 distinct family members, involved in mitogenic, chemotactic and angiogenic responses in cells of mesodermal and neuroectodermal origin (discussed in detail in chapter 10).[28]

So far, it has been demonstrated that exogenous administration of

FGF-1, FGF-2 and, to some extent, FGF-4 increased the number of arteries and improved blood flow, demonstrating that these factors are highly potent in arteriogenesis.[29-31] The data, however, regarding the role of FGFs and PDGFs in SMCs during collateral growth (arteriogenesis) are far from being complete. Thus, we focused our attention on the actions of FGF-2 on SMCs and compared them with those elicited by one of the PDGF family member, PDGF-AB.

Porcine aortic SMCs in culture as a model system for arteriogenesis

To obtain more insight into the proliferative mechanisms and signaling events in SMCs during the process of arteriogenesis, SMCs from porcine aortic tissue were isolated and stimulated with growth factors FGF-2 or PDGF-AB from 10 minutes to 24 hours for studying signaling pathways and up to 7d to elucidate morphological and phenotypical changes (Fig. 1). To exclude contamination with other cell types, the expression of smooth muscle specific marker proteins such as α-smooth muscle actin, tropomyosin and desmin was tested by immunostaining and FACS analysis. As a measure of proliferative activity, DNA-synthesis induction was determined by $3^{[H]}$ thymidine incorporation. To assess the phosphorylation and activation of signaling pathway components in response to these growth factors, Western blot analysis using phospho-specific antibodies was performed. Egr1 expression was analyzed by means of Northern and Western blotting.

Control

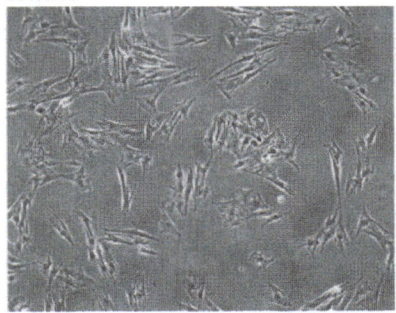

Fig. 1a

PDGF-AB

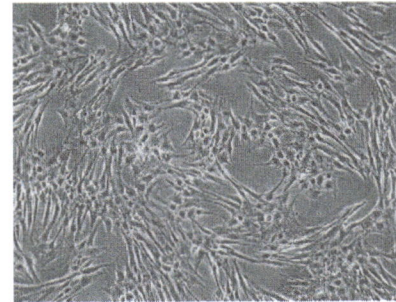

Fig. 1b

FGF-2

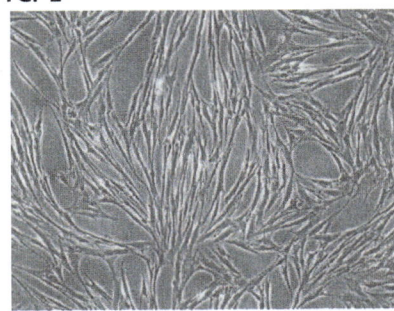

Fig. 1c

Phase contrast micrograph of SMCs in culture after stimulation with PDGF-AB (1b) or FGF-2 (1c) for 7 days. Stimulation of SMCs with these mitogens augments the cell number and leads to morphological/phenotypical changes compared to untreated controls (1a).

Growth factors of the FGF and PDGF family bind to their corresponding membrane-associated receptors, which belong to a family of receptor tyrosine kinases (RTKs). The catalytic activity of the receptor kinase is significantly increased by phosphorylation of a specific, conserved tyrosine residue in the catalytic domain of the receptor.

The autophosphorylation of tyrosine residues outside the catalytic domain creates docking sites for signal transduction molecules. The interaction between FGF and PDGF receptors with down-stream signaling effectors occurs predominantly through a specific domain termed Src homology 2 (SH2) domain harbored in downstream effector molecules.

Four members of the FGF receptor family have been described and termed FGFR1-FGFR4. FGF-2 preferentially binds to FGFR1, which itself is the predominant FGFR form expressed by proliferating SMCs.[32] FGFR1 is, therefore, the likely candidate to mediate signal transduction in FGF-2-stimulated SMCs, whereby phosphorylation of tyrosine residues 653 and 654 activates the kinase domain of the receptor. In addition, FGFR1 activation was detected in growing collateral vessels in the rabbit model of femoral artery occlusion.[33]

In our hands, FGF-2 stimulation led to a pronounced increase in receptor activation within 2 minutes.

Members of the PDGF growth factor family display their function by binding to PDGFRα and PDGFRβ. PDGFRβ was shown to be expressed on the surface of SMCs.[34] Since PDGF-AB binds with high affinity to αβ-receptor heterodimers, we analyzed the temporal phosphorylation pattern of PDGFRβ. Stimulation of SMCs with PDGF-AB did not increase the total amount of the PDGFRβ but led to a rapid phosphorylation of a conserved residue, Tyr857, which was described to be essential for receptor activation.[35] Within 2 minutes of stimulation the receptor reached its peak activation, followed by a rapid decrease towards control value after 10 minutes. Receptor phosphorylation as well as the activation of downstream signaling mediators ERK1/2 and Akt in response to both factors was efficiently counteracted by RTK inhibitor genistein.

Co-transcription factor Egr1 was found to be up-regulated in growing collateral vessels after femoral artery occlusion in mice. Differential expression of this factor in the very early phase of collateral growth (mRNA was up-regulated 6 and 12 hours, the protein 24 hours following occlusion) points to a role for this gene during the initial stage of arteriogenesis. Strong immunostaining was found in endothelial cells and some smooth muscle cells of arterioles including collateral arteries, however, not in veins or capillaries. Furthermore, some staining in nerves and very rarely in myocyte nuclei was observed. Mutational analysis of putative transcription factor binding sites in the Egr-1 promoter revealed that the activation of Egr-1 in response to shear stress is predominantly mediated by three serum response elements located upstream of the transcriptional start site.[36] Studies by Lowe and co-workers using DNAzymes provided clear evidence that abrogation of Egr1 expression significantly inhibited SMC proliferation and their response to vascular injury.[37] Since SMCs play a pivotal role in the process of arteriogenesis, we investigated whether stimulation of cultured SMCs with FGF-2 or PDGF-AB also triggers Egr1 induction. Whereas Egr1 expression proved to be poor in quiescent porcine aortic SMCs, both mRNA and protein levels of Egr1 were highly increased within 1 hour of stimulation with FGF-2 or PDGF-AB. Egr1 expression was not only rapid but also of a transient nature since the transcript vanished by 2 hours. This could be due to the subsequent binding of transcription factors, which downregulate the transcription of this gene or raises the possibility of a rapid mRNA degradation by an enzyme.

To define key signaling mediators of FGF- and PDGF-induced mitogenesis and Egr1 expression, the activation of an array of signaling pathways was analyzed (Fig. 2). The proliferative response in many cell types depends on the activation of the Ras-Raf-MEK-ERK signaling module. This cascade is employed ubiquitously in the transduction of growth and differentiation signals from RTKs and G-protein coupled receptors.

In adult porcine SMCs, MEK displayed a rapid and transient pattern of activation in response to both factors, returning to control levels after approximately 10 minutes. This was followed by a strong activation of ERK1/2, which decreased gradually over 12 hours. Furthermore, both growth factors increased the phosphorylation of transcription factor c-Myc, which, after being activated, transactivates genes predominantly involved in cellular proliferation and differentiation.[38,39] This activation culminated within 10 minutes of stimulation and decreased to control level after 20 minutes, thus correlating with previous findings that this nuclear phosphoprotein has a short life-span. Transcriptional induction of c-Myc did not occur during this initial stage of growth factor stimulation.

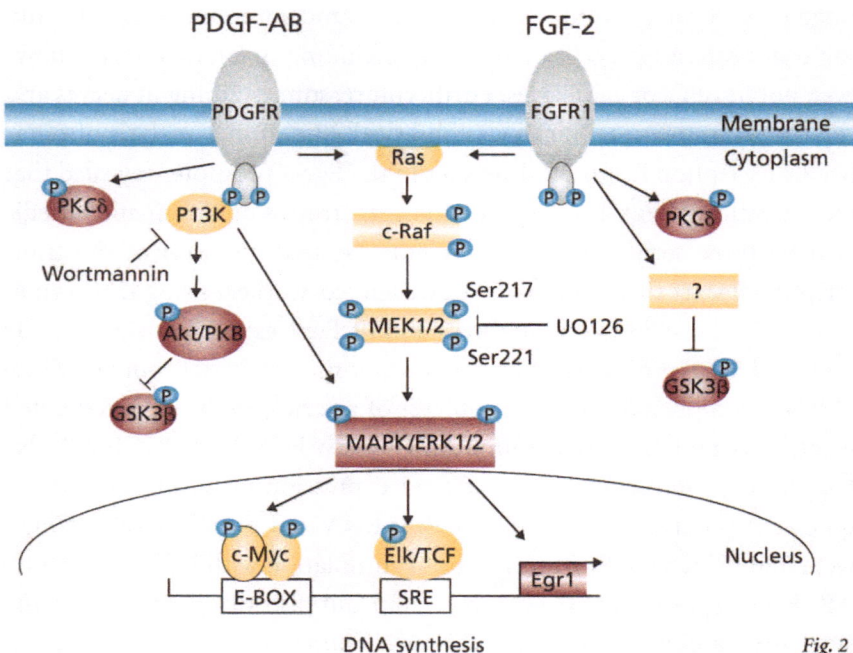

Fig. 2

DNA synthesis

Schematic presentation to summarise the network of signaling pathways elicited by PDGF-AB or FGF-2 in proliferating vascular SMCs. The figure also depicts the regulatory mechanisms of Egr1 expression in this particular cell type.

Apart from the already described ERK1/2 (p44/p42), two additional kinases of the MAPK family were demonstrated to be implicated in various cellular responses: SAPK/JNK and p38. Both kinases control cellular responses to cytokines and stress[40-42] and to some extent to growth factors. Previous studies demonstrated that these two kinases also participate in signaling cascades initiated by FGF and PDGF.[24,43,44]

We were interested whether these kinases acquire an activation status when SMCs were stimulated with FGF-2 or PDGF-AB. In porcine aortic SMCs no activation of these kinases could be detected either in response to FGF-2 or PDGF-AB between 10 minutes and 24 hours. Significant divergence may, however, exist between different animal species. In support of this notion, Yamaguchi et al. showed that in rat aortic SMCs signaling of all PDGF isoforms depends on p38 activation, but also found no indication for SAPK/JNK involvement.[44]

Protein kinase C (PKC) plays a central role in signal transduction, cellular growth and differentiation.[45] The family of structurally related PKC isoforms can be classified into three subfamilies based on their Ca2$^+$ and phorbol ester sensitivities. We differentiate between classical PKCs (α, β, γ), novel PKCs (δ, ϵ, η, θ), and atypical PKCs (ζ, ι, λ).[46] In many cell types, the mitogenic effects of FGF and PDGF are dependent on PKC activation, but which PKC isoforms are involved, particularly in SMCs, remains to be elucidated.

We analyzed the activation status of various classical, novel and atypical PKC isoforms within the time frame of 10 minutes to 12 hours. Our results revealed that only novel isoforms PKCδ and PKCθ were phosphorylated in SMCs upon stimulation with FGF-2 or PDGF-AB. Interestingly, although being rapidly activated, the PKCδ and PKCθ activity did not return to control levels even after 12 hours, suggesting that cross-regulation with other signaling molecules may determine the response outcome.

We further focused our interest on the PI3K/Akt cascade, which takes a central place in intracellular signaling events ranging from growth, differentiation, chemotaxis, and actin reorganization to anti-apoptosis (reviewed in [47]). To assess the involvement of this cascade in FGF-2- and PDGF-AB-induced mitogenesis of SMCs, activation of PKB/Akt was analyzed.

Our studies demonstrated that in SMCs only PDGF-AB induced rapid activation of PKB/Akt with concomitant phosphorylation of an important downstream target, GSK3β. Peak levels at 10 minutes were followed by a continuous decrease towards basal level after 12 hours. In FGF-2-stimulated SMCs no PKB/Akt activation was observable at any time point tested. Interestingly though, FGF-2 phosphorylated GSK3β in the same manner as PDGF-AB. These findings suggest different regulatory mechanisms of GSK3β inactivation in SMCs depending on the initial proliferative stimulus.

To examine the contribution of individual signaling pathways to SMC proliferation and Egr1 expression, specific inhibitors of particular key molecules were used. The most common way to inhibit the Ras-Raf-MEK-ERK cascade in living cells is to block the key mediator MEK. Two specific inhibitors of MEK, UO126 and PD98059, have been successfully used both in *in vitro* and *in vivo* systems. Preincubation of SMCs with UO126 prevented the phosphorylation of components ERK1/2 (Fig. 3) and c-Myc. In the presence of UO126, growth factor stimulated SMCs

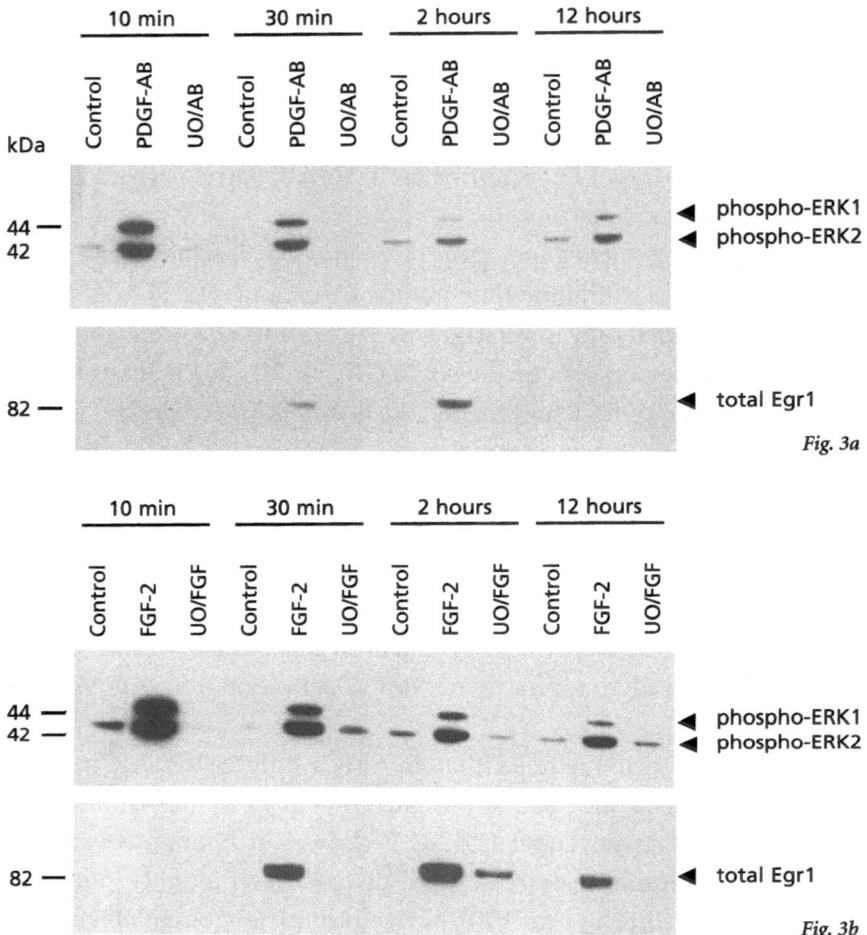

Western blot analysis of ERK1/2 phosphorylation and Egr1 protein expression in response to PDGF-AB (3a) or FGF-2 (3b). Pre-treatment of SMCs with 10μM UO126, a specific in-hibitor of MEK, abolished ERK1 and ERK2 phosphorylation induced by PDGF-AB or FGF-2 (upper panel in 3a and 3b) and counteracted the transcriptional induction of Egr1 (lower panel in 3a and 3b). Note that the effect of FGF-2 on ERK1/2 phos-phorylation and Egr1 ex-pression is more pronounced compared to PDGF-AB. Abbreviations: AB=PDGF-AB; FGF= FGF-2; UO=UO126

ceased to proliferate as evidenced by a complete abolishment of the DNA-synthesis rate. Finally, induction of Egr1 expression was counter-acted by this MEK inhibitor, suggesting that this particular signaling cas-cade plays a pivotal role in inducing DNA synthesis and Egr1 expression in FGF-2- or PDGF-AB-stimulated SMCs (Fig. 3).

MEK itself, however, became highly phosphorylated in the presence of UO126, an effect that lasted for several hours. The intensity of these phosphorylation signals exceeded by far those observed with growth factor stimulation alone. The specificity of this hyper-phosphorylation effect was confirmed by means of PD98059. Furthermore, inhibitor induced hyper-phosphorylation of MEK was not an artefact of SMCs but was also detected in vascular endothelial and microvascular endothelial cells. The fact that MEK inhibition by UO126 and PD98059 closely correlates with its hyper-phosphorylation is an important finding because it demonstrates that a phosphorylation is not only a necessary prerequisite for kinase activation but also for its inhibition.

To obtain more insight into the role of the PI3K/Akt cascade in pro-life-rating SMCs, PI3K was inactivated by wortmannin. In PDGF-AB-stimulated cells wortmannin abolished PKB/Akt and GSK3β phosphorylation, i.e., inactivation. In FGF-2-stimulated SMCs wortmannin had no inhibitory effect on GSK3β phosphorylation. These results demonstrate that whereas the classical PI3K/Akt cascade is utilized to inactivate GSK3β in PDGF-AB stimulated SMCs, other signaling molecules are required to mediate this effect when FGF-2 is the proliferative stimulus for SMCs.

Experiments using wortmannin provided an important finding that the inhibition of the PI3K/Akt cascade also leads to induction of Egr1 expression. Exposure of cells to wortmannin followed by a long term stimulation with PDGF-AB (14–24 hours) resulted in a dramatic increase of ERK1/2 activity with concomitant up-regulation of Egr1. This indicates that the loss of PI3K signaling switches the cellular response towards the mitogenic Ras pathway. We aimed to determine the consequence of this switch on DNA-synthesis induction but obtained controversial results. One set of experiments (performed in triplicates) demonstrated a clear increase in DNA-synthesis rate when SMCs were pre-incubated with wortmannin, whereas in the second experimental set wortmannin did not influence the level of DNA synthesis. Since inhibition of PI3K counteracts the survival processes, this discrepancy may result from the balance between apoptotic and proliferative responses. It is also tempting to speculate that some not yet identified factor(s) may influence this balance in our model system.

In addition to porcine aortic SMCs, evidence for a similar cross-regulation between the PI3K/Akt and the Ras-Raf-MEK-ERK signaling cascades has been reported in rat neonatal SMCs.[48]

Apart from identifying signaling pathways we tested the influence of FGF-2 and PDGF-AB on desmin expression. One of the early hallmarks of arteriogenesis is the loss of this intermediate filament protein in phenotypically modulated SMCs of the neointima of growing collateral arteries.[18] We observed a similar effect in cultured SMCs stimulated with FGF-2. The effect of PDGF-AB was modest by only 25 % downregulation, whereas FGF-2 dramatically diminished the level of desmin by 80 % compared to controls.

Our results point to a close correlation between Egr1 expression and collateral growth. In an attempt to delineate the major signal transducers that activate the Egr1 promoter, we demonstrated the complete abolishment of Egr1 expression by UO126, indicating that the Ras-Raf-MEK-ERK cascade plays the predominant role in the transcriptional induction of this factor in FGF-2- and PDGF-AB-stimulated SMCs. In contrast to endothelial cells, in SMCs SAPK/JNK and p38 are not likely to be involved. Switching the response from the PI3K-initiated cascade to the mitogenic Ras module provides an additional pathway of inducing Egr1 promoter activity.

The MAP kinase pathway was potently activated in FGF-2- or PDGF-AB-treated SMCs as shown by the phosphorylation of prominent members MEK, ERK1/2 and c-Myc. Inhibition of MEK correlated with the inhibition of ERK1/2 and c-Myc phosphorylation and, importantly, with the inhibition of DNA-synthesis, suggesting a crucial role of the Ras-Raf-MEK-ERK signaling cascade in mediating proliferative events in porcine SMCs.

Important links between the MEK/ERK pathway and the cell cycle machinery is the induction of cyclin D1 expression[49], activation of carbamoyl phosphate synthetase II (CPSII), the key regulatory enzyme of *de novo* pyrimidine nucleotide synthesis[50] as well as enhancement of protein synthesis by ERK1/2. Furthermore, ERK1/2 facilitate gene transcription by directly phosphorylating transcription factors c-jun, c-fos and c-Myc or by modifying chromatin structure.[51] Finding ways to influence and regulate this pathway would provide a valuable therapeutic tool in the clinical management of excessive SMC proliferation correlating with several pathological disorders.

The PI3K/Akt signaling cascade represents a cellular pathway impli-cated in a wide range of cellular functions ranging from proliferation to anti-apoptosis. In vascular SMCs, FGF-2 and PDGF-AB display distinct effects on the activation of this pathway. Whereas PDGF-AB triggered a rapid and long lasting activation of Akt, this effect was completely absent when cells were stimulated with FGF-2. Importantly, however, both fac-tors led to a phosphorylation and therefore inactivation of GSK3β, which is an essential step towards Cyclin D1 stabilisation and cell cycle entry.[52] Since both PDGF-AB and FGF-2 are potent mitogens for SMCs, it is not surprising that their action consists in the inactivation of those molecules that would attenuate proliferative responses. In studies using wortmannin we demonstrated that PDGF-AB utilises the classical PI3K pathway to inac-tivate GSK3β, whereas FGF-2 transmits the signal most likely via p70S6K.

Nevertheless, the experiments with UO126 do not lead to the conclu-sion that the prime importance of the PI3K/Akt pathway in our system lies in the mediation of proliferative signals. This role should rather be at-tributed to the Ras mitogenic signaling because the PI3K signaling could not compensate the abolishment of DNA synthesis by UO126. The MAPK pathway seems to act in a "conditio sine qua non" fashion, orchestrating downstream events required for smooth muscle cell cycle entry. Although cell viability was seriously impaired in SMCs treated with wortmannin, the role of PI3K/Akt in our model is not likely to be restricted solely to survival regulation and suppression of apoptotic effects. Rather, PI3K/Akt were shown to regulate important aspects of glycogen metabolism by inhibiting GSK3β,[53] protein synthesis by indirectly activating eIF2B,[54] and energy-dependent processes, all of them contributing to prepare cells for passing the restrictive proliferative points. Furthermore, PI3K signaling influences changes in cytoskeletal organisation.[55] It thereby contributes to the regulation of actin dynamics and cell movement, processes required for physiological migration of SMCs during arteriogenesis.[18]

Importantly, normal cell functioning depends on the fact that these signaling pathways never work in isolation; they are integrated in com-plex cellular networks and the final response represents an outcome of a cross-regulation of multiple, interconnected signaling molecules (Fig. 2).

In addition, using growth factors we simulated the arteriogenic behav-iour of cultured SMCs and found key similarities to the SMC responses during collateral growth. ERK1/2 activation (unpublished observations),

Egr1 expression and the drastic reduction in desmin amount are important features observed in growing collateral arteries. In our *in vitro* system we could demonstrate that particularly FGF-2 was very efficient in eliciting these responses. PDGF-AB effects were similar but less pronounced.

It is not surprising that FGF-2 simulated the arteriogenic SMC performance so convincingly. Given the fact that the corresponding receptor, FGFR1, was found to be up-regulated and activated early during arteriogenesis[33] and FGF-1 and FGF-2 clearly detected (although not differentially regulated) in collateral vessels, we assume a potential role for this growth factors in arteriogenesis *in vivo*. By contrast, PDGF receptors as well as the ligands were neither detected nor found to be up-regulated in growing collaterals (E. Deindl, unpublished). Although PDGF-AB proved to be an important mitogen for SMCs, exactly which contribution the PDGF family makes to the process of arteriogenesis is currently not clear.

However, recent studies in our laboratory using shear-stress stimulated collateral arteries showed activities very similar observed to those in SMC cultures: a marked constitutive activation of the RAS/ERK pathway but no activity of the JNK/SAPK and the p38 pathway. This is common to both the FGF-2 as well as to the PDGF-AB effects. However, the factors differ in that only FGF-2 strongly downregulates desmin and destrin, just like in SMC culture. The mild activation of Rho found in collateral vessels may be due to the direct stimulation by shear stress activated integrins. In conclusion, we can say that although FGF-2 may not be the only growth factor, it certainly plays a prominent part in the concerted action called arteriogenesis.

A summary of the findings described is presented in figure 4.

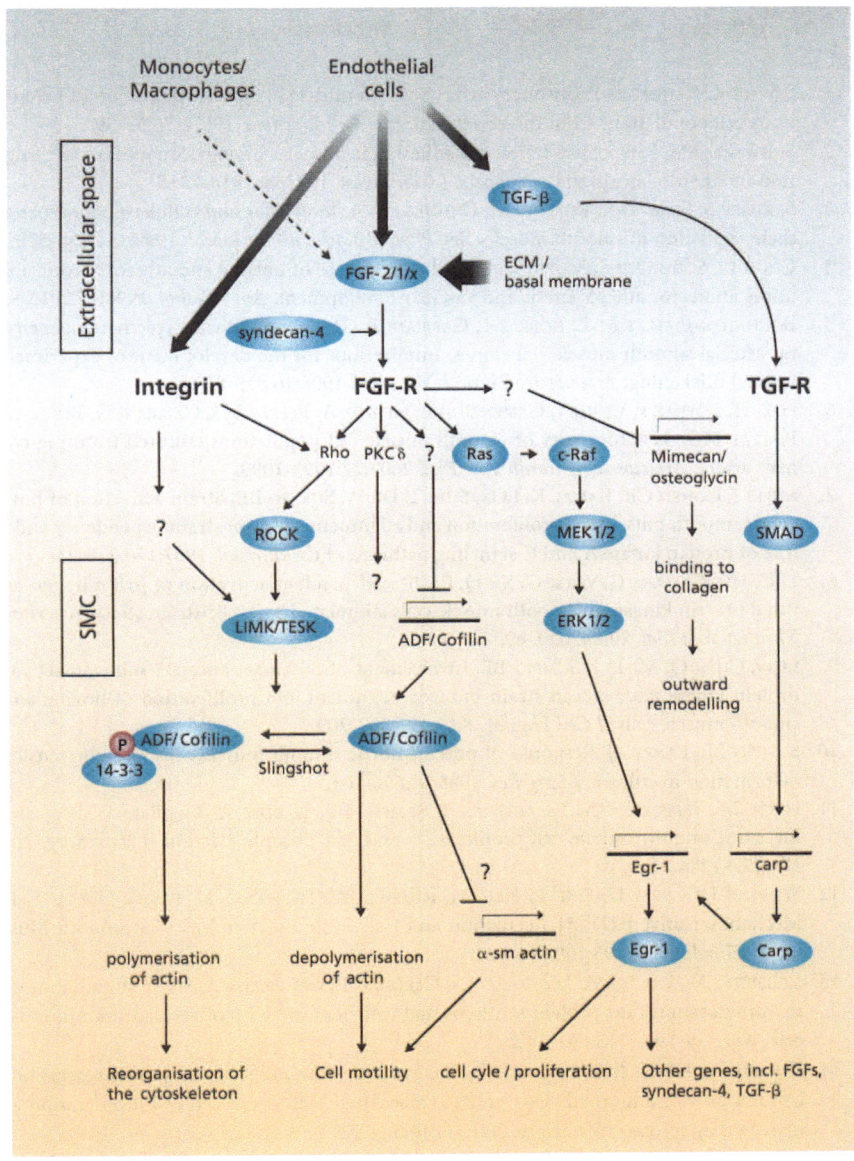

Fig. 4

Schematic representation of growth factor signaling pathways in smooth muscle cells during arteriogenesis/collateral growth.

References

1. SAWARD L, ZAHRADKA P. Coronary artery smooth muscle in culture: migration of heterogenous cell populations from the vessel wall. *Mol Cell Biochem.* 1997;176:53-59.
2. SCHWARTZ SM. Perspective series: cell adhesion in vascular biology. Smooth muscle migration in atherosclerosis and restenosis. *J Clin Invest.* 1997;99:2814-2816.
3. SARTORE S, FRANCH R, ROELOFS M, CHIAVEGATO A. Molecular and cellular phenotypes and their regulation in smooth muscle. *Rev Physiol Biochem Pharmacol.* 1999;134:235-320.
4. CHUNG I, SCHWARTZ S, MURRY C. Clonal architecture of normal and atherosclerotic aorta: implications for atherogenesis and vascular development. *Am J Pathol.* 1998;152:913-923.
5. BOCHATON-PIALLAT M-L, ROPRAZ P, GABBIANI F, GABBIANI G. Phenotypic heterogeneity of rat arterial smooth muscle cell clones. Implications for the development of experimental intimal thickening. *Arterioscler Thromb Vasc Biol.* 1996;16:815-820.
6. HAO H, ROPRAZ P, VERIN V, CAMENZIND E, GEINOZ A, PEPPER MS, GABBIANI G, BOCHATON-PIALLAT M-L. Heterogeneity of smooth muscle cell populations cultured from pig coronary artery. *Arterioscler Thromb Vasc Biol.* 2002;22:1093-1099.
7. MILLS I, COHEN CR, KAMAL K, LI G, SHIN T, DU W, SUMPIO BE. Strain activation of bovine aortic smooth muscle cell proliferation and alignment: study of strain dependency and the role of protein kinase A and C signaling pathways. *J Cell Physiol.* 1997;170:228-234.
8. LI C, HU Y, STURM G, WICK G, XU Q. Ras/Rac-dependent activation of p38 mitogen-activated protein kinases in smooth muscle cells stimulated by cyclic strain stress. *Arterioscler Thromb Vasc Biol.* 2000;20:e1-e9.
9. LI W, CHEN Q, MILLS I, SUMPIO BE. Involvement of S6 kinase and p38 mitogen activated protein kinase pathways in strain-induced alignment and proliferation of bovine aortic smooth muscle cells. *J Cell Physiol.* 2003;195:202-209.
10. SUMPIO BE, BANES AJ. Response of porcine aortic smooth muscle cells to cyclic tensional deformation in culture. *J Surg Res.* 1988;44:696-701.
11. HAGA M, YAMASHITA A, PASZKOWIAK J, SUMPIO BE, DARDIK A. Oscillatory shear stress increases smooth muscle cell proliferation and Akt phosphorylation. *J Vasc Surg.* 2003;37:1277-1284.
12. SEDDING DG, SEAY U, FINK L, HEIL M, KUMMER W, TILLMANNS H, BRAUN-DULLAEUS RC. Mechanosensitive p27Kip1 Regulation and Cell Cycle Entry in Vascular Smooth Muscle Cells. *Circulation.* 2003;108:616-622.
13. STERPETTI AV, CUCINA A, D'ANGELO LS, CARDILLO B, CAVALLARO A. Shear stress modulates the proliferation rate, protein synthesis and mitogenic activity of arterial smooth muscle cells. *Surgery.* 1993;113:691-699.
14. BERCELI SA, DAVIES MG, KENAGY RD, CLOWES AW. Flow-induced neointimal regression in baboon polytetrafluoroethylene grafts is associated with decreased cell proliferation and increased apoptosis. *J Vasc Surg.* 2002;36:1248-1255.
15. SCHAPER W. The collateral circulation of the heart, Amsterdam: *North-Holland Publishing Company,* 1971.
16. THYBERG J, PALMBERG L, NILSSON J, KSIAZEK T, SJOELUND M. Phenotype modulation in primary cultures of arterial smooth muscle cells. On the role of platelet-derived growth factor. *Differentiation.* 1983;25:156-167.
17. HEDIN U, ROY J, TRAN PK, LUNDMARK K, RAHMAN A. Control of smooth muscle cell proliferation-the role of the basement membrane. *Thromb Haemost.* 1999;82 Suppl 1:23-26.

18. WOLF C, CAI W-J, VOSSCHULTE R, KOLTAI S, MOUSAVIPOUR D, SCHOLZ D, AFSAH-HEDJRI A, SCHAPER W, SCHAPER J. Vascular remodeling and altered protein expression during growth of coronary collateral arteries. *J Mol Cell Cardiol.* 1998;30:2291-2305.

19. SOBUE K, KEN'ICHIRO H, NISHIDA W. Expressional regulation of smooth muscle cell-specific genes in association with phenotypic modulation. *Mol Cell Biochem.* 1999;190:105-118.

20. HULTGAARDH-NILSSON A, LOEVDAHL C, BLOMGREN K, KALLIN B, THYBERG J. Expression of phenotype- and proliferation-related genes in rat aortic smooth muscle cells in primary culture. *Cardiovasc Res.* 1997;34:418-430.

21. CAI W-J, VOSSCHULTE R, AFSAH-HEDJRI A, KOLTAI S, KOCSIS E, SCHOLZ D, KOSTIN S, SCHAPER W, SCHAPER J. Altered balance between extracellular proteolysis and antiproteolysis is associated with adaptive coronary arteriogenesis. *J Mol Cell Cardiol.* 2000;32:997-10111.

22. ROY J, KAZI M, HEDIN U, THYBERG J. Phenoypic modulation of arterial smooth muscle cells is associated with prolonged activation of ERK1/2. *Differentiation.* 2001;67:50-58.

23. HEDIN U, THYBERG J, ROY J, DUMITRESCU A, TRAN PK. Role of tyrosine kinases in extracellular matrix-mediated modulation of arterial smooth muscle cell phenotype. *Arterioscler Thromb Vasc Biol.* 1997;17:1977-1984.

24. HAYASHI K, TAKAHASHI M, KIMURA K, NISHIDA W, SAGA H, SOBUE K. Changes in the balance of phosphoinositide 3-kinase/protein kinase B (Akt) and the mitogen-activated protein kinases (ERK/p38 MAPK) determine a phenotype of visceral and vascular smooth muscle cells. *J Cell Biol.* 1999;145:727-740.

25. BROWN DM, HONG SP, FARRELL CL, PIERCE GF, KHOURI RK. Platelet-derived growth factor BB induces functional vascular anastomoses *in vivo. Proc Natl Acad Sci.* 1995;92:5920-5924.

26. LINDAHL P, JOHANSSON BR, LEVEEN P, BETSHOLTZ C. Pericyte loss and microaneurysm formation in PDGF-B-deficient mice. *Science.* 1997;277:242-245.

27. ROSS R. The pathogenesis of atherosclerosis: A perspective for the 1990s. *Nature.* 1993; 362:801-809.

28. BASILICO C, MOSCATELLI D. The FGF family of growth factors and oncogenes. *Adv Cancer Res.* 1992;59:115-165.

29. YANG HT, DESCHENES MR, OGILVIE RW, TERJUNG RL. Basic fibroblast growth factor increases collateral blood flow in rats with femoral arterial ligation. *Circ Res.* 1996;79:62-69.

30. DOUKAS J, BLEASE K, CRAIG D, MA C, CHANDLER LA, SOSNOWSKI BA, PIERCE GF. Delivery of FGF genes to wound repair cells enhances arteriogenesis and myogenesis in skeletal muscle. *Molecular Therapy.* 2002;5:517-527.

31. RISSANEN TT, MARKKANEN JE, ARVE K, RUTANEN J, KETTUNEN MI, VAJANTO I, JAUHIAINEN S, CASHION L, GRUCHALA M, NARVANEN O, TAIPALE P, KAUPPINEN RA, RUBANYI GM, YLA-HERTTUALA S. Fibroblast growth factor 4 induces vascular permeability, angiogenesis and arteriogenesis in a rabbit hind limb ischemia model. *FASEB J.* 2003;17:100-102.

32. XIN X, JOHNSON AD, SCOTT-BURDEN T, ENGLER D, CASSCELLS W. The predominant form of fibroblast growth factor receptor expressed in proliferating human arterial smooth muscle cells in culture is type I. *Biochem Biophys Res Commun.* 1994;204:557-564.

33. DEINDL E, HOEFER IE, FERNÁNDEZ B, BARANCIK M, HEIL M, STRNISKOVA M, SCHAPER W. Involvement of the Fibroblast Growth Factor System in Adaptive and Chemokine-Induced Arteriogenesis. *Circ Res.* 2003;92:561-568.

34. SJOLUND M, RAHM M, CLAESSON-WELSH L, SEJERSEN T, HELDIN CH, THYBERG J. Expression of PDGF alpha- and beta-receptors in rat arterial smooth muscle cells is phenotype and growth state dependent. *Growth Factors.* 1990;3:191-203.

35. BAXTER RM, SECRIST JP, VAILLANCOURT RR, KAZLAUSKAS A. Full activation of the platelet-derived growth factor beta receptor kinase involves multiple events. *J Biol Chem.* 1998; 273:17050-17055.

36. SCHWACHTGEN J-L, HOUSTON P, CAMPBELL C, SUKHATME V, BRADDOCK M. Fluid Shear Stress Activation of Egr-1 Transcription in Cultured Human Endothelial and Epithelial Cells Is Mediated via the Extracellular Signal-related Kinase 1/2 Mitogen-activated Protein Kinase Pathway. *J Clin Invest.* 1998;101:2540-2549.

37. LOWE HC, FAHMY RG, KAVURMA MM, BAKER A, CHESTERMAN CN, KHACHIGIAN LM. Catalytic oligodeoxynucleotides define a key regulatory role for early growth response factor-1 in the porcine model of coronary in-stent restenosis. *Circ Res.* 2001;89:670-677.

38. HENRIKSSON M, BAKARDJIEV A, KLEIN G, LUSCHER B. Phosphorylation sites mapping in the N-terminal domain of c-myc modulate its transforming potential. *Oncogene.* 1993; 8:3199-3209.

39. LUTTERBACH B, HANN SR. Hierarchial phosphorylation at N-terminal transformation-sensitive sites in c-Myc protein is regulated by mitogens and in mitosis. *Mol Cell Biol.* 1994; 14:5510-5522.

40. DERIJARD B, HIBI M, WU IH, BARRETT T, SU B, DENG T, KARIN M, DAVIS R. JNK: a protein kinase stimulated by UV light and Ha-Ras that binds and phosphorylates the c-Jun activation domain. *Cell.* 1994;76:1025-1037.

41. KYRIAKIS JM, BANERJEE P, NIKOLAKAKI E, DAI T, RUBIE EA, AHMAD MF, AVRUCH J, WOODGETT JR. The stress-activated protein kinase subfamily of c-Jun kinases. *Nature.* 1994;369:156-160.

42. RAINGEAUD J, GUPTA S, ROGERS JS, DICKENS M, HAN J, ULEVITCH RJ, DAVIS RJ. Proinflammatory cytokines and environmental stress cause mitogen-activated protein kinase activation by dual phosphorylation on tyrosine and threonine. *J Biol Chem.* 1995; 270:7420-7426.

43. HAZZALIN CA, LE PANSE R, CANO E, MAHADEVAN LC. Anisomycin selectively desensitizes signaling components involved in stress kinase activation and fos and jun induction. *Mol Cell Biol.* 1998;18:1844-1854.

44. YAMAGUCHI H, IGARASHI M, HIRATA A, TSUCHIYA H, SUSA S, TOMINAGA M, DAIMON M, KATO T. Characterisation of platelet-derived growth factor-induced p38 mitogen-activated protein kinase activation in vascular smooth muscle cells. *Eur J Clin Invest.* 2001;31:672-680.

45. ZHOU W, TAKUWA N, KUMADA M, TAKUWA Y. Protein kinase C-mediated bidirectional regulation of DNA synthesis, RB protein phosphorylation and cyclin -dependent kinases in human vascular endothelial cells. *J Biol Chem.* 1993;268:23041-23048.

46. NEWTON AC. Regulation of protein kinase C. *Curr Opin Cell Biol.* 1997;9:161-167.

47. VANHAESEBROECK B, LEEVERS SJ, PANAYOTOU G, WATERFIELD MD. Phosphoinositide 3-kinases: a conserved family of signal transducers. *Trends Biochem Sci.* 1997;22:267-272.

48. REUSCH HP, ZIMMERMANN S, SCHAEFER M, PAUL M, MOELLING K. Regulation of Raf by Akt controls growth and differentiation in vascular smooth muscle cells. *J Biol Chem.* 2001; 276:33630-33637.

49. LAVOIE JN, L'ALLEMAIN G, BRUNET A, MUELLER R, POUYSSEGUR J. Cyclin D1 expression is regulated positively by the p42/p44 MAPK and negatively by the p38/HOG MAPK pathway. *J Biol Chem.* 1996;271:20608-20616.

50. GRAVES LM, GUY HI, KOZLOWSKI P, HUANG M, LAZAROWSKI E, POPE RM, COLLINS MA, DAHLSTRAND EN, EARP HS, EVANS DR. Regulation of carbamoyl phosphate synthetase by MAP kinase. *Nature.* 2000;403:328-332.

51. ZHOU X, RICHON VM, WANG AH, YANG X-J, RIFKIND RA, MARKS PA. Histone deacetylase 4 associates with extracellular signal-regulated kinases 1 and 2, and its cellular localisation is regulated by oncogenic Ras. *Proc Natl Acad Sci USA.* 2000;97:14329-14333.

52. DIEHL JA, CHENG M, ROUSSEL MF, SHERR CJ. Glycogen synthase kinase-3β regulates cyclin D1 proteolysis and subcellular localisation. *Genes Dev.* 1998;12:3499-3511.

53. CROSS DA, ALESSI DR, COHEN P, ANDJELKOVICH M, HEMMINGS BA. Inhibition of glycogen synthase kinase-3 by insulin mediated by protein kinase B. *Nature.* 1995;378:785-789.

54. WELSH GI, PROUD GC. Glycogen synthase kinase-3 is rapidly inactivated in response to insulin and phosphorylates eukaryotic initiation factor eIF-2B. *Biochem J.* 1993;294:625-629.

55. JIMENEZ C, PORTELA RA, MELLADO M, RODRIGUEZ-FRADE JM, COLLARD J, SERRANO A, MARTINEZ-A C, AVILA J, CARRERA AC. Role of the PI3K regulatory subunit in the control of actin organisation and cell migration. *J Cell Biol.* 2000;151:249-261.

Chapter 12

Expression Profiling of Growing Collateral Arteries/ Hunting for New Genes

René Zimmermann, Kerstin Boengler,
Andreas Kampmann, Borja Fernández,
Elisabeth Deindl and Wolfgang Schaper

The number of genes involved in arteriogenesis is rapidly growing. We and others have identified several growth factors (e.g. FGF-1, FGF-2, FGF-4, NGF, TNF-α)[1-7], growth factor-associated genes (Notch1 and Dll4, DANCE)[8-10], cytokines (MCP-1)[11], as well as genes involved in the composition of the extracellular matrix (ECM)[12,13] and in the reorganization of the cytoskeleton (e.g. cofilin2)[14] as participants in these processes. Furthermore, our studies indicate that hypoxia and the expression of hypoxia-regulated genes like VEGF do not play an important role in arteriogenesis[15], implying that the basic mechanisms of collateral growth differ from those of angiogenesis[3,16-18].

In order to identify additional molecules involved in this process we initiated molecular studies in our rabbit and mouse hind limb femoral artery occlusion models as well as in the pig model of arteriovenous shunt, which are still ongoing. Techniques used include Differential Display RT-PCR, Suppression Subtractive Hybridization, Serial Analysis of Gene Expression (SAGE), micro-arrays and 2D gel electrophoresis followed by mass spectrometry.

The techniques

Differential Display Reverse Transcriptase PCR (DDRT-PCR) is based on the amplification of cDNA, generated from RNA isolated from the tissue of interest[19]. For amplification anchored oligo-dT primers and short (~10-14bp) arbitrary PCR primers are used. Because these primers contain an arbitrary sequence, DDRT-PCR is capable of isolating unknown transcripts[20]. In short, the technique involves the amplification of first strand cDNA by PCR and separation of the PCR products on a gel (for review:[21]). In our experiments we used 48 different combinations to analyze RNA samples from control vessels and from growing collaterals after 3 and 7 days of femoral artery occlusion. These combinations can theoretically cover 62% of the transcribed genes in a given cell-type or tissue. Because DDRT-PCR is based on the amplification of cDNA, results obtained with this method are only preliminary. It is necessary to confirm the differential expression of the isolated clones with independent, reliable methods like Northern blot analysis or quantitative Real-Time PCR.

In order to perform Suppression Subtractive Hybridization (SSH), collateral arteries were isolated, the mRNA extracted and amplified by means of the SMART technique. SSH is a technique especially designed for the detection of rare transcripts, which vary in their expression pattern between two experimental setups[22]. SSH allows a synchronous normalization and subtraction of two cDNA pools in one step and has the advantage that it does not rely on the availability of specific sequences as do DNA-microarrays. However, background molecules can arise via unspecific annealing during the adapter-ligation or represent non-subtracted cDNAs and have to be excluded from the cDNA libraries. To identify truly differentially expressed genes different strategies can be applied: background molecules can be eliminated by application of mirror orientation selection[23] or cDNAs from the subtracted libraries can be screened for differential expression via spotting them on glass-slides and hybridizing with fluorescent labeled cDNAs derived from experimental or control RNAs.

Serial analysis of gene expression (SAGE) was first described in 1995[24] and later adapted for the use in complex tissues[25]. SAGE is a powerful method to examine the expression profile of a certain tissue, disease state or growth process because it allows the quantitative and simultaneous analysis of a large number of transcripts. The method is based on short (approximately 10bp) tags, which are diagnostic for a transcript. RNA isolated from the tissue of interest is reverse transcribed into cDNA, which is then cleaved by two restriction enzymes to generate short 10bp tags. These tags are ligated to form concatemers, cloned and analyzed by sequencing. SAGE is a quantitative method because it does not involve any PCR step. The number of the appearance of a certain tag in a SAGE-library is a direct measurement for the expression of the corresponding gene in a given context, e.g. arteriogenesis. SAGE libraries in combination with appropriate statistical methods provide a reliable and comparable overview of gene expression. The comparison of two different libraries is done by comparing the tags-counts of these two libraries. This numerical analysis does not necessarily require the direct comparison of two libraries; in fact, it is possible to perform it separately. Therefore, genes that are differentially expressed may be identified just by counting the tags from two independent libraries.

Genes involved in arteriogenesis

Osteoglycin/Mimecan

By means of DDRT-PCR we cloned a gene, which was downregulated after day 3 and 7 of femoral artery occlusion. The originally isolated DDRT-PCR fragment of approximately 250bp showed no homology to any known gene. However, after the cloning of the rabbit full-length cDNA, we found that this cDNA has a homology of 89% to human osteoglycin (Acc. No. XM 011797.3), also known as osteoinductive factor or mimecan. The protein was originally isolated as osteoinductive factor, because of its ability to induce bone formation [26]. This activity was later shown to be due to a contamination of the analyzed protein preparation by bone-morphogenetic-protein-1 and 2 [27]. Because of the possible confusions associated with the name osteoglycin it was renamed mimecan [28].

Mimecan/osteoglycin is a member of the family of the small leucine-rich proteoglycans [29] with a molecular weight of approximately 34kDa and it maps to human chromosome 9q22 [30]. The small leucine-rich proteoglycans are characterized by tandem leucine repeats, six of them can be found in the central domain of mimecan/osteoglycin. They play a role in the organization of tissues and of collagen fibers, both during normal and pathological conditions [29,31].

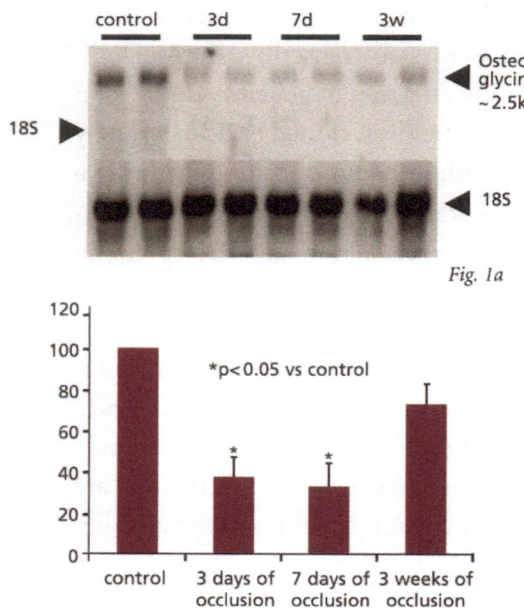

Fig. 1a

*p<0.05 vs control

Fig. 1b

Northern blot hybridization of osteoglycin.
mRNA levels were 37% of control value after 3 days of femoral artery occlusion and 33% after 7 days, respectively. After 3 weeks of occlusion the expression was 72% of the control value

Our results show that osteoglycin is downregulated in response to the occlusion of a major artery (Fig. 1). mRNA expression levels decreased to 37% and 33% of control (expression in non growing collaterals) after 3d and 7d of femoral artery occlusion, respectively. Three weeks after femoral artery occlusion, when collateral growth has stopped due to near normal shear stress levels in the growing collaterals, osteoglycin is expressed on a level comparable to resting collaterals (approximately 72%). Comparable changes were seen when osteoglycin protein levels were analyzed: three days after femoral artery occlusion protein levels were 44% of the control value while at 7d they reached 51%. However, at 3 weeks the protein level did not reach the original level in control vessels, as seen with the mRNA, but stayed at low levels (44%) (Fig. 2).

These findings are in accordance with reports in the literature, which show that osteoglycin is downregulated in proliferating smooth muscle cells and after vascular injury (also a process characterized by proliferating smooth muscle cells)[32]. Our own *in vitro* data show that osteoglycin mRNA expression can be influenced by different cytokines, including FGF-2, which leads to a strong downregulation of mRNA levels after 48h and 72h. FGF-2 is of special interest because it was shown that it can stimulate arteriogenesis[3]. Furthermore, our own data showed that administration of PAS (polyanetholsulfonic acid) – a substance blocking the action of FGFs via complex formation – almost completely abolished the downregulation of osteoglycin in rabbits after femoral artery occlusion (E. Deindl, unpublished).

Immunohistochemical analysis of normal rabbit tissues revealed localization of osteoglycin protein in the adventitia of all arteries and veins.

In the aorta, osteoglycin mRNA was expressed by smooth muscle cells and adventitial fibroblasts, but not by endothelial cells. Heart and skeletal muscles showed focal osteoglycin accumulation in the extracellular matrix surrounding myocytes, whereas intestine and uterus showed homogenous distribution of the protein. Non-muscular tissues like brain, kidney, liver, and lung showed low levels or no expression of osteoglycin in the parenchyma, although the protein was always present in the arterial adventitia.

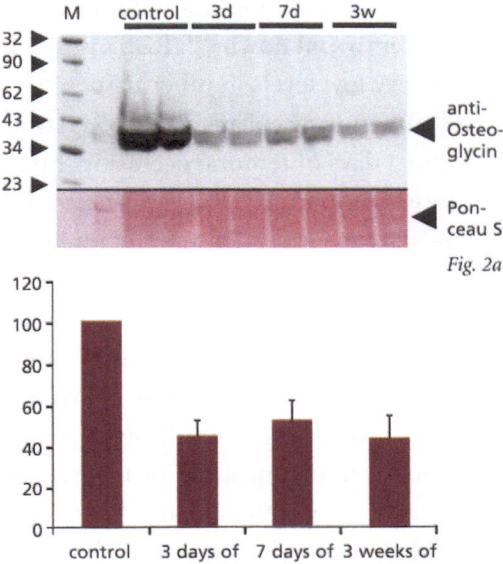

Fig. 2a

Fig. 2b

During collateral artery growth osteoglycin mRNA was localized in smooth muscle cells of proliferating and non-proliferating vessels as well as in nerve fibers. The protein accumulated in the adventitia of all vessels, was less abundant in the media and appeared in the intima of a few big vessels. After 7 days

Western blot analysis of osteoglycin.
Two forms of the protein were detected: the complete core protein (app. 34kDa) and the protein after removal of the signal peptide (app. 31kDa). The changes in protein expression were comparable to the changes on the mRNA level. The expression was 44 % when compared to the control value after 3 days of femoral artery occlusion and 51 % after 7 days, respectively. After 3 weeks of occlusion the expression was 44 % of the control value.

of femoral artery occlusion the protein was significantly reduced in the adventitia of growing collaterals when compared to quiescent vessels.

We therefore conclude that osteoglycin plays an important role during the growth of collateral arteries. It is a key component for remodeling of the extracellular matrix (ECM). Downregulation of its expression allows proliferation of smooth muscle cells and a partial breakdown of the ECM while in mature collaterals it seems to be involved in keeping them functional and preventing that the vessels get leaky.

RGS5

RGS is an acronym for <u>R</u>egulator of <u>G</u>-protein <u>S</u>ignaling and it is one member of a larger family of proteins. The core function of RGS-proteins is to regulate G-protein signaling strength and duration by binding to and dephosphorylating Gα-subunits. The exact function of RGS5, however, is currently unknown [33,34]. RGS5 is highly expressed in heart and aorta, but at very low levels in other tissues [35-37].

In growing collaterals RGS5 is strongly downregulated between 6 hours and 3 days of femoral occlusion, but upregulated in the same setting at 3 weeks, implicating an important role of G-proteins and their regulators in arteriogenesis (Zimmermann, unpublished).

Cofilin2

Arteriogenesis, which is mainly induced by fluid shear stress, is promoted by growth factors and cytokines supplied by monocytes [38]. It was shown that both stimuli, shear stress as well as growth factor binding, cause a re-organization of the cytoskeleton [39]. Among the proteins contributing to actin dynamics, cofilin is well-characterized [40,41]. Previous studies demonstrated that cofilin depolymerizes and severs actin in a pH-dependent manner [42] whereby the activity of the protein is controlled by its phosphorylation status. LIM-kinases, effectors of Rho-GTPases, phosphorylate cofilin, thereby converting it to the inactive form [43,44], while the dephosphorylation of cofilin via the phosphatase slingshot activates the protein [45]. In mouse and human, two cofilin genes are described: cofilin1, which is widely expressed in non-muscle tissues, whereas cofilin2 is found in muscle tissue as well as in smooth muscle cells [46].

By immunohistochemistry endothelial cells and smooth muscle cells of collateral arteries of the rabbit m. quadriceps were positive for both isoforms, i.e., cofilin1+2 [14]. Additionally, the proteins were detected in the nuclei of skeletal myocytes as well as in some interstitial cells. In contrast, cofilin1 expression was restricted to endothelial cells of collaterals, capillaries and veins. These data indicated that cofilin2 is mainly localized in the smooth muscle cells of collateral vessels.

The mRNA and protein levels of cofilin2 increased in collateral arteries 24 hours and 3 days after femoral artery ligation compared to sham operated animals, but not in the m. quadriceps devoid of collateral arteries. However, the protein level of cofilin1 was unchanged in collaterals between experimental and control animals (Fig. 3). These data make it likely that cofilin2 is the isoform involved in the early phase of arteriogenesis.

Interestingly, there are data indicating that the expression of the different isoforms of cofilin is characteristic for the species studied: in a pig model of chronical shear stress due to arteriovenous shunting, cofilin expression in the collateral vessels differs from that in the 7d rabbit model by the fact that increased levels of cofilin1 were detected while cofilin2 was decreased (S. Boehm, unpublished; see also chapter 5).

We hypothesize that the two cofilin isoforms play distinct roles in the turnover of actin in specific cell types during specific stages of collateral artery growth. Previous studies already have demonstrated that cofilin1 and 2 differ in their ability to depolymerize actin[47].

Furthermore, the phenotype of smooth muscle cells changes from contractile to synthetic, a process associated with a decrease of the α-smooth muscle actin protein level[48]. Our results indicate that the mRNA level of α-smooth muscle actin is also downregulated, namely at a point of time,

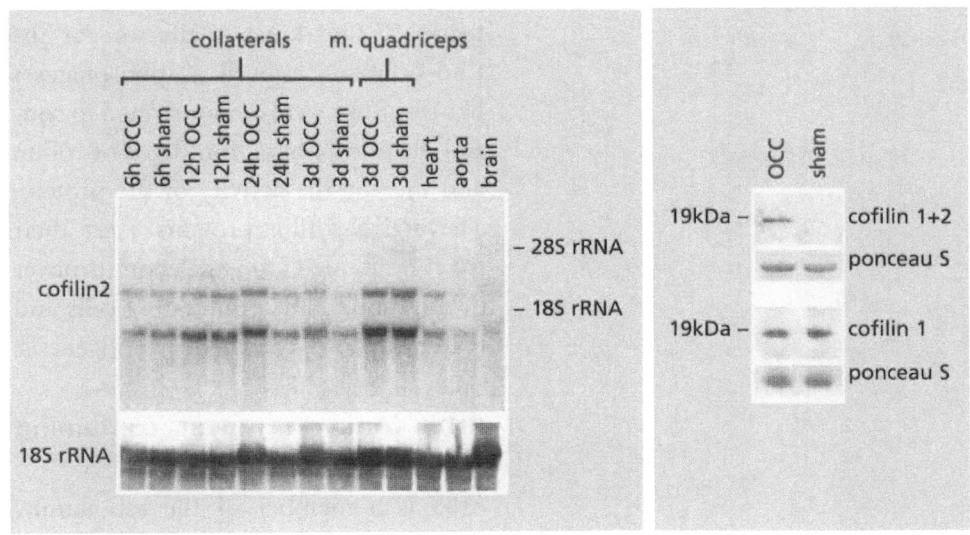

Fig. 3a   Fig. 3b

Expression pattern of cofilin2.
3a: Northern blot analysis of cofilin2 mRNA expression in collaterals at distinct experimental intervals (6h–3d), in the m. quadriceps, and in rabbit organs. Positions of the 18S and 28S rRNA are indicated (top). To control for RNA loading, the blot was rehybridized with an 18S rRNA specific probe (bottom). 3b: Western blot analysis of cofilin1 and cofilin2 in collateral arteries. Protein extracts were probed with an antibody against cofilin1+2 (top) or against cofilin1 (bottom). To control for equal loading, a representative ponceau S stained band is shown (reprinted from[14] with permission).

when cofilin2 is upregulated. These data suggest a common mechanism for the regulation of the cofilin2 and α-smooth muscle actin mRNA expression in collateral artery growth.

Based on our findings we hypothesize that cofilin2 is associated with the integrin signaling network (Fig. 4). Mechanical stress like fluid shear stress, the main stimulus of arteriogenesis, induces a remodeling of the focal adhesions, which are complexes of integrins. The integrins are also differentially expressed during arteriogenesis. Studies from our laboratory demonstrated increased protein levels of $\alpha_v\beta_3$ integrin in the endothelium as well as in the media of collateral arteries after femoral ligation (K. Broich, unpublished; see chapter 9). Previous studies showed that on the one hand the integrins regulate the Rho family GTPases, and on the other hand the Rho-GTPases are influencing the integrins[49]. LIM-kinases, effectors of the Rho-GTPases, as well as phosphatases like slingshot were demonstrated to control the phosphorylation status of cofilin and thereby the activity of the protein. The active cofilin proteins exert their function in regulating the actin turnover of migrating and proliferating cells and thereby the progression of arteriogenesis.

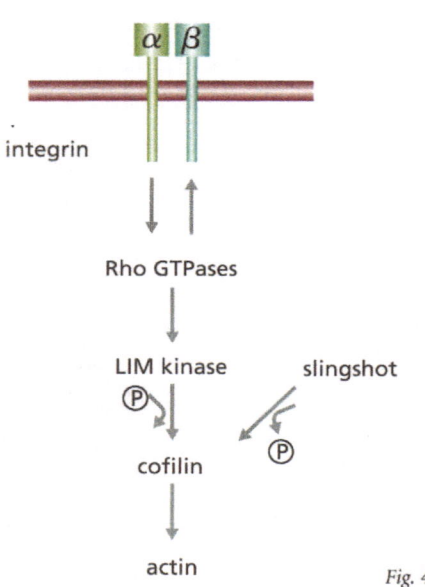

Fig. 4

Schematic representation of the putative signal transduction cascade regulating the level of actin polymerization in growing collateral arteries. The clustering of the heterodimeric integrins located at the focal adhesion is regulated by mechanical stress. The integrins and Rho-GTPases interact with each other. The phosphorylation status of cofilin is either controlled by kinases like the LIM-kinases or via phosphatases like slingshot. The active cofilin is able to depolymerize actin filaments. ECM = extracellular matrix

Asb5 (Ankyrin repeat containing SOCS box protein 5)

Asb5 is a member of the asb family, which comprises 18 members[50]. The asb proteins – not well characterized up to now – are depicted by a non-conserved N-terminus, a various number of ankyrin repeat motifs as well as a C-terminal SOCS box (suppressors of cytokine signaling). The SOCS box, a conserved motif of 39 amino acids, was originally identified in the proteins SOCS1-3, which are implicated in the inhibition of cytokine signaling via a negative feedback mechanism[51]. The exact functions of asb proteins in physiological processes remain to be elucidated. We cloned the rabbit asb5 cDNA, which is highly conserved (~96%) compared to the human and mouse cDNAs[52]. Analysis of the asb5 amino acid sequence revealed a putative N-terminal transmembrane domain, six ankyrin repeats, which are mediating protein-protein interactions, and a C-terminal SOCS box (Fig. 5).

Asb5 mRNA is expressed in rabbit heart as well as in skeletal muscle, but not in brain, lung, kidney, thyroid gland or uterus. This expression pattern is similar to that of asb2 and asb10, which both are predominantly expressed in heart and muscle. Immunohistochemical data showed that endothelial cells and smooth muscle cells of collateral arteries as well as the endothelial cells of capillaries stained positive for asb5. Additionally, asb5 was localized in the satellite cells of striated myocytes, but not in the myocytes themselves (Fig. 6).

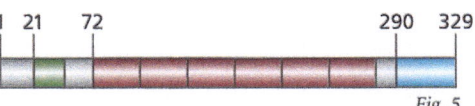

Fig. 5

Schematic representation of the functional domains of the rabbit asb5 protein.

The putative transmembrane domain is marked in green, the ankyrin repeat motifs in red and the SOCS box in blue. Numbers are indicating the position of the respective amino acids (reprinted with permission from[52]).

Asb5 was increased in collateral arteries on mRNA as well as on protein level 6, 12 and 24 hours after occlusion of the femoral artery. However, in the m. quadriceps devoid of collaterals asb5 was not differentially expressed, indicating that asb5 is specifically upregulated in collateral arteries. Furthermore, asb5 mRNA levels were decreased in collateral vessels after infusion of the anti-tumor agent doxorubicin, but not after infusion of TGF-β1 or MCP-1, both substances known to promote arteriogenesis. We speculate that the downregulation of asb5 mRNA by doxorubicin may inhibit arteriogenesis, since it has been shown that the delivery of doxorubicin in rats inhibits vascular smooth muscle cell proliferation[53].

In summary, our results show that asb5 is a novel protein associated with collateral artery growth. However, the exact function of asb5 in arteriogenesis remains unclear. We speculate that asb5 interacts via its ankyrin repeat motifs with target proteins (Fig. 7). The SOCS box of asb5 may contact the elongin BC complex, as it was shown for asb2[54]. E3 ubiquitin ligase was also demonstrated to be part of the elongin BC complex

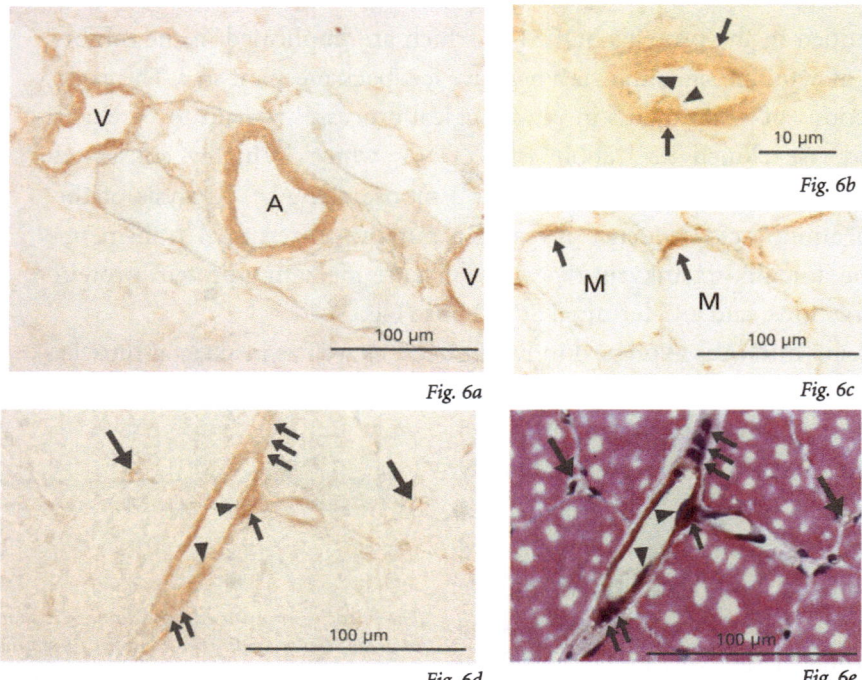

Fig. 6b

Fig. 6a

Fig. 6c

Fig. 6d

Fig. 6e

*Immunoperoxidase localization of asb5 (a-d) and hematoxilin/eosin
counterstaining (e) of rabbit m. quadriceps.
6a: Asb5 immunoreactivity was found in the wall of collateral arteries (A) and veins (V).
6b: both endothelial cells (arrowheads) and smooth muscle cells (arrows) stained positive for
asb5. 6c: Some satellite cells (arrows) were found positive, but myocytes (M) were negative.
6d,e: asb5 stained the cytosol of ECs and SMCs of arteries (arrowheads and small arrows).
Capillaries were also positive (big arrows). (reprinted with permission from[52])*

and was shown to transfer polyubiquitin chains to a target protein, thereby labeling it for proteasomal degradation (Fig. 7). Asb5 might therefore play a role in the termination of a specific signal transduction pathway by targeting itself and specific signaling molecules for degradation. It remains to be elucidated, which factors represent specific asb5 targets. However, it is unlikely that substrates of asb5 are members of the JAK/STAT family, which are described to interact with SOCS proteins, since asb5 does not contain the SH2 domain necessary for this protein-protein interaction[55].

Carp (cardiac ankyrin repeat protein)

The rabbit carp cDNA encodes a 36 kDa protein containing a PEST like sequence, which targets proteins for rapid degradation, four ankyrin repeats, shown to mediate protein-protein interactions, as well as nuclear localization signals (Fig. 8).

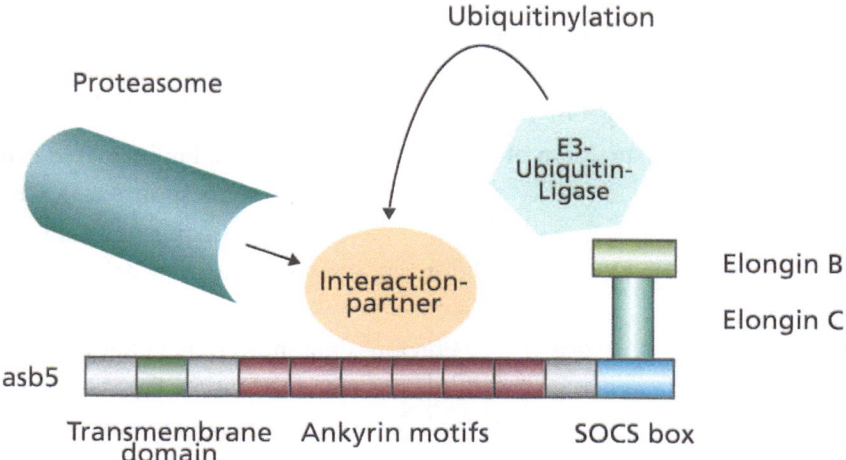

Fig. 7

Model of the asb5 function in terminating a signal transduction cascade.

Asb5 may contact an interaction-partner via the ankyrin motifs. The SOCS box can interact with elongin BC and the E3 ubiquitin ligase, which may ubiquitinylate the interaction-partner, thereby targeting it for proteasomal degradation.

Carp mRNA is expressed in a segment-specific manner during embryonic heart development[56] and elevated levels are a marker of cardiac hypertrophy[57,58]. Carp is localized in the nucleus where it functions as a transcriptional co-factor[59]. Additionally, previous data indicated that carp functions in the negative regulation of cardiac gene expression[60].

Our data[61] showed increased levels of the carp mRNA in rabbit collateral arteries 6, 12 and 24h after femoral ligation compared to sham operated animals. Furthermore, an upregulation of the carp transcript was detected in a similar arteriogenesis model in mice. Carp, also enhanced on protein level, was shown to be localized in endothelial cells as well as in smooth muscle cells of collateral arteries by immunohistochemistry. The expression of carp was not restricted to the nuclei, but was found throughout the whole cells. In contrast, in striated myocytes only the nuclei stained positive for carp.

The mRNA level of carp was further increased by infusion of TGF-β1 in rabbits, but was not affected by the application of doxorubicin – shown to downregulate the carp mRNA *in vitro* – or by

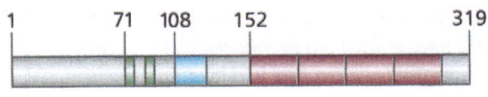

Fig. 8

Schematic representation of the functional domains of the rabbit carp protein.

The nuclear localization signals are marked in green, the PEST-like sequence in blue and the ankyrin repeat motifs in red. Numbers are indicating the positions of the respective amino acids.

infusion of MCP-1. These data suggest that during arteriogenesis, in which both, MCP-1 or TGF-β1 are involved, carp represents a specific downstream target of TGF-β1.

The overexpression of carp in cos-1 cells resulted in increased expression of the early growth response factor Egr-1, thereby indicating that carp is not only able to inhibit but also to enhance protein expression (Fig. 9).

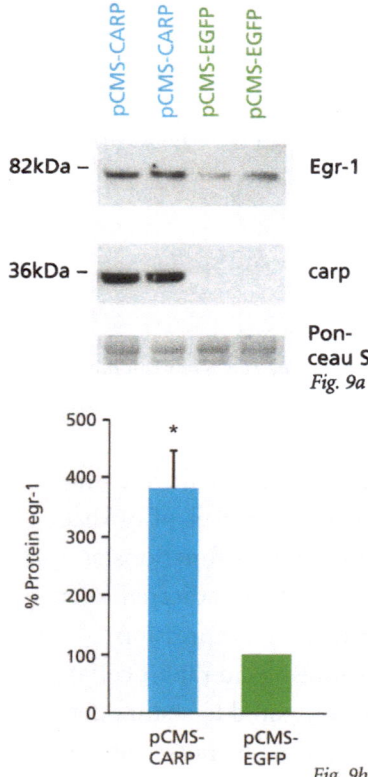

Previous data showed that after the onset of fluid shear stress, mRNAs for Egr-1, carp as well as for TGF-β_1 were upregulated *in vitro*[62-64] and induced during collateral artery growth. We hypothesize that TGF-β_1, known to increase the number of collaterals as well as their conductance, activates carp via the SMAD proteins, which were shown to bind to the carp promoter[65]. Carp itself may – among other genes – induce Egr-1, a protein functioning in regulating the expression of target genes like bFGF or TGF-β1[66,67]. Therefore, we suggest a putative feedback mechanism, in which carp controls the mRNA levels of genes associated with the process of arteriogenesis as shown in Fig. 10.

Influence of carp overexpression on the Egr-1 protein level in vitro.
9a: Cos-1 cells were transfected with a carp expression plasmid (pCMSCARP) or with the vector pCMS-EGFP as control. The protein level of carp and Egr-1 2d after transfection were monitored in the nuclear fractions by Western blot analysis. To demonstrate equal loading, a representative ponceau S stained protein signal is shown. 9b: Quantification of the Egr-1 expression. The values of the control vector pCMS- EGFP were set as 100%. Each transfection was performed 6 times independently.

Cytochrome b

In the forward subtracted library we found a high number of mitochondrial encoded genes [14]. We confirmed the upregulation exemplary for the cytochrome b, where we detected a minor, but significant increase of the mRNA levels in collateral arteries 24h after surgery. We suggest that the high quantity of mitochondria in cells and the therefore over-representation of the transcripts in comparison to nuclear encoded genes was presumably responsible for the numerous mitochondrial encoded genes in the subtracted

libraries. We furthermore hypothesize that an upregulation of
the cytochrome b mRNA and
perhaps of other mitochondrial
encoded genes is most likely
needed for the increased energy
demands of the proliferating
cells during arteriogenesis.

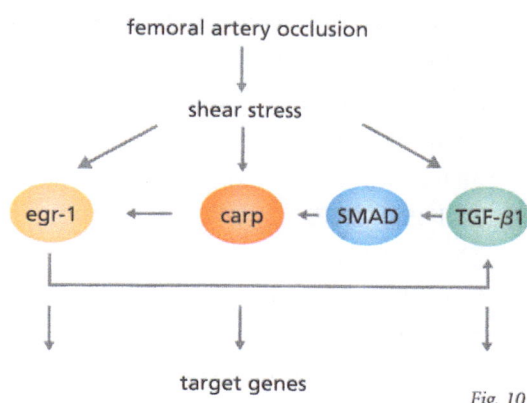

Lsm5

Lsm5 was found to be upregulated in growing collaterals 24h
after femoral artery occlusion[14].
Lsm5 encodes a protein binding
to the 3' end of the U6 snRNA
that contributes to the spliceo-
somal complex and is thereby
involved in the regulation of
transcription.

Fig. 10

Schematic representation of the putative role of carp in arteriogenesis.
Occlusion of the femoral artery results in elevated levels of shear stress in the collateral arteries. Shear stress increases the expression of Egr-1, carp, and TGF-β_1, which may target carp via the SMAD proteins. Carp itself may induce Egr-1, which can re-act on TGF-β_1, thereby providing the possibility of a feedback mechanism, regulating the expression of target genes associated with the process of arteriogenesis.

Preliminary findings from gene chips

Affymetrix chips were used for expression profiling of mouse and rabbit mRNA obtained from collateral vessels at various stages of development. The C57Bl6 strain was used because collaterals grow after femoral artery occlusion in an ischemia-free surrounding. However, skeletal muscle contamination could not be entirely avoided given the extremely small size of the collateral vessels. Although no rabbit-specific chip is currently available from Affymetrix, we used the human one with good results. A total of 724 genes were positively identified from the mRNA obtained from shear-stressed collaterals (see chapter 5) at day 7. Of the 724 sequences 303 were upregulated, 89 showed no change of expression compared to 7 day old collaterals not under high shear stress, and 332 exhibited downregulation. Many of the upregulated genes reflected the ongoing (rabbit) or restarted (pig) shear stress induced proliferative activity. Of note is the strong upregulation of FGF-7, which, of all the screens used so far, was the first time that a growth factor of the FGF-family appeared.

Most of the changes in SMC gene expression (mRNA from the rabbit shunt experiments) encompass the proteins of the cytoskeleton, of signaling and transcription. About 22 transcription factors are down- and 14 are upregulated in states of high shear stress, several of them incompletely studied zinc finger proteins (ZNF142, ZNF7, ZNF pT3, ZNF28, ZNF258, ZNF286, ZNF177, ZNF138, ZNF 259 (all down), ZFHX 1B, ZNFN1A3, ZFHX 1B, ZNFN1A3, ZNF184, HKR3, and the homeobox gene PAX 9). Other transcription factors with differential expression between high- and normalized shear stress are the homeobox C10, forkhead box 11, sonic hedgehog homolog, distal-less homeobox DLX2, VSX-1, helix-loop-helix TF4, homeobox B6, human kruppel-like zinkfinger ZNF184, GLI Kruppel family member HKR3.

In the endothelium as well in the SMC layers the dominant signaling system is the RAS system with phosphorylation of the ERK-1 and 2- proteins. This is easy to understand in view of the active proliferation going on in these cells during the early phases of arteriogenesis. However, the MAPkinases are in itself a complex system and we found the MAPK 11 and the MAP4K5 genes downregulated by shear stress, whereas MAP3K2, MAP3K7, and the MAP2K1 genes upregulated. Other signaling pathways may also be also involved like the WNT-system: the WNT 10A precursor and WNT inducible signaling pathway protein WISP-3 were found upregulated. In tune with this the "secreted frizzle like" SFRP1and SFRP5 were also differentially regulated. The toll-like receptor 7 was down- whereas the toll-like receptor 3 was upregulated. We found evidence for the marked involvement of the Rho pathway with its association with the cytoskeleton (see destrin and cofilin in preceding chapters) supported by the upregulation by shear stress of the Rho-guanine nucleotide exchange factor. Feeding into this signaling chain are the proto-oncogenes vav2 and vav3 both of which we found strongly upregulated by high shear stress. Vav 3 is co-localized with actin, which it is able to rearrange. Ephrin A3 and Ephrin B3 are downregulated but the importance of this is at present unclear.

In our gene hunting projects the classical vascular growth factors did not show up probably because of their very low transcript concentration: no FGFs (with the notable but unexpected exception of FGF-7 and angiopoietin-2, the Tie-2 antagonist, which were upregulated), no members of the VEGF-family, and none of the PDGF-family. However, a strong case for the role of a ligand of the FGF-family exists because of the findings discussed in previous chapters: upregulation of the FGF-receptor 1, which is phosphorylated after femoral occlusion even in FGF-2 knockout mice. Also of interest is the differential regulation of the the bone morphogenic proteins BMP 3 and –5 (the latter up-, the former down regulated), the interleukins IL3 and –15, the chemotactic peptides MCP-1 and –3 together with the receptor CCR-6.

In the mouse screen over 3000 genes were identified of which 243 showed differential expression. At day 1 after femoral artery occlusion, 7 genes were upregulated and 4 were downregulated. At day 3 (the peak of mitotic activity) 45 genes were up- and 187 were downregulated. Due to skleletal muscle contamination the number of collateral-specific genes will probably be much smaller. However, it was reassuring to note that carp, detected by other screens in uncontaminated rabbit collaterals, was strongly upregulated.

References

1. UNGER EF, BANAI S, SHOU M, LAZAROUS DF, JAKLITSCH MT, SHEINOWITZ M, CORREA R, KLINGBEIL C, EPSTEIN SE. Basic fibroblast growth factor enhances myocardial collateral flow in a canine model. *Am J Physiol.* 1994;266:H1588-H1595.
2. FERNÁNDEZ B, BUEHLER A, WOLFRAM S, KOSTIN S, ESPANION G, FRANZ WM, NIEMANN H, DOEVENDANS PA, SCHAPER W, ZIMMERMANN R. Transgenic myocardial overexpression of fibroblast growth factor-1 increases coronary artery density and branching. *Circ Res.* 2000;87:207-213.
3. SCHOLZ D, ZIEGELHOEFFER T, HELISCH A, WAGNER S, FRIEDRICH C, PODZUWEIT T, SCHAPER W. Contribution of arteriogenesis and angiogenesis to postocclusive hind limb perfusion in mice. *J Mol Cell Cardiol.* 2002;34:775-787.
4. DEINDL E, HOEFER IE, FERNÁNDEZ B, BARANCIK M, HEIL M, STRNISKOVA M, SCHAPER W. Involvement of the fibroblast growth factor system in adaptive and chemokine-induced arteriogenesis. *Circ Res.* 2003;92:561-568.
5. RISSANEN TT, MARKKANEN JE, ARVE K, RUTANEN J, KETTUNEN MI, VAJANTO I, JAUHIAINEN S, CASHION L, GRUCHALA M, NARVANEN O, TAIPALE P, KAUPPINEN RA, RUBANYI GM, YLA-HERTTUALA S. Fibroblast growth factor-4 induces vascular permeability, angiogenesis, and arteriogenesis in a rabbit hind limb ischemia model. *FASEB J.* 2002;02-0377.
6. EMANUELI C, SALIS MB, PINNA A, GRAIANI G, MANNI L, MADEDDU P. Nerve growth factor promotes angiogenesis and arteriogenesis in ischemic hind limbs. *Circulation.* 2002;106: 2257-2262.,
7. HOEFER IE, VAN ROYEN N, RECTENWALD JE, BRAY EJ, ABOUHAMZE Z, MOLDAWER LL, VOSKUIL M, PIEK JJ, BUSCHMANN IR, OZAKI CK. Direct Evidence for tumor necrosis factor-(alpha) signaling in arteriogenesis. *Circulation.* 2002;105:1639-1641.
8. LIU Z-J, SHIRAKAWA T, LI Y, SOMA A, OKA M, DOTTO GP, FAIRMAN RM, VELAZQUEZ OC, HERLYN M. Regulation of Notch1 and Dll4 by vascular endothelial growth factor in arterial endothelial cells: Implications for modulating arteriogenesis and angiogenesis. *Mol Cell Biol.* 2003;23:14-25.
9. NAKAMURA T, RUIZ-LOZANO P, LINDNER V, YABE D, TANIWAKI M, FURUKAWA Y, KOBUKE K, TASHIRO K, LU Z, ANDON NL, SCHAUB R, MATSUMORI A, SASAYAMA S, CHIEN KR, HONJO T. DANCE, a novel secreted RGD protein expressed in developing, atherosclerotic and balloon-injured arteries. *J Biol Chem.* 1999;274:22476-22483.
10. NAKAMURA T, LOZANO PR, IKEDA Y, IWANAGA Y, HINEK A, MINAMISAWA S, CHENG C-F, KOBUKE K, DALTON N, TAKADA Y, TASHIRO K, ROSS JR. J, HONJO T, CHIEN KR. Fibulin-5/DANCE is essential for elastogenesis *in vivo. Nature.* 2002;415:171-175.
11. ITO WD, ARRAS M, WINKLER B, SCHOLZ D, SCHAPER J, SCHAPER W. Monocyte chemotactic protein-1 increases collateral and peripheral conductance after femoral artery occlusion. *Circ Res.* 1997;80:829-837.
12. CAI W-J, VOSSCHULTE R, AFSAH-HEDJRI A, KOLTAI S, KOCSIS E, SCHOLZ D, KOSTIN S, SCHAPER W, SCHAPER J. Altered balance between extracellular proteolysis and antiproteolysis is associated with adaptive coronary arteriogenesis. *J Mol Cell Cardiol.* 2000;32:997-10111.
13. KAMPMANN A, FERNÁNDEZ B, KUBIN T, VON DER AHE D, SCHAPER W, ZIMMERMANN R. Osteoglycin: a potential new target for the promotion of arteriogenesis? *Circulation.* 2001; 104:II-235.
14. BOENGLER K, PIPP F, BROICH K, FERNÁNDEZ B, SCHAPER W, DEINDL E. Identification of differentially expressed genes like cofilin2 in growing collateral arteries. *Biochem Biophysic Res Comm.* 2003;300:751-756.
15. DEINDL E, BUSCHMANN I, HOEFER IE, PODZUWEIT T, BOENGLER K, VOGEL S, VAN ROYEN N, FERNÁNDEZ B, SCHAPER W. Role of ischemia and of hypoxia-inducible genes in arteriogenesis after femoral artery occlusion in the rabbit. *Circ Res.* 2001;89:779-786.
16. BUSCHMANN I, SCHAPER W. Arteriogenesis versus angiogenesis: two mechanisms of vessel growth. *News Physiol Sci.* 1999;14:121-125.

17. CARMELIET P. Mechanisms of angiogenesis and arteriogenesis. *Nat Med.* 2000;6:389-395.
18. HERSHEY JC, BASKIN EP, GLASS JD, HARTMAN HA, GILBERTO DA, ROGERS IT, COOK JJ. Revascularization in the rabbit hind limb: dissociation between capillary sprouting and arteriogenesis. *Cardiovasc Res.* 2001;49:618-625.
19. LIANG P, PARDEE AP. Differential display of eukaryotic messenger RNA by means of the polymerase chain reaction. *Science.* 1992;257:967-971.
20. LIANG P, BAUER D, AVERBOUKH L, WARTHOE P, ROHRWILD M, MULLER H, STRAUSS M, PARDEE AB. Analysis of altered gene expression by differential display, in (eds.): *Methods in Enzymology.* New York: Academic Press; 1995:304-321.
21. LIANG P, PARDEE AB. *Differential display methods and protocols.* Totowa, N.J.: Humana Press;1997.
22. DIATCHENKO L, LAU Y-F, CAMPBELL AP, CHENCHIK A, MOQADAM F, HUANG B, LUKYANOV S, LUKYANOV K, GURSKAYQA N, SVERDLOV ED, SIEBERT PD. Suppression substratctive hybridization: a method for generating differentially regulated or tissue-specific cDNA probes and libraries. *Proc Natl Acad Sci USA.* 1996;93:6025-6030.
23. BOENGLER K, PIPP F, SCHAPER W, DEINDL E. Rapid identification of differentially expressed genes by combination of SSH and MOS. *Lab Invest.* 2003;83:759-761.
24. VELCULESCU VE, ZHANG L, VOGELSTEIN B, KINZLER KW. Serial analysis of gene expression. *Science.* 1995;270:484-487.
25. VIRLON B, CHEVAL L, BUHLER J-M, BILLON E, DOUCET A, ELALOUF J-M. Serial microanalysis of renal transcriptomes. *Proc Natl Acad Sci USA.* 1999;96:15286-15291.
26. BENTZ H, NATHAN R, ROSEN D, ARMSTRONG R, THOMPSON A, SEGARINI P, MATHEWS M, DASCH J, PIEZ K, SEYEDIN S. Purification and characterization of a unique osteoinductive factor from bovine bone. *J Biol Chem.* 1989;264:20805-20810.
27. BENTZ H, THOMPSON AY, ARMSTRONG R, CHANG RJ, PIEZ KA, ROSEN DM. Transforming growth factor-beta 2 enhances the osteoinductive activity of a bovine bone-derived fraction containing bone morphogenetic protein-2 and -3. *Matrix.* 1991;11:269-275.
28. FUNDERBURGH JL, CORPUZ LM, ROTH MR, FUNDERBURGH ML, TASHEVA ES, CONRAD GW. Mimecan, the 25-kDa corneal keratan sulfate proteoglycan, is a product of the gene producing osteoglycin. *J Biol Chem.* 1997;272:28089-28095.
29. IOZZO R. The family of small leucine-rich proteoglycans: key regulators of matrix assembly and cellular growth. *Crit Rev Biochem Mol Biol.* 1997;32:141-174.
30. TASHEVA ES, PETTENATI M, VON KAP-HER C, CONRAD GW. Assignemant of mimemacan gene (OGN) to human chromosome band 9q22 by *in situ* hybridization. *Cytogenet Cell Genet.* 1999;88:326-327.
31. TASHEVA ES, KOESTER A, PAULSEN AQ, GARETT AS, BOYLE DL, DAVIDSON HJ, SONG M, FOX N, CONRAD GW. Mimecan/osteoglycin-deficient mice have collagen fibril abnormalities. *Mol Vision.* 2002;8:407-415.
32. SHANAHAN CM, CARY NRB, OSBOURN JK, WEISSBERG PL. Identification of osteoglycin as a component of the vascular matrix. Differential expression during neointima formation and in atherosclerotic plaques. *Arterioscler Thromb Vasc Biol.* 1997;17:2437-2447.
33. ADAMS LD, GEARY RL, MCMANUS B, SCHWARTZ SM. A Comparison of aorta and vena cava medial message expression by cDNA array analysis identifies a set of 68 consistently differentially expressed genes, all in aortic media. *Circ Res* 2000;87:623-615.
34. BONDJERS C, KALEN M, HELLSTROM M, SCHEIDL SJ, ABRAMSSON A, RENNER O, LINDAHL P, CHO H, KEHRL J, BETSHOLTZ C. Transcription profiling of platelet-derived growth factor-B-deficient mouse embryos identifies RGS5 as a novel marker for pericytes and vascular smooth muscle cells. *Am J Pathol.* 2003;162:721-729.
35. MITTMANN C, CHUNG CH, HOPPNER G, MICHALEK C, NOSE M, SCHULER C, SCHUH A, ESCHENHAGEN T, WEIL J, PIESKE B. Expression of ten RGS proteins in human myocardium: functional characterization of an upregulation of RGS4 in heart failure. *Cardiovascr Res.* 2002;55:778-786.

36. WANG Q, LIU M, MULLAH B, SIDEROVSKI DP, NEUBIG RR. Receptor-selective Effects of Endogenous RGS3 and RGS5 to regulate mitogen-activated protein kinase activation in rat vascular smooth muscle cells. *J Biol Chem.* 2002;277:24949-24958.
37. CHO H, KOZASA T, BONDJERS C, BETSHOLTZ C, KEHRL JH. Pericyte-specific expression of Rgs5: implications for PDGF and EDG receptor signaling during vascular maturation. *FASEB J.* 2003;02-0340.
38. ARRAS M, STRASSER R, MOHRI M, DOLL R, ECKERT P, SCHAPER W, SCHAPER J. Tumor necrosis factor-alpha is expressed by monocytes/macrophages following coronary microembolization and is antagonized by cyclosporine. *Basic Res Cardiol.* 1998;93:97-107.
39. GALBRAITH CG, SKALAK R, CHIEN S. Shear stress induces spatial reorganization of the endothelial cell cytoskeleton. *Cell Motil Cytoskeleton.* 1998;40:317-330.
40. MOON A, DRUBIN DG. The ADF/cofilin proteins: stimulus-responsive modulators of actin dynamics. *Mol Biol Cell.* 1995;6:1423-1431.
41. THERIOT JA. Accelerating on a Treadmill: ADF/cofilin promotes rapid actin filament turnover in the dynamic cytoskeleton. *J Cell Biol.* 1997;136:1165-1168.
42. YONEZAWA N, NISHIDA E, SAKAI H. pH control of actin polymerization by cofilin. *J Biol Chem.* 1985;260:14410-14412.
43. ARBER S, BARBAYANNIS FA, HANSER H, SCHNEIDER C, STANYON CA, BERNARD H, CARONI P. Regulation of actin dynamics through phosphorylation of cofilin by LIM-kinase. *Nature.* 1998;393:805-809.
44. TOSHIMA J, TOSHIMA JY, AMANO T, YANG N, NARUMIYA S, MIZUNO K. Cofilin Phosphorylation by protein kinase testicular protein kinase 1 and its role in integrin-mediated actin reorganization and focal adhesion formation. *Mol Biol Cell.* 2001;12:1131-1145.
45. NIWA R, NAGATA-OHASHI K, TAKEICHI M, MIZUNO K, UEMURA T. Control of actin reorganization by slingshot, a family of phosphatases that dephosphorylate ADF/cofilin. *Cell.* 2002; 108:233-246.
46. ONO S, MINAMI N, ABE H, OBINATA T. Characterization of a novel cofilin isoform that is predominantly expressed in mammalian skeletal muscle. *J Biol Chem.* 1994;269:15280-15286.
47. VARTIAINEN MK, MUSTONEN T, MATTILA PK, OJALA PJ, THESLEFF I, PARTANEN J, LAPPALAINEN P. The three mouse actin-depolymerizing factor/cofilins evolved to fulfill cell-type-specific requirements for actin dynamics. *Mol Biol Cell.* 2002;13:183-194.
48. WOLF C, CAI WJ, VOSSCHULTE R, KOLTAI S, MOUSAVIPOUR D, SCHOLZ D, AFSAH-HEDJRI A, SCHAPER W, SCHAPER J. Vascular remodeling and altered protein expression during growth of coronary collateral arteries. *J Mol Cell Cardiol.* 1998;30:2291-2305.
49. SCHWARTZ MA, SHATTIL SJ. Signaling networks linking integrins and Rho family GTPases. *Trends Biochem Sci.* 2000;25:388-391.
50. KILE BT, SCHULMAN BA, ALEXANDER WS, NICOLA NA, MARTIN HME, HILTON DJ. The SOCS box: a tale of destruction and degradation. *Trends Biochem Sci.* 2002;27:235-241.
51. KILE BT, ALEXANDER WS. The suppressors of cytokine signaling (SOCS). *Cell Mol Life Sci.* 2001;58:1627-1635.
52. BOENGLER K, PIPP F, FERNÁNDEZ B, RICHTER A, SCHAPER W, DEINDL E. The ankyrin repeat containing SOCS box protein 5: a novel protein associated with arteriogenesis. *Biochem Biophysl Res Comm.* 2003;302:17-22.
53. UWATOKU T, SHIMOKAWA H, ABE K, MATSUMOTO Y, HATTORI T, OI K, MATSUDA T, KATAOKA K, TAKESHITA A. Application of nanoparticle technology for the prevention of restenosis after balloon injury in rats. *Circ Res.* 2003;92:62e-69.
54. ZHANG JG, FARLEY A, NICHOLSON SE, WILLSON TA, ZUGARO LM, SIMPSON RJ, MORITZ RL, CARY D, RICHARDSON R, HAUSMANN G, KILE BJ, KENT SBH, ALEXANDER WS, METCALF D, HILTON DJ, NICOLA NA, BACA M. The conserved SOCS box motif in suppressors of cytokine signaling binds to elongins B and C and may couple bound proteins to proteasomal degradation. *Proc Natl Acad Sci.* 1999;96:2071-2076.

55. NICHOLSON SE, WILLSON TA, FARLEY A, STARR R, ZHANG J-G, BACA M, ALEXANDER WS, METCALF D, HILTON DJ, NICOLA NA. Mutational analyses of the SOCS proteins suggest a dual domain requirement but distinct mechanisms for inhibition of LIF and IL-6 signal transduction. *EMBO J.* 1999;18:375-385.

56. KUO H, CHEN J, RUIZ-LOZANO P, ZOU Y, NEMER M, CHIEN K. Control of segmental expression of the cardiac-restricted ankyrin repeat protein gene by distinct regulatory pathways in murine cardiogenesis. *Development.* 1999;126:4223-4234.

57. AIHARA Y, KURABAYASHI M, ARAI M, KEDES L, NAGAI R. Molecular cloning of rabbit CARP cDNA and its regulated expression in adriamycin-cardiomyopathy. *Biochimt Biophys Acta (BBA).* 1999;1447:318-324.

58. ZOLK O, FROHME M, MAURER A, KLUXEN F-W, HENTSCH B, ZUBAKOV D, HOHEISEL J, ZUCKER IH, PEPE S, T. E. Cardiac ankyrin repeat protein, a negative regulator of cardiac gene expression is augmented in human heart failure. *Biochem Biophys Res Comm.* 2002;293:1377-1382.

59. ZOU Y, EVANS S, CHEN J, KUO H, HARVEY R, CHIEN K. Carp, a cardiac ankyrin repeat protein, is downstream in the Nkx2-5 homeobox gene pathway. *Development.* 1997;124:793-804.

60. JEYASEELAN R, POIZAT C, BAKER RK, ABDISHOO S, ISTERABADI LB, LYONS GE, KEDES L. A novel cardiac-restricted target for doxorubicin. Carp, a nuclear modulator of gene expresion in cardiac progenitor cells and cardiomyocytes. *J Biol Chem.* 1997;272:22800-22808.

BOENGLER, K., PIPP, F., FERNÁNDEZ, B., ZIEGELHOEFFER, T., SCHAPER, W., DEINDL, E. Arteriogenesis is associated with an induction of the cardiac ankyrin repeat protein (carp). *Cardiovasc Res* 2003, 59, 573-581

62. SCHWACHTGEN J-L, HOUSTON P, CAMPBELL C, SUKHATME V, BRADDOCK M. Fluid shear stress activation of Egr-1 transcription in cultured human endothelial and epithelial cells Is mediated via the extracellular signal-related kinase 1/2 mitogen-activated protein kinase pathway. *J Clin Invest.* 1998;101:2540-2549.

63. YOSHISUE H, SUZUKI K, KAWABATA A, OHYA T, ZHAO H, SAKURADA K, TABA Y, SASAGURI T, SAKAI N, YAMASHITA S. Large scale isolation of non-uniform shear stress-responsive genes from cultured human endothelial cells through the preparation of a subtracted cDNA library. *Atherosclerosis.* 2002;162:323-334.

64. NEGISHI M, LU D, ZHANG YQ, SAWADA Y, SASAKI T, KAYO T, ANDO J, IZUMI T, KURABAYASHI M, KOJIMA I, MASUDA H, TAKEUCHI T. Upregulatory expression of furin and transforming growth factor-ß by fluid shear stress in vascular endothelial cells. *Arterscler Thromb Vasc Biol.* 2001;21:785-790.

65. KANAI H, TANAKA T, AIHARA Y, TAKEDA S-I, KAWABATA M, MIYAZONO K, NAGAI R, KURABAYASHI M. Transforming Growth Factor-{beta}/SMADs signaling induces transcription of the cell type-restricted ankyrin repeat protein carp gene through CAGA motif in vascular smooth muscle cells. *Circ Res.* 2001;88:30-29.

66. LIU C, YAO J, DE BELLE I, HUANG R-P, ADAMSON E, MERCOLA D. The Transcription factor Egr-1 suppresses transformation of human fibrosarcoma HT1080 cells by coordinated induction of transforming growth factor-beta 1, fibronectin, and plasminogen activator inhibitor-1. *J Biol Chem.* 1999;274:4400-4411.

67. BIESIADA E, RAZANDI M, LEVIN ER. Egr-1 activates basic fibroblast growth factor transcription. Mechanistic implications for astrocyte proliferation. *J Biol Chem.* 1996;271:18576-18581.

Chapter 13

Theory of Arteriogenesis

Wolfgang Schaper

The scheme presented in figure 1 shows the time relationship of changes observed during arteriogenesis. It is descriptive and the only suggestion of causality is precedence: later ones cannot have caused early events. In figure 2 causality is expressed and dependencies had been tested for causality either by transgenic studies or by pharmacological interventions. As said several times during the course of this book: shear stress acting on the endothelium starts the entire arteriogenic cascade. Shear stress increases when the pressure in the reentry part of a preexisting arteriole falls which is the case with tight stenoses or acute arterial occlusions. Shear stress must be present for several hours before the endothelium becomes activated, which manifests itself in swelling and edema. The endothelial cell tries to correct the partial loss of volume regulation by changing the open probability of anion-, (later by kation-) channels. Interfering with that process (regaining of volume control, blockade with T-type Ca++ channel blockers) inhibits arteriogenesis. The signaling of the activated endothelium starts at channel activation (and probably reactive oxygen species), proceeds via the MAPKinases and results in upregulation of a number of genes, mainly of cell adhesion proteins (ICAM, VCAM, osteopontin), in chemo-attractants (MCP-1), chemo-repellents (eNOS), and proteases (u-PA). The resulting adhesion and invasion of monocytes leads to the production of growth factors and proteases (MMPs) and starts remodeling and growth by lysis of the extracellular matrix, thereby releasing again growth factors (released FGF-2 increases the transcription of FGF-7) and upregulating growth factor receptors. The MMPs are activated by u-PA and elastolysis is probably one of the most important steps of outward remodeling: the breakdown of the tension-bearing skeleton increases the circumferential wall tension for the SMCs, a proliferative stimulus which is increased by the growth-induced increase in radius and becomes normal again (by negative feedback) only after the final step of remodeling, the increase in wall thickness. Elastin fragments attract new monocytes, they downregulate the elastin transcription in SMCs that change phenotype, become mobile, move toward the intima and proliferate. That proliferation becomes directional and results in a larger vessel is probably caused by the expression of eNOS which, by NO production, directs the intimal smooth muscle cells towards the media and outer layers. Smooth muscle cells, normally devoid of a junctional system, develop one during the process of arteriogenesis (connexin 37). Meanwhile changes occur in the expression of a number of cytoskeletal proteins as well as proteins of the extracellular matrix which are first downregulated and, at later mature stages, upregulated again. Signaling proceeds via the MAPKinases and via Rho and starts with the upregulation of the FGF receptor 1 and with downregulation of RGS-5 which opens the chain of signals processed via G-protein coupled receptors. Prominent transcription factors are Egr-1, Mef2A and carp, together with a number of not very closely studied (within the context of arteriogenesis) zink finger and homeobox factors. The larger dimensions of the remodeled collateral vessel together with the restitution of normal blood flow reduce shear stress and the endothelial activation stops and with it all endothelial-dependent changes in gene expression. Smooth muscle proliferation continues for some time until the wall thickness has reached values that are compatible with normal circumferential wall tension.

Therapeutic Considerations, the Bottom Line

From what is presented in this book arteriogenesis stimulation is a realistic goal and almost normal maximal blood flow values can be obtained after arterial occlusion in animal models. It is difficult to foresee whether similar results can be obtained in patients with atherosclerosis. However, the small arterioles from which large collateral vessels develop are usually free from atherosclerotic lesions with the exception of diabetic vasculopathy. From our studies we would predict that a solution containing a proteolytic enzyme that digests the extracellular matrix including elastin, plus a chemotactic peptide that attracts monocytes, together with a non-specific mitogen and a potent vasodilator should be successful in restoring blood flow reserve. Such a solution should be infused at a strategically chosen place in the arterial system. The clinical feasibility of such a treatment is at present unknown.

A summary of the findings described is presented in figure 1 and 2.

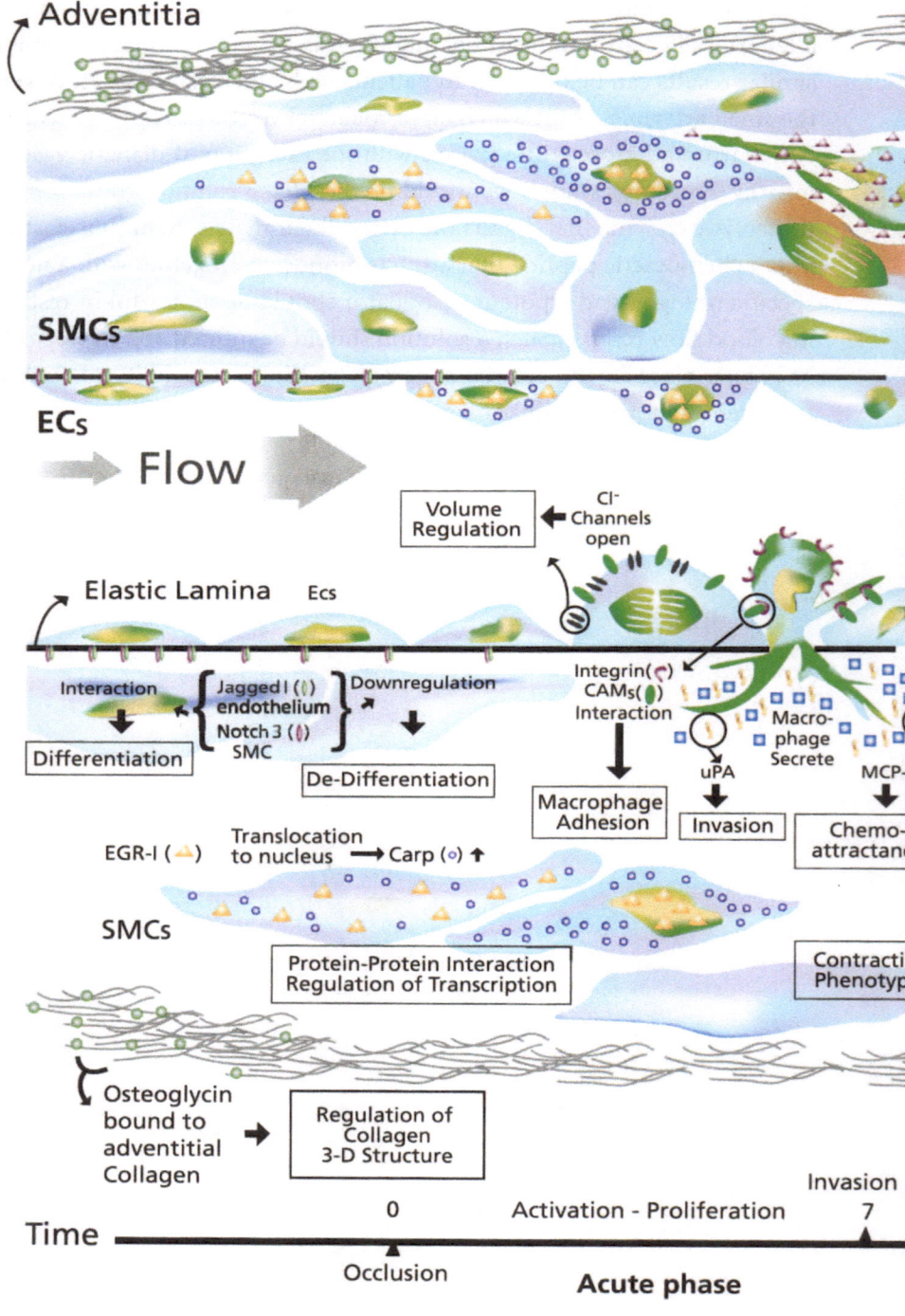

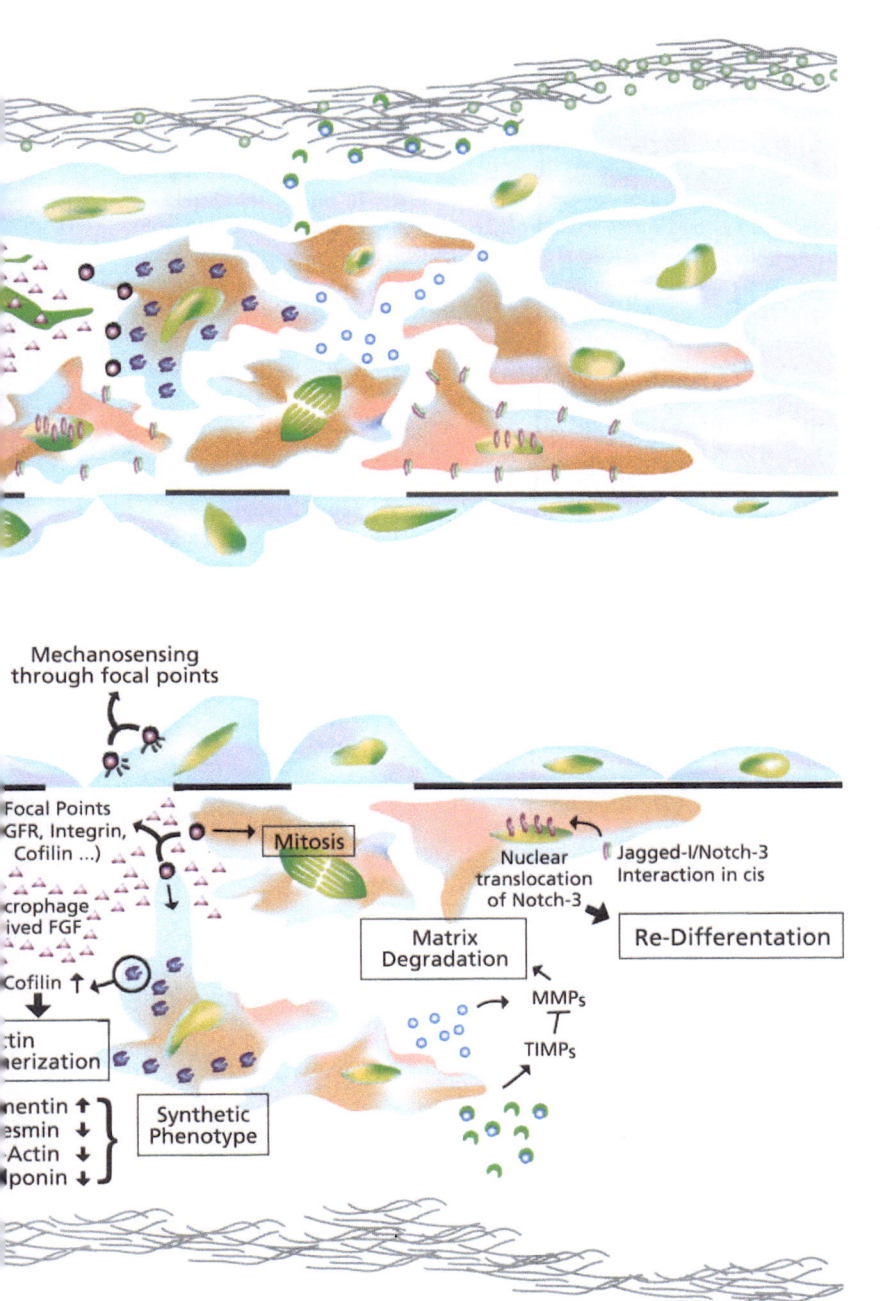

Mechanosensing
through focal points

Focal Points
GFR, Integrin,
Cofilin ...)

Mitosis

Nuclear
translocation
of Notch-3

Jagged-I/Notch-3
Interaction in cis

crophage
ived FGF

Re-Differentiation

Cofilin ↑

**Matrix
Degradation**

ctin
erization

MMPs
⊤
TIMPs

mentin ↑
esmin ↓
-Actin ↓
ponin ↓

**Synthetic
Phenotype**

ima Formation   14   Maturation   21 ▲ Days

Remodeling

1) Time course of arteriogenesis. Molecular to cellular events.

Arteriogenesis is initiated by a sudden increase in the blood flowing from the stem to the reentry segments of the collateral artery (left to right). The first molecular events concentrate in the endothelium, where chloride channels (⊗) open, regulating volume overload that leads to endothelial cell hypertrophy, the first morphological sign in arteriogenesis. Early responding genes like EGR-1 (▲) are upregulated and translocated to the nucleus, inducing the expression of ankirin repeating proteins like CARP (○), responsible for protein-protein interactions that regulate gene transcription. Endothelium to SMC interactions through Jagged (❘) and Notch (❘) are reduced, what probably leads to activation and de-differenti-ation of SMCs. The same pathway may be responsible for later re-differentiation of the newly formed media. Integrins (ϛ) and cell adhesion molecules (❘) in the surface of endothelial cells and monocytes respectively, facilitate leukocyte transmigration through the collateral wall. Activated macrophages secrete then growth factors like FGF-2 (▲), which bind to re-ceptors clustered to focal points (❡ː) in the smooth muscle and endothelial cell membrane, leading to proliferation and migration. SMCs change phenotype (from contractile to synthetic), creating a neointimal layer that constitutes the backbone of the regenerating collateral media. Matrix degradation, crucial for intimal remodeling, is mediated by matrix metalloproteinases (MMPs) (○) and their inhibitors (TIMPs) (◥). The final increase in size of the collateral artery is facilitated by adventitial remodeling, where downregulation of osteoglycin (○) seems to play a key role. The whole arteriogenic process takes place in several weeks, and can be divided in three overlapping basic stages: activation/proliferation; intima formation; maturation.

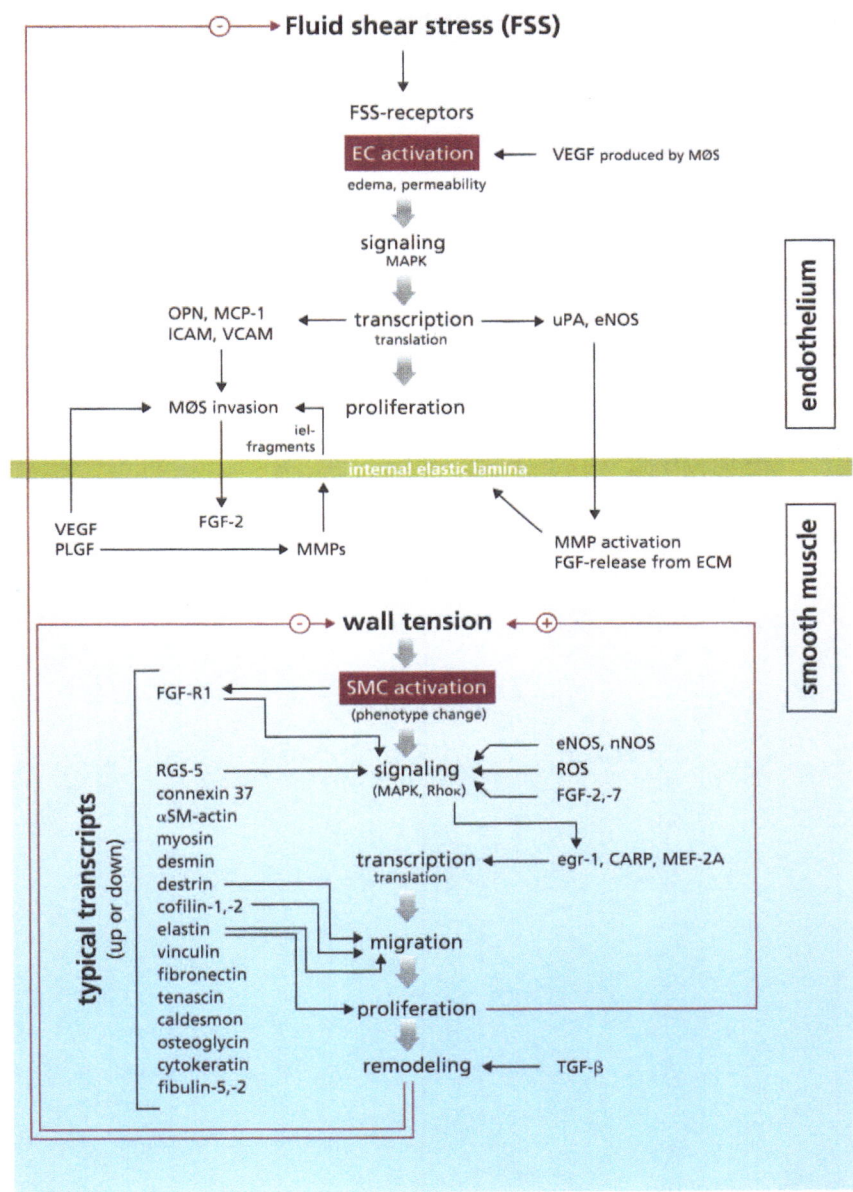

Fig. 2

Scheme to illustrate possible causal relationships and the cascade originating at the fluid shear stressed endothelium, which ends with the enlarged (remodeled) collateral vessels. Note the positive and negative feedback loops, which tend to restore physiological strains to normal values.

Chapter 14

Effects of Physical Activity

Swen Wolfram

Background

One of the first studies that explored the role of exercise for the treatment of peripheral arterial obstructive disease (PAOD) was done by Foley in 1957[1]. He reported faster healing of gangrenous feet when patients were subjected to a walking program. The German clinician Schoop focussed mainly on the importance of the collateral circulation[2]. He hypothesized that the speed of blood flow, but not ischemia, causes an increase in the collateral circulation and that exercise is the simplest, most effective method for increasing blood flow. He even suggested a precise interval training program for the treatment of PAOD. Unfortunately, these studies were mainly based on clinical impressions and little data were presented to prove the hypothesis and the effect of exercise on PAOD in general and on the collateral circulation in particular. In 1967, Skinner and Strandness[3] investigated the effect of a walking exercise program on three different parameters in patients with PAOD. Systolic pressure at the ankle after exercise, maximal walking time, and the time of the onset of claudication pain were significantly improved in all of the five study subjects. They concluded, without supplying further data, that a significant increase in collateral circulation of long-term exercised patients is improving the blood supply to the obstructed leg. In 1969, Alpert et al.[4] observed a significant correlation between the improvement in maximal walking time and the increase in calf blood flow during exercise after a six months walking regimen. The authors concluded that functional factors (e.g. better coordination of the working muscles) as well as anatomic factors (increase in the number and/or size of collateral vessels) are involved in the improvement of performance of patients after regular physical activity.

In 1968, Sanne and Sivertsson[5] performed one of the first experimental studies with regard to exercise and PAOD. After unilateral ligation of the femoral artery cats were trained for five weeks on a treadmill. The collateral resistance at maximal vasodilation was significantly reduced in trained cat, when compared to sedentary controls. They also reported that the flow resistance in the distal vascular bed was not changed after occlusion and not affected by exercise. Even though not providing any histological evidence they suggested that the "spontaneous" growth of the collateral vessels in the occluded limb was excellent. Five weeks after occlusion, the collateral resistance during maximal vasodilation decreased almost exactly threefold in the untrained animals. The authors hypothesized that the "normal" stimuli for collateral development, whatever their nature would be, are very efficient. They concluded that physical exercise is a very potent additional stimulus, which further enhances the development of collateral vessels. This study, being very elegant for its time, was pointing into a new direction. From there on, more attention was paid to collateral vessel development as a therapeutic mechanism for the treatment of PAOD.

Exercise-induced arteriogenesis in the rat

Terjung and coworkers mainly established the rat model of PAOD and exercise as a stimulus for arteriogenesis. In 1986, the results of their first study about the influence of exercise on rat hind limbs with femoral artery occlusion were reported[6]. Their results indicate a clear beneficial effect of exercise on maximal running duration and intensity. Functional performance of the gastrocnemius-plantaris-soleus muscles in trained animals with femoral artery occlusion was similar to control rats but reduced in sedentary animals. However, blood flow measurements with microspheres did not yet provide conclusive results about the exercise-induced arteriogenesis with subsequent increase in skeletal muscle perfusion during exercise.

Four years later this work was continued with slightly modified techniques[7]. After an endurance exercise program of six weeks no significant difference in total hind limb blood flow was observed between acutely occluded, sedentary occluded, and trained occluded animals. Total hind limb blood flow reached only 46-63 % when compared to unoperated control rats. However, a significant difference could be observed when blood flow distribution was analyzed. Animals with acute occlusion showed a markedly reduced blood flow to the gastrocnemius-plantaris-soleus muscle group relative to proximal blood flow. In sedentary animals, distal blood flow partially recovered and further increased in trained animals with occlusion. The authors suggested that the increase in blood flow to the distal hind limb in trained animals is due to better collateral vessel function. However, it is important to state that the total hind limb perfusion could not be recovered by exercise alone.

In the same year, Terjung and colleagues detected a significant increase in total hind limb blood flow in rats with occlusion and trained for up to eight weeks[8]. Again a significantly greater redistribution of blood flow to the gastrocnemius-plantaris-soleus muscles was observed in trained rats with occlusion compared to sedentary rats.

In 1993, the same group reported increased blood flow to the total hind limb, to the proximal muscles, and to the distal muscles, when the femoral artery was occluded after treatment with an ACE inhibitor for up to seven days[9]. The authors hypothesized that a larger diameter of the collateral vessels due to ACE inhibition is responsible for the increased blood flow. In a follow-up study[10], it was observed that long-term administration of an ACE inhibitor combined with physical activity for three weeks elevated total hind limb blood flow and exercise tolerance to a greater extent than physical activity or ACE inhibition alone.

The next pharmacological intervention in the same model was heparin treatment[11]. It was demonstrated that heparin treatment further enhanced blood flow to the entire hind limb, to proximal muscles, and to distal muscles. Heparin treatment in combination with physical activity also increased contractile force of the gastrocnemius-plantaris-soleus muscle group as well as exercise capacity as compared to sedentary heparin treated animals. This study is particularly interesting because heparin is known to interact with angiogenic growth factors. Through its high-affinity binding, heparin aids in the storage and possibly in the mobilization of growth factors in and from the extracellular matrix. It interacts with cell surface receptors and growth factors initiating the growth factor signaling. Therefore, it is not surprising that heparin enhances the process of collateral artery growth by possibly potentiating the effects of growth factors released due to physical activity.

In 1996, these investigators determined the influence of FGF-2 on collateral artery dependent blood flow[12]. FGF-2 infusion via osmotic pumps for four weeks markedly increased blood flow to the total hind limb, to proximal muscles, and to distal muscles. Muscle performance of the gastrocnemius-plantaris-soleus muscle group was enhanced and capillary-to-fiber ratio of FGF-2 infused rats was increased in high-oxidative fiber regions but not in a predominantly low-oxidative region as compared to rats with acute ligation and to heparin infused control animals. Postmortem angiograms revealed more collateral arteries and a better filling of the femoral artery distal to the point of occlusion. Thus, the authors proved FGF-2 treatment to be very efficient in inducing arteriogenesis upon femoral artery ligation.

When the stimulating effect of FGF-2 was combined with physical activity, a more pronounced increase in collateral artery dependent blood flow could be observed[13]. Hind limb blood flow measurements compared to the sedentary carrier group revealed an increase in the following order: trained carrier group, sedentary FGF-2 group, trained FGF-2 group. Interestingly, blood flow to the proximal hind limb muscles was especially enhanced in the trained FGF-2 group indicating a significant treatment interaction. However, when muscle performance was analyzed, the two sedentary groups could not maintain the tension as well as the trained carrier group. Again, the interaction of training and FGF-2 application led to the highest increase of muscle performance. These data indicate that muscle performance is not just determined by blood flow to the working muscle. But, other factors must also have contributed. Unfortunately, the investigators did not determine blood flow and muscle performance in unoperated control animals. It would be very interesting to compare the potency of the combined treatment with the physiological conditions. This could reveal whether blood flow to the occluded limb is partially or even totally restored and thus, the true significance of the combined treatment. Additionally, capillary-to-fiber ratio increased only in the low-oxidative gastrocnemius section of trained rats opposing their findings of the previous FGF-2 infusion study[12].

In 2000, the efficacy and specificity of FGF-2 application on the increase in collateral artery blood flow were determined[14]. The investigators found similar increases in the intraarterially infused group when compared to the intravenously infused group or the subcutaneously injected group as long as similar amounts were administered. There was no obvious difference in collateral artery blood flow when FGF-2 application was short-term or prolonged and continuous or intermittent. Chronic FGF-2 treatment did not alter blood flow upon acute femoral artery occlusion compared to untreated or carrier treated control rats. Therefore, the authors conclude that FGF-2-induced arteriogenesis requires vascular occlusion and can be restricted to short-term application through different routes to be effective.

In the same year, Yang et al.[15] evaluated the influence of an endurance exercise program before acute occlusion of the femoral artery on collateral artery blood flow. Prior endurance exercise training increased blood flow to the hind limb in the distal as well as in the proximal segment in comparison to sedentary control rats. Blood flow to the gastrocnemius-plantaris-soleus muscles was significantly increased but did not nearly reach the level of trained FGF-2 infused rats as shown earlier[13]. These results indicate that prior exercise training is effective in increasing blood flow to the distal hind limb muscles upon acute occlusion of the femoral artery. But since there is no need for an excessive use of the preexistent collateral arterioles during exercise with intact legs the increase in shear stress is just enough to induce a moderate growth of these vessels.

The most recently published study by Terjung and colleagues indicates that nitric oxide (NO) is implicated in arteriogenesis induced by FGF-2 as well as VEGF[16]. Nitric oxide synthase (NOS) inhibition abolished the effect of both FGF-2 and VEGF on arteriogenesis. Both growth factors alone were capable of increasing blood flow to the total hind limb, to proximal muscles, and to distal muscles to a similar extent when compared to untreated control rats. However, NOS inhibition together with FGF-2 or VEGF treatment resulted in unchanged blood flow when compared to untreated control rats. Thus, reduced NO production, availability, and/or responsiveness, which are frequent phenomena in patients with PAOD and CHF[17-19], could inhibit the arteriogenic response to FGF-2 and VEGF treatments.

Summarizing the results of Terjung and colleagues, one could speculate that the ideal treatment for rats with an arterial occlusion would
begin even before the onset of occlusion with at least six weeks of treadmill running and possibly ACE inhibition. After femoral artery occlusion
FGF-2 application via different routes has proven to be extremely effective when combined with an endurance regimen for at least four weeks.
In this model, exercise appears to potentiate the effect of FGF-2 via further increase in shear stress and increased release of NO (for review see[20]).
It has also been shown that FGF-2 application to vascular smooth muscle cells *in vitro* upregulates the expression of VEGF[21]. A marked synergistic effect on VEGF expression could be observed when hypoxia was
combined with FGF-2 application. This study suggests that FGF-2 and
skeletal muscle hypoxia during exercise could have promoted among
other factors an amplified VEGF response in trained FGF-2 treated rats.

Exercise-induced arteriogenesis in the dog

In the late 1970s, researchers and clinicians paid much more attention to
the possible effect of exercise on the development of the collateral circulation upon occlusion of a major coronary artery. Arteriosclerosis had
become the leading cause of death some years ago and cardiovascular
medicine was looking for ways to increase perfusion in areas distal to the
site of occlusion. The dog model had been shown to be useful for clinicians, surgeons, and researchers at the time for three reasons:

- Surgical techniques used for humans could be applied with slight
  modifications.
- Dogs develop impressive coronary collaterals that could be visualized
  by angiography.
- Last but not least dogs proved to be very good runners.

In 1978, Heaton et al.[22] reported that exercise enhanced blood flow only
to the endocardium of the collateral dependent zone in dogs with occlusions of the left circumflex coronary artery and of the distal part of the
left anterior descending artery. The enhanced endocardial blood flow
could only be observed during exercise. The training program of six
weeks was sufficient to induce a decrease in heart rate at a given workload. In sedentary control animals blood flow did not change over the
same period, which would indicate that no significant arteriogenic re-

sponse occurred. However, the baseline measurements were performed two weeks after the initial operation, which is the period were the main arteriogenic adaptation occurs. Thus, these results are not indicative for the entire process of arteriogenesis.

Neill and Oxendine[23] reported that trained dogs with occlusion of the left circumflex coronary artery had a higher retrograde flow from the distal part of the occluded artery when compared to their sedentary controls. However, the retrograde flow method does not indicate the true tissue perfusion by collaterals. The greater pressure drop across the coronary collaterals observed in sedentary dogs is most likely due to increased scar formation in the collateral dependent zone of the myocardium. There was no apparent difference in the angiographic images of trained and sedentary dogs. Furthermore, the microsphere technique demonstrated that there was no beneficial effect of physical activity on blood flow to the collateral dependent zone of the myocardium.

In 1981[24], it was reported that exercise promotes collateral dependent blood flow after a three months convalescent period after occlusion of the left circumflex coronary artery. Again, the retrograde perfusion method used in this study does not allow conclusions about the tissue perfusion provided by collateral arteries. Daily low intensity exercise for six weeks did not alter collateral dependent blood flow in control dogs with normal coronary arteries.

In 1982, our group at the Max-Planck-Institute in Bad Nauheim conducted a study to precisely determine the role of exercise in the induction of collateral coronary growth[25]. For this purpose, we used a standardized isolated heart model to determine regional blood flows with tracer microspheres during maximal vasodilation and under a wide range of perfusion pressures (40-140mm Hg). The dogs performed a vigorous exercise program (up to three months) before the left circumflex and the right coronary arteries were slowly occluded with ameroid constrictors (one-vessel occlusion was used in most of the aforementioned studies). After a recovery period of two weeks the dogs continued the exercise program for another 12 weeks. The workloads used in this study were the highest reported so far. At the end of the training period the dogs achieved a very high level of physical fitness. They were able to run at an inclination of 22% and a speed of eight miles per hour for one hour. However, there was neither a difference in coronary nor in collateral blood flow in exercised dogs when compared to the sedentary control animals. Collateral conductance in trained and sedentary dogs reached only about 40% of that of the replaced coronary artery. Calculated total collateral resistance of trained dogs was not different from sedentary animals. No significant change in mortality was observed. This study was mainly designed to precisely determine the influence of physical activity on coronary collateral arteries of the dog. The isolated heart preparation allowed the use of fixed pressures under maximal vasodilation and the determination of the corresponding blood flow via use of radiolabled microspheres. The study demonstrated that a very high level of physical activity does not produce an increase in coronary collateral blood flow in dogs and thus, did not provide a further stimulus for arteriogenesis. Because of the advanced techniques used in our study the observations are at variance with other studies that reported beneficial effects of physical activity on collateral dependent blood flow. Nevertheless, we cannot exclude the possibility that treadmill running at a certain workload could have produced differences in collateral blood flow when comparing the highly trained dogs and their sedentary controls. Note that the beneficial effect of exercise on final infarct size that was previously reported by our group[26] was not again assessed in this study.

A study that partially confirmed this assumption was conducted in the same year[27]. Dogs with a stenosed left circumflex coronary artery were trained for 12 weeks on a treadmill in sprints and endurance running. In comparison to sedentary controls trained dogs exhibited less evidence of left ventricular failure (higher cardiac output, lower left atrial pressure) upon total occlusion of the left circumflex coronary artery during a single exercise session. Trained dogs showed improved collateral dependent blood flow at rest and during exercise while there was virtually no improvement in the sedentary control dogs. The authors concluded that running exercise stimulates the development of collateral vessels in dogs with a stenosed coronary artery, and that the enhanced collateral flow has salutary effects on myocardial function. However, compared with our findings regarding myocardial blood flow these results could also be interpreted differently. Physical activity induced beneficial changes of myocardial function during exercise, leading to enhanced perfusion of the myocardium upon total occlusion during a given level of exercise.

In 1985, Cohen and Steingart reported their findings on coronary collateral development after occlusion of the left circumflex coronary artery in dogs submitted to an endurance exercise program for six weeks[28]. Using thallium-201 scintigraphy during exercise, the investigators revealed a significant improvement in scintigraphic measurements over the first four weeks. Microsphere measurements showed a good recovery of perfusion distal to the site of occlusion. Serial angiographic studies showed the development of collateral vessels and the increase in collateral circulation to the left circumflex coronary artery. Cardiac output during exercise increased and left atrial pressure decreased significantly during the study period. However, the lack of a real control group makes it difficult to ascribe these beneficial effects to the exercise regimen used in this study. Nevertheless, this study demonstrated that collateral coronary artery development is a dynamic process and that exercise hemodynamic measurements improve with progression of arteriogenesis.

Two years later, the same model was used to investigate the effect of an exercise program prior to occlusion of the left circumflex coronary artery on the degree of infarction and collateral dependent blood flow[29]. No significant change in infarct size was observed. The effect of exercise on collateral dependent blood flow did not reach the level of significance. Evaluating the parameters used in this study, no clear beneficial role of prior exercise in cardioprotection was observed.

Cohen and coworkers[30] investigated the role of exercise training in collateral vessel development in dogs with normal coronary arteries. Ten to 12 weeks of endurance exercise resulted in significant adaptations of the cardiovascular system and skeletal muscle. However, the increase in collateral dependent blood flow was not significant, suggesting that exercise is not an appropriate stimulus for arteriogenesis in dogs with normal coronary arteries.

In 1990, it was reported that endurance training does not induce changes in collateral development in dogs with normal coronary arteries[31]. After an endurance exercise regimen of 12 weeks collateral blood flow determined by microspheres was not different from sedentary animals. The author concluded that exercise in dogs with normal coronary arteries does not alter the development of collateral vessels. This suggests that arteriogenesis is not an adaptation mechanism to an exercise program of 12 weeks in dogs with normal coronary arteries.

Weiss et al.[32] investigated the effect of treadmill walking on collateral dependent blood flow in dogs with unilateral occlusion of the femoral artery and its branches for over one year. At the end of the exercise period, blood flow during resting conditions as well as immediately after exercise was determined using microspheres. Interestingly, there was no difference in blood flow between the control leg and the leg with occlusion under both conditions, suggesting that walking exercise induced an immense increase in collateral dependent blood flow to hind limb muscles. However, due to the lack of a sedentary control group no definite conclusion can be drawn about the true role of physical activity in this study.

In summary, dogs with occlusion of one or two coronary arteries develop large and well visible collateral arteries. The collateral conductance reaches only about 40 % of that of the replaced coronary artery leaving room for therapeutic intervention. Exercise has failed to induce arteriogenesis. Increases in tissue perfusion in exercised dogs have mainly been observed during exercise but not under pressure controlled ex vivo conditions. Cardiac output increases, heart rate and atrial filling pressure decrease at a given workload. Therefore, regular physical activity could lead to either increased myocardial perfusion at a certain workload due to the increased cardiac output and/or to reduced myocardial oxygen demand due to enhanced oxidative metabolism. These questions remain to be solved.

Furthermore, there are no studies that undoubtedly prove the acceleration of arteriogenesis due to exercise in dogs with femoral artery occlusion. However, regular physical activity causes beneficial changes of hemodynamic parameters. Applying these results to the human should not result in questioning the importance of physical activity. Even without paying attention to the anatomical and physiological species differences it should be encouraging for us that trained dogs with coronary occlusions can develop an impressive physical fitness even though their collateral conductance remains similar to that of sedentary controls.

Exercise-induced arteriogenesis in the pig

Bloor and coworkers made major contributions to the knowledge of development of coronary arteries due to exercise. In 1984, Bloor et al.[33] investigated the effects of exercise on coronary collateral artery development in pigs with occlusion of the left circumflex coronary artery. The investigators have chosen pigs as study species because it has sparse innate coronary collaterals like in humans. Two weeks after placing an ameroid constrictor around the left circumflex coronary artery, the pigs were assigned to an endurance exercise regimen for five months. Physical activity resulted in an increase of exercise capacity, a reduction of infarct size, and an increase in collateral blood flow to the noninfarcted jeopardized myocardium as compared to sedentary control animals. Therefore, with respect to the utilized exercise regimen and the experimental protocol, it appears that collateral vessels develop primarily in or near the ischemic zone of the myocardium and served in tissue salvage.

The influence of strenuous exercise on cardiac hypertrophy as well as capillary and arteriolar density of pig myocardium was assessed in a later study[34]. A reduction in capillary density and an increase in arteriolar density were reported. However, densities were assessed in number per mm^2 and since myocyte cross sectional area was increased by 21% in the trained group, these data are not conclusive. Nevertheless, the increase in arteriolar density would be more meaningful when expressed as capillary-to-fiber ratio. Blood flow was not significantly different at rest, during exercise, and during exercise under maximal vasodilation. The only change that could be detected in trained pigs was an increase in epicardial blood flow during exercise and exercise under maximal vasodilation.

In 1987, these investigators reported similar results considering capillary and arteriolar densities[35]. Additional measurements revealed increased maximal oxygen consumption, and increased stroke volume and end-diastolic volume during exercise. The initial reduction in left ventricular end-diastolic diameter during progressive exercise was abolished after the strenuous training regimen. This study is again highlighting the importance of functional adaptations of the myocardium to exercise stimuli. In addition, arteriolar growth had been induced by strenuous physical activity in pig myocardium.

Four years later, another study was carried out to determine the effect of exercise on myocardial blood flow and function after occlusion of the left circumflex coronary artery[36]. An increase in systolic wall thickening during exercise could be observed after a running regimen of 25 days. The effect of the training regimen on myocardial blood flow was best visible during severe exercise. Subepicardial, submyocardial, and subendocardial blood flow ratios increased significantly when compared to the initial blood flow measurements prior to training. Neither systolic wall thickening nor blood flow changed during exercise in sedentary control animals over the study period. The authors concluded that exercise improved myocardial function and blood flow to the collateral dependent myocardium.

There are no data available regarding the effect of exercise on arteriogenesis after femoral artery occlusion in the pig.

In summary, pigs with occlusion of the left circumflex coronary artery respond to regular physical activity with improved myocardial performance. Blood flow to the jeopardized myocardium is increased at a given workload suggesting that arteriogenesis has taken place. Nevertheless, these results are in need of confirmation by other techniques. The isolated heart preparation could be useful to detect if the increase in blood flow during exercise is induced by growth of collaterals or by enhanced myocardial performance. However, exercise has been demonstrated to induce the growth of arterioles in hypertrophied myocardium of pigs. This growth appears to be merely a mechanism for blood flow maintenance.

Exercise-induced arteriogenesis in the mouse

To the best of our knowledge, there are no studies concerning the effect of exercise on arteriogenesis in mice. In recent years it has been a major issue in our department to develop a mouse model of PAOD. This was especially important because the availability of different transgenic mice provides the possibility to explore the underlying mechanisms of arteriogenesis. The small size of the animal allows the use of very expensive and rare compounds. After investing a lot of time and effort, we were able to develop a mouse model of PAOD together with techniques to detect changes in collateral dependent blood flow via Laser Doppler Imaging (LDI) [37] and Magnetic Resonance Imaging (MRI). We adapted our histological methods to visualize arteriogenesis in tissue. Angiography of the hind limbs depicts the growth pattern of the collateral vessels. Furthermore, we developed a technique to quantify reactive hyperemia in mice with femoral artery occlusion and we found that Balb/C mice displayed significantly greater reactive hyperemia in the legs with arterial occlusion compared to two other mouse strains (129/Sv and C57BL/6) (Helisch et al. unpublished data). The fact that reactive hyperemia was similar in the normal legs among all three strains suggests that the legs with occlusion of 129/Sv and C57BL/6 mice were fully vasodilated at this stage.

Determination of exercise capacity provides us with information about functional relevance of arteriogenesis (see Appendix)[38]. We developed a progressive, moderate intensity exercise program for mice with femoral artery ligation to determine the influence of physical activity on arteriogenesis in mice.

The first study was carried out in mice overexpressing FGF-2 and their nontransgenic littermates[39]. In a preliminary study we have observed the beneficial effect of constant FGF-2 infusion on collateral dependent blood flow as well as on the size of collateral arteries. We hypothesized that subjecting FGF-2 transgenic mice to regular physical activity would result in accelerated growth of collateral arteries and that this would possibly lead to total recovery of the blood flow deficit caused by femoral artery occlusion. After unilateral occlusion of the femoral artery 12 FGF-2 transgenic mice and 12 nontransgenic littermates were randomly divided into sedentary and trained groups. The exercise program was started at day 3 post occlusion. Initially, mice ran at a speed of 10 m/min at an inclination of 9° for 30 minutes. Every day speed and duration were increased by 1 m/min and 5 minutes, respectively, until the animals were able to run for one hour at a speed of 25 m/min. The trained groups exercised six days per week for five weeks while the sedentary mice were restricted to cage activity. The trained mice never reached the point of fatigue during an exercise session. Therefore, we considered the intensity of our exercise regimen to be moderate.

Collateral dependent blood flow of the foot determined by LDI increased significantly in trained transgenic animals when compared to sedentary wildtype animals and trained wildtype mice (Fig 1). A trend towards an increase in foot blood flow of sedentary transgenic mice was noted.

MRI measurements revealed that both trained and sedentary FGF-2 transgenic animals showed a dramatic increase in gastrocnemius blood flow of the leg with femoral artery occlusion, which reached the blood flow level of the normal leg of sedentary wildtype mice (Fig 2). This suggests that FGF-2 overexpression causes a total compensation of the blood flow impairment due to femoral artery occlusion. In transgenic mice,

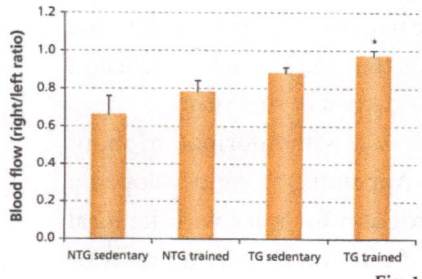

Fig. 1

*Collateral dependent blood flow to the foot (determined by LDI) of sedentary nontransgenic (NTG sedentary), trained nontransgenic (NTG trained), sedentary FGF-2 transgenic (TG sedentary), and trained FGF-2 transgenic (TG trained) mice at day 39 post occlusion. Data are means ± SEM. * p < 0.05 vs. sedentary nontransgenic mice.*

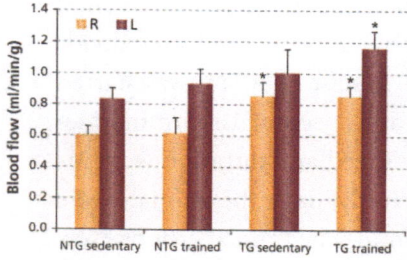

Fig. 2

*Collateral dependent blood flow to the gastrocnemius (determined by MRI) of sedentary nontransgenic (NTG sedentary), trained nontransgenic (NTG trained), sedentary FGF-2 transgenic (TG sedentary), and trained FGF-2 transgenic (TG trained) mice at day 39 post occlusion (R = right occluded femoral artery, L = left normal leg). Data are means ± SEM. * p < 0.05 vs. sedentary nontransgenic mice.*

endurance exercise training even led to a significant increase in gastrocnemius blood flow of the normal leg. These results imply that the combination of FGF-2 overexpression and exercise promotes skeletal muscle blood flow not only under disease conditions but also under physiological conditions.

Much to our surprise we did not detect an increase in the number or in the diameter of collateral arteries in transgenic and/or trained mice. However, angiographs of the hind limb vasculature suggested that exercise training causes growth of straight collateral vessels rather than the regular corkscrew growth pattern observed in untrained mice (Fig 3).

Interestingly, capillarity of the gastrocnemius muscle in the leg with femoral artery occlusion was similar among all groups. However, capillarity in the normal leg was increased by expression of the transgene and by exercise (Fig 4). The greatest capillary density was observed in trained transgenic mice, which coincides with pronounced staining of skeletal muscle (i.e. tissue perfusion with contrast agent) observed in angiographs of this group. Note that femoral artery occlusion alone caused an increase in capillarity.

FGF-2 overexpression seemed to protect skeletal muscle as we did not observe a fiber type shift towards the oxidative type I skeletal muscle fibers displayed by wildtype mice (Fig 5).

The most impressive finding of the study was the pronounced increase in functional performance due to training (Fig 6). When compared to sedentary wildtype mice, trained transgenic mice demonstrated the greatest exercise capacity followed by trained wildtype mice. Trained transgenic mice improved exercise capacity to more than 300% while trained wildtype animals improved to more than 200%. Interestingly, there was no significant difference between the sedentary groups.

These findings are important for various aspects of the treatment of PAOD. They suggest that FGF-2 might be an important treatment option for patients with PAOD. In our mouse model, FGF-2 caused improved blood flow to distal tissues. It increased capillarity of skeletal muscle and prevented the fiber type shift due to femoral artery occlusion. However, these changes might not be sufficient to cause an increase in functional performance. On the other hand, exercise alone did only moderately affect blood flow and skeletal muscle fiber type composition but resulted in a pronounced increase in treadmill performance. When FGF-2 was combined with exercise the greatest improvement in treadmill performance was observed. Our findings strongly emphasize that evaluating the success of growth factor therapy has to involve blood flow measurements and determination of structural changes of vasculature and skeletal muscle.

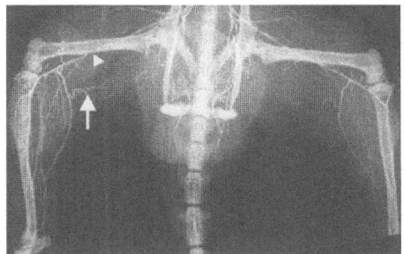

Fig. 3a

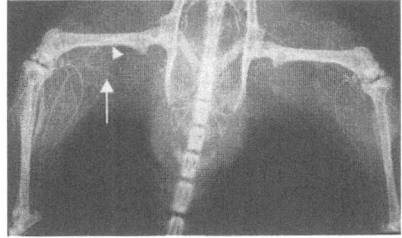

Fig. 3b

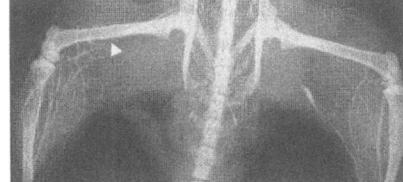

Fig. 3c

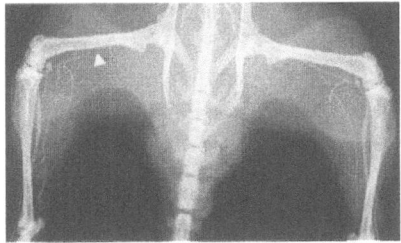

Fig. 3d

Representative angiographies of a) of sedentary nontransgenic mice, b) sedentary FGF-2 transgenic mice, c) trained nontransgenic mice, and d) trained FGF-2 transgenic mice. Note the site of occlusion (arrowhead) and the typical corkscrew growth pattern of the collateral arteries in sedentary mice (arrow). In trained mice, collateral arteries display a straight growth pattern.

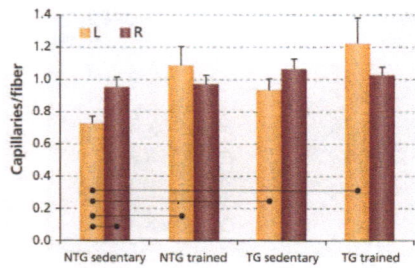

Fig. 4

Capillary-to-fiber ratio in gastrocnemius muscle of sedentary nontransgenic (NTG sedentary), trained nontransgenic (NTG trained), sedentary FGF-2 transgenic (TG sedentary), and trained FGF-2 transgenic (TG trained) mice at day 39 post occlusion (R=right occluded femoral artery, L=left normal leg). Data are means ± SEM, •—• p < 0.05 vs. left normal leg of sedentary nontransgenic mice.

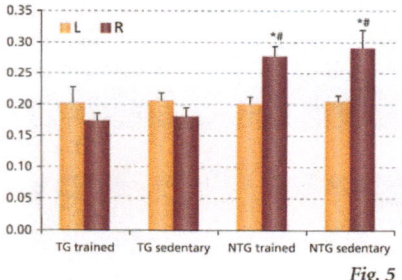

Fig. 5

*Gastrocnemius area occupied by myosin heavy chain 1-positive fibers of sedentary nontransgenic (NTG sedentary), trained nontransgenic (NTG trained), sedentary FGF-2 transgenic (TG sedentary), and trained FGF-2 transgenic (TG trained) mice at day 39 post occlusion. Data are means ± SEM. * p < 0.05 vs. left normal leg, # p < 0.05 vs. right leg with occlusion of corresponding transgenic group.*

Exercise and arteriogenesis in humans

There are numerous studies that demonstrate the beneficial effect of exercise on increase in both pain free walking distance and maximal walking distance in patients with PAOD (for reviews see [40,41]). However, results are conflicting considering increased blood flow due to regular physical activity in patients with PAOD. There are some studies that report increased blood flow [3,4,42-44], some that demonstrate unaltered perfusion [45-50], and one study that even reports a decreased resting perfusion [51].

Two recently published studies can be used as examples for the existing diversity. Gardner et al. [52] reported that calf blood flow was increased in elderly patients with PAOD after taking part in a six months treadmill exercise program. Blood flow was slightly elevated under resting conditions and more pronounced under reactive hyperemic conditions. The increase in reactive hyperemic blood flow correlated with the increase in pain free walking distance. On the other hand, Tan et al. [53] reported that three months of exercise training did not result in an increase in femoral artery blood flow.

Explanations for the opposite findings might involve the methodological differences in assessing blood flow. Furthermore, blood flow was determined at various time points and under different conditions. The duration and the intensity of the exercise regimen differ markedly. There is no consensus whether blood flow should be assessed under resting conditions, during or immediately after exercise, or during reactive hyperemia. These studies were conducted over a period of almost 40 years, which might explain the use of different methods. Nevertheless, establishing a widely accepted standard for measuring blood pressure in the human could solve this problem for further studies.

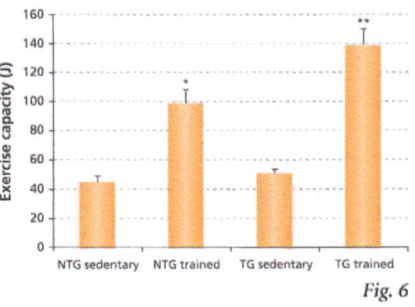

Fig. 6

Exercise capacity of sedentary nontransgenic (NTG sedentary), trained nontransgenic (NTG trained), sedentary FGF-2 transgenic (TG sedentary), and trained FGF-2 transgenic (TG trained) mice at day 36 post occlusion. Data are means ± SEM. * p < 0.05 vs. sedentary nontransgenic mice, ** p < 0.05 vs. trained nontransgenic mice.

Exercise proved to exert beneficial effects on the endothelial function of patients with heart failure[54]. Therefore, the beneficial effect of exercise training on blood flow could also be ascribed to enhanced endothelial function in some of the experimental settings. Restoration of the normal vasodilatory response due to endurance exercise is extremely relevant to achieve sufficient blood flow to skeletal muscle. This fact has to be considered for all studies investigating the influence of exercise on blood flow recovery in subjects with PAOD, especially if definite conclusions about the contribution of angiogenesis, arteriogenesis, or various treatments to increase blood flow can be drawn.

Furthermore, exercise influences a variety of other factors that are likely to contribute to the increase in maximal walking distance. These factors include skeletal muscle metabolism and morphology, blood rheology, development of atherosclerosis, walking economy, pain perception, and cardiac adaptations (for review see[55]). It is worth mentioning that a 2003 textbook on "Peripheral Artery Disease" states that exercise is the only proven therapy in PAOD[56].

Growth factors therapies for cardiovascular diseases are presently evaluated in clinical studies mainly focusing on coronary collateral development. However, many unresolved issues appear as these trials proceed (for review see[57]). An answer to the question which growth factor is effective in the induction of arterial growth in different cardiovascular diseases cannot be given with certainty. There is no study investigating the combined effect of regular physical activity and growth factor treatment.

Despite all efforts to introduce other treatment options for patients with PAOD endurance exercise training is still superior to any other therapy. One possible explanation is the increased shear stress in response to exercise. Skeletal muscle is rarely utilized for substantial work in patients with PAOD. On the other hand, the heart of patients with an occluded coronary artery is still incessantly contracting. Thus, an increase in physical activity is more likely to exert a beneficial effect on skeletal muscle than on the heart. However, more patients with PAOD could and should take advantage of the improvement potential of endurance exercise training.

In conclusion, there is no definite evidence for induction of arteriogenesis in patients with PAOD by exercise. However, exercise has been proven to be beneficial for maximal walking distance and quality of life of these patients. Further studies are needed to investigate the role of exercise in arteriogenesis in humans suffering from PAOD.

Appendix

As mentioned above (Exercise-induced arteriogenesis in the mouse) we investigated whether a relationship between collateral artery development and functional performance after femoral artery occlusion exists[38]. We observed that the recovery of collateral dependent foot blood flow under resting conditions differs markedly among three strains of mice with unilateral femoral artery occlusion. When compared to Balb/C mice, 129/Sv and C57BL/6 mice displayed a pronounced improvement in collateral dependent foot blood flow (Fig 7). At the end of the study foot blood flow in the leg with occlusion reached the level of the normal leg in 129/Sv and C57BL/6 mice. In contrast, in Balb/C mice resting foot blood flow of the leg with occlusion reached only 51 % of the normal leg after the 28-day study period.

In order to determine whether the observed differences in collateral dependent resting foot blood flow are reflected by differences in functional capacity we quantified exercise capacity of the three mouse strains. A graded exercise test on a rodent treadmill was carried out every seven days over the course of four weeks after bilateral femoral artery occlusion.

The pattern of recovery of exercise capacity after femoral artery occlusion was similar to the pattern of recovery of foot blood flow (Fig 8). In 129/Sv and C57BL/6 mice, exercise capacity recovered significantly faster and to a greater extent than in Balb/C mice. Thus, we conclude that the recovery of exercise capacity resembles the arteriogenic growth process as depicted by the recovery in foot blood flow. In our mouse model of PAOD, the determination of exercise capacity serves as a physiological marker for the severity of blood flow limitation due to femoral artery occlusion. Additionally, the recovery of exercise capacity reflects the increase in blood flow due to arteriogenesis on the functional level.

Furthermore, we noted several important details. The increase in collateral dependent resting foot blood flow precedes the increase in exercise capacity. Even though resting foot blood flow has totally recovered 28 days after femoral artery occlusion in 129/Sv and C57BL/6 mice exercise capacity was only partially restored. This suggests that skeletal muscle blood flow during exercise is still significantly impaired in our mouse model of PAOD, thereby closely resembling the situation in human patients with PAOD.

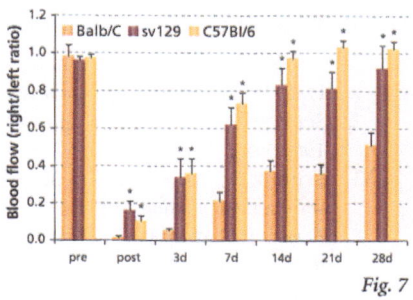

Fig. 7

*Collateral dependent blood flow to the foot (right/left ratio) determined by LDI of Balb/C, 129/Sv, and C57BL/6 mice with unilateral femoral artery occlusion immediately before and after occlusion and at days 3, 7, 14, 21, and 28. Data are means ± SEM. * p < 0.05 vs. Balb/C.*

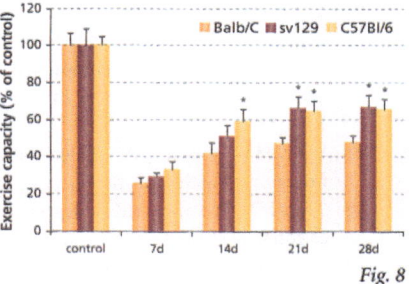

Fig. 8

*Recovery (% of control mice) of exercise capacity of Balb/C, 129/Sv, and C57BL/6 mice with bilateral femoral artery occlusion and at days 7, 14, 21, and 28 post occlusion. Data are means ± SEM. * p < 0.05 vs. Balb/C.*

References

1. FOLEY W. Treatment of gangrene of the feet and legs by walking. *Circulation.* 1957;15:689-700.
2. SCHOOP W. Bewegungstherapie bei peripheren Durchblutungsstörungen. *Med Welt Part 1.* 1964;502-.
3. SKINNER JS, STRANDNESS DE. Exercise and intermittent claudication.II. Effect of physical training. *Circulation.* 1967;36:23-9.
4. ALPERT JS, LARSEN OA, LASSEN NA. Exercise and intermittent claudication. Blood flow in the calf muscle during walking studied by the xenon-133 clearance method. *Circulation.* 1969;39:353-9.
5. SANNE H, SIVERTSSON R. The effect of exercise on the development of collateral circulation after experimental occlusion of the femoral artery in the cat. *Acta Physiol Scand.* 1968; 73:257-63.
6. MATHIEN GM, TERJUNG RL. Influence of training following bilateral stenosis of the femoral artery in rats. *Am J Physiol.* 1986;250:H1050-9.
7. MATHIEN GM, TERJUNG RL. Muscle blood flow in trained rats with peripheral arterial insufficiency. *Am J Physiol.* 1990;258:H759-65.
8. YANG HT, DINN RF, TERJUNG RL. Training increases muscle blood flow in rats with peripheral arterial insufficiency. *J Appl Physiol.* 1990;69:1353-9.
9. YANG HT, TERJUNG RL. Angiotensin-converting enzyme inhibition increases collateral-dependent muscle blood flow. *J Appl Physiol.* 1993;75:452-7.
10. YANG HT, TERJUNG RL. Angiotensin-converting enzyme inhibition increases exercise tolerance and muscle blood flow in rats with peripheral arterial insufficiency. *J Clin Pharmacol.* 1994;34:345-55.
11. YANG HT, OGILVIE RW, TERJUNG RL. Heparin increases exercise-induced collateral blood flow in rats with femoral artery ligation. *Circ Res.* 1995;76:448-56.
12. YANG HT, DESCHENES MR, OGILVIE RW, TERJUNG RL. Basic fibroblast growth factor increases collateral blood flow in rats with femoral arterial ligation. *Circ Res.* 1996;79:62-9.
13. YANG HT, OGILVIE RW, TERJUNG RL. Exercise Training Enhances Basic Fibroblast Growth Factor-Induced Collateral Blood Flow. *Am J Physiol.* 1998;43:H2053-H2061.
14. YANG HT, FENG Y, ALLEN LA, PROTTER A, TERJUNG RL. Efficacy and specificity of bFGF increased collateral flow in experimental peripheral arterial insufficiency. *Am J Physiology Heart & Circulatory Physiology.* 2000;278:H1966-73.
15. YANG HT, LAUGHLIN MH, TERJUNG RL. Prior exercise training increases collateral-dependent blood flow in rats after acute femoral artery occlusion. *Am J Physiol.* 2000;279:H1890-7.
16. YANG HT, YAN Z, ABRAHAM JA, TERJUNG RL. VEGF(121)- and bFGF-induced increase in collateral blood flow requires normal nitric oxide production. *Am J Physiol.* 2001;280: H1097-104.
17. KATZ SD, KHAN T, ZEBALLOS GA, MATHEW L, POTHARLANKA P, KNECHT M, WHELAN J. Decreased activity of the L-arginine-nitric oxide metabolic pathway in patients with congestive heart failure. *Circulation.* 1999;99:2113-7.
18. ARIMURA K, EGASHIRA K, NAKAMURA R, IDE T, TSUTSUI H, SHIMOKAWA H, TAKESHITA A. Increased inactivation of nitric oxide is involved in coronary endothelial dysfunction in heart failure. *Am J Physiol.* 2001;280:H68-75.

19. MOMBOULI JV, VANHOUTTE PM. Endothelial dysfunction: from physiology to therapy. *J Mol Cell Cardiol.* 1999;31:61-74.

20. RADEGRAN G, HELLSTEN Y. Adenosine and nitric oxide in exercise-induced human skeletal muscle vasodilatation. *Acta Physiol Scand.* 2000;168:575-91.

21. STAVRI GT, ZACHARY IC, BASKERVILLE PA, MARTIN JF, ERUSALIMSKY JD. Basic fibroblast growth factor upregulates the expression of vascular endothelial growth factor in vascular smooth muscle cells. Synergistic interaction with hypoxia. *Circulation.* 1995;92:11-4.

22. HEATON WH, MARR KC, CAPURRO NL, GOLDSTEIN RE, EPSTEIN SE. Beneficial effect of physical training on blood flow to myocardium perfused by chronic collaterals in the exercising dog. *Circulation.* 1978;57:575-81.

23. NEILL WA, OXENDINE JM. Exercise can promote coronary collateral development without improving perfusion of ischemic myocardium. *Circulation.* 1979;60:1513-1519.

24. SCHEEL KW, INGRAM LA, WILSON JL. Effects of exercise on the coronary and collateral vasculature of beagles with and without coronary occlusion. *Circ Res.* 1981;48:523-30.

25. SCHAPER W. Influence of physical exercise on coronary collateral blood flow in chronic experimental two-vessel occlusion. *Circulation.* 1982;65:905-912.

26. SCHAPER W, FLAMENG W, SNOECKX L, JAGENEAU A. Der Einfluß körperlichen Trainings auf den Kollateralkreislauf des Herzens. *Verh Dt Ges Kreislaufforschg.* 1971;37:112-121.

27. COHEN MV, YIPINTSOI T, SCHEUER J. Coronary collateral stimulation by exercise in dogs with stenotic coronary arteries. *J Appl Physiol.* 1982;52:664-71.

28. COHEN MV, STEINGART RM. Exercise thallium-201 scintigraphy in dogs: effects of long-term coronary occlusion and collateral development on early and late scintigraphic images. *Circulation.* 1985;72:881-91.

29. COHEN MV, STEINGART RM. Lack of effect of prior training on subsequent ischaemic and infarcting myocardium and collateral development in dogs with normal hearts. *Cardiovasc Res.* 1987;21:269-78.

30. COHEN MV, YIPINTSOI T, MALHOTRA A, PENPARGKUL S, SCHEUER J. Effect of exercise on collateral development in dogs with normal coronary arteries. *J Appl Physiol.* 1978;45:797-805.

31. COHEN MV. Training in dogs with normal coronary arteries: lack of effect on collateral development. *Cardiovasc Res.* 1990;24:121-8.

32. WEISS T, FUJITA Y, KREIMEIER U, MESSMER K. Effect of intensive walking exercise on skeletal muscle blood flow in intermittent claudication. *Angiology.* 1992;43:63-71.

33. BLOOR CM, WHITE FC, SANDERS TM. Effects of exercise on collateral development in myocardial ischemia in pigs. *J Appl Physiol.* 1984;56:656-65.

34. BREISCH EA, WHITE FC, NIMMO LE, MCKIRNAN MD, BLOOR CM. Exercise-induced cardiac hypertrophy: a correlation of blood flow and microvasculature. *J Appl Physiol.* 1986;60:1259-67.

35. WHITE FC, MCKIRNAN MD, BREISCH EA, GUTH BD, LIU YM, BLOOR CM. Adaptation of the left ventricle to exercise-induced hypertrophy. *J Appl Physiol.* 1987;62:1097-110.

36. ROTH DM, WHITE FC, NICHOLS ML, DOBBS SL, LONGHURST JC, BLOOR CM. Effect of long-term exercise on regional myocardial function and coronary collateral development after gradual coronary artery occlusion in pigs. *Circulation.* 1990;82:1778-89.

37. SCHOLZ D, ZIEGELHOEFFER T, HELISCH A, WAGNER S, FRIEDRICH C, PODZUWEIT T, SCHAPER W. Contribution of arteriogenesis and angiogenesis to postocclusive Hind limb perfusion in mice. *J Mol Cell Cardiol.* 2002;34:775-787.

38. WOLFRAM S, ZIEGELHOEFFER T, SCHOLZ D, FERNÁNDEZ B, SCHAPER W. Exercise capacity precisely reflects arteriogenic adaptation to femoral artery occlusion in mice. *J Am Coll Cardiol.* 2001;37:A180.

39. WOLFRAM S, ZIEGELHOEFFER T, FERNÁNDEZ B, COFFIN JD, WAGNER S, HELISCH A, ZIMMERMANN R, SCHAPER W. Arteriogenesis on demand in exercising mice expressing FGF-2 under the control of the phosphoglycerate kinase promoter. *J Am Coll Cardiol.* 2002;39:A204.

40. GARDNER AW, POEHLMAN ET. Exercise rehabilitytion progrmas for the treatment of claudicatio pain-a metaanalysis [Review]. *J Am Med Ass.* 1995;274:975-980.

41. GIROLAMI B, BERNARDI E, PRINS MH, TEN CATE JW, HETTIARACHCHI R, PRANDONI P, GIROLAMI A, BULLER HR. Treatment of intermittent claudication with physical training, smoking cessation, pentoxifylline, or nafronyl - A meta-analysis [Review]. *Arch Int Med.* 1999;159:337-345.

42. JONASON T, RINGQVIST I. Effect of training on the post-exercise ankle blood pressure reaction in patients with intermittent claudication. *Clin Physiol.* 1987;7:63-9.

43. HIATT WR, REGENSTEINER JG, HARGARTEN ME, WOLFEL EE, BRASS EP. Benefit of exercise conditioning for patients with peripheral arterial disease. *Circulation.* 1990;81:602-9.

44. FEINBERG RL, GREGORY RT, WHEELER JR, SNYDER SO, JR., GAYLE RG, PARENT FN, 3RD, PATTERSON RB. The ischemic window: a method for the objective quantitation of the training effect in exercise therapy for intermittent claudicatio. *J Vasc Surg.* 1992;16:244-50.

45. LARSEN OA, LASSEN NA. Effect of daily muscular exercise in patients with intermittent claudication. *Lancet.* 1966;2:1093-6.

46. ZETTERQUIST S. The effect of active training on the nutritive blood flow in exercising ischemic legs. *Scand J Clin Lab Invest.* 1970;25:101-11.

47. DAHLLOF AG, BJORNTORP P, HOLM J, SCHERSTEN T. Metabolic activity of skeletal muscle in patients with peripheral arterial insufficiency. *Eur J Clin Invest.* 1974;4:9-15.

48. SORLIE D, MYHRE K. Effects of physical training in intermittent claudication. *Scand J Clin Lab Invest.* 1978;38:217-22.

49. RUELL PA, IMPERIAL ES, BONAR FJ, THURSBY PF, GASS GC. Intermittent claudication. The effect of physical training on walking tolerance and venous lactate concentration. *Eur J Appl Physiol Occup Physiol.* 1984;52:420-5.

50. CARTER SA, HAMEL ER, PATERSON JM, SNOW CJ, MYMIN D. Walking ability and ankle systolic pressures: observations in patients with intermittent claudication in a short-term walking exercise program. *J Vasc Surg.* 1989;10:642-9.

51. PANCERA P, PRIOR M, ZANNONI M, LUCCHESE L, DE MARCHI S, AROSIO E. Micro- and macro-circulatory, and biohumoral changes after a month of physical exercise in patients with intermittent claudication. *Scand J Rehabil Med.* 1995;27:73-6.

52. GARDNER AW, KATZEL LI, SORKIN JD, KILLEWICH LA, RYAN A, FLINN WR, GOLDBERG AP. Improved functional outcomes following exercise rehabilitation in patients with intermittent claudication. *J Gerontol Series A Biol Sci &Med Sci.* 2000;55:M570-M577.

53. TAN KH, COTTERRELL D, SYKES K, SISSONS GRJ, DE COSSART L, EDWARDS PR. Exercise training for claudicants: Changes in blood flow, cardiorespiratory status, metabolic functions, blood rheology and lipid profile. *Eur J Vasc Endovasc Surg.* 2000;20:72-78.

54. LINKE A, SCHOENE N, GIELEN S, HOFER J, ERBS S, SCHULER G, HAMBRECHT R. Endothelial dysfunction in patients with chronic heart failure: Systemic effects of lower-limb exercise training. *J Am Coll Cardiol.* 2001;37:392-397.

55. REMIJNSE-TAMERIUS HCM, DUPREZ D, DE BUYZERE M, OESEBURG B, CLEMENT DL. Why is training effective in the treatment of patients with intermittent claudication? [Review]. *Int Angiol.* 1999;18:103-112.

56. COFFMAN JD, EBERHARDT RT (2003). Pripheral Arterial Disease. *Humana Press*

57. SIMONS M, BONOW RO, CHRONOS NA, COHEN DJ, GIORDANO FJ, HAMMOND HK, LAHAM RJ, LI W, PIKE M, SELLKE FW, STEGMANN TJ, UDELSON JE, ROSENGART TK. Clinical trials in coronary angiogenesis: issues, problems, consensus: An expert panel summary. *Circulation.* 2000;102:E73-86.

Chapter 15

Cerebral Arteriogenesis

Ivo R. Buschmann, Joerg Busch, Edda Schneeloch
and Konstantin-Alexander Hossmann

Introduction

The previous chapters of this book have focused on the physiological, cellular, molecular and developmental aspects of myocardial and peripheral arteriogenesis. However, in the cerebrovascular system, similar studies have not been carried out.

This is surprising because a multitude of extra- and intracranial collateral systems, such as the leptomeningeal anastomoses of Heubner or the anastomotic pathways via the ophthalmic artery or the circle of Willis, provide the chance of improving blood supply under conditions of slowly progressing vascular occlusion [1]. In fact, there is evidence that the hemodynamic reserve of the cerebrovascular system correlates inversely with the severity of cerebral infarction and, in turn, seems to rely on the efficacy of the collateral circulation [2-5].

Amelioration of the cerebrovascular hemodynamic reserve by improving collateral cerebral circulation via induced arteriogenesis is therefore a promising approach for the prevention of cerebrovascular disorders [6]. We addressed this question using different experimental models of brain ischemia.

In the first part of our experiments we used Sprague-Dawley rats which were randomly assigned to uni- or bilateral common carotid and vertebral artery occlusions in different combinations for the development of an extracranial vascular occlusion model (Fig. 1). Common carotid arteries were exposed by ventral cervical midline incision, and ligated either unilaterally or bilaterally. Vertebral arteries were electrocoagulated via a paravertebral access[7,8]. This study led to the identification of a 3-vessel-occlusion model (3-VO, left common carotid and bilateral vertebral artery occlusion), for induction of non-lethal brain hypoperfusion, which was subsequently used for the investigation of cerebral arteriogenesis. Bilateral common carotid artery occlusion reduced cerebral blood flow to about 30% of control. By combining bilateral vertebral with unilateral carotid artery occlusion the collateral system comes close to its limits. Kawata and coworkers reported in an earlier study in Wistar rats[9] that resting cerebral blood flow was not impaired, but the hemodynamic reserve tested by azetazolamide application was distinctly reduced. In the present study in which Sprague-Dawley rats were used, blood flow was reduced to levels of about 50%, and the hemodynamic reserve was completely abolished, indicating that in this strain the collateral system is less efficient. However, even under this more critical condition ischemia did not produce morphological lesions, indicating that oxygen supply still remained above the threshold of structural integrity[6].

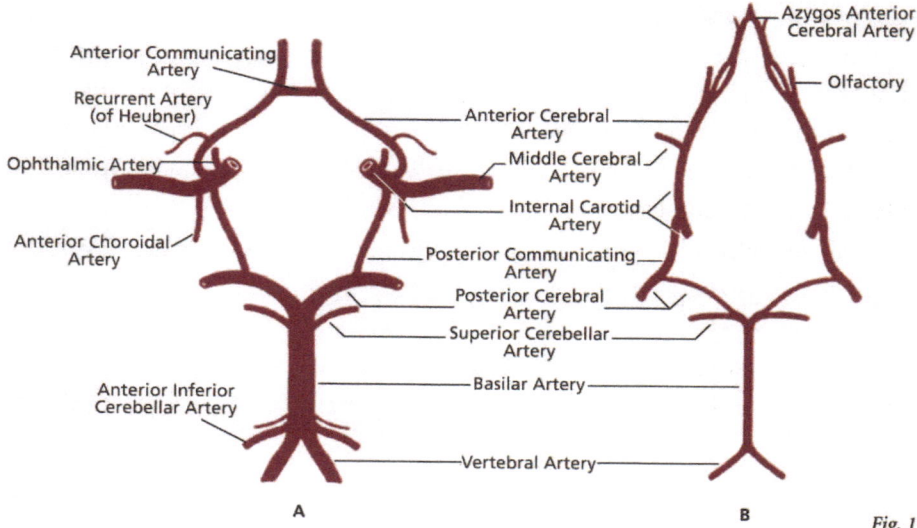

A   B   *Fig. 1*

Arterial circle of Willis of the rat.

Identification of collateral proliferation upon 3-VO

Once we had identified a stable experimental setting of arterial occlusion in the rat model we were uncertain about the site of collateral proliferation after 7 days. Our first idea was that upon 3-VO Heubner's anastomoses should be at least partially recruited and show typical patterns of collateral proliferation (increased tortuosity, increased diameters).

We used the cerebrovascular latex perfusion method (Fig. 2), which visualized the arterial vasculature upon complete vasodilation (papaverine). (We had learned form our studies in the periphery, that a complete vasodilation is the key to achieve stable values of blood flow and pressure and thus to calculate the conductance of the collateral circulation. In the rabbit *in-vivo* hind limb model, the slow vasodilatory effect of papaverine (even under high concentrations) was disadvantageous and less effective compared with adenosine. In the brain model, however, this was not the case.)

The common carotid artery ligated for 3-VO was cannulated with a polyethylene tubing (internal diameter 0.75 mm), and a lethal dose of papaverine hydrochloride (40-50 mg/kg) was intra-arterially injected to produce maximal vasodilatation. Undiluted warm (37°C) latex was mixed with a small amount of carbon black. Of this solution, 3.5-4 ml/kg were injected through the intracarotid catheter at 150 mmHg pressure. Thoracotomy was performed, and the right atrium was incised to facilitate venous outflow. To harden the latex, animals were placed on crushed ice for 15 minutes. Subsequently, brains were carefully removed and fixed by immersion in 4% paraformaldehyde.

The external diameter of the main supplying arteries of the brain was measured at the various survival times after 3-VO and compared with non-ischemic control animals (Fig. 3). Immediately after 3-VO no changes were observed, demonstrating that the application of high dose of papaverine prior to latex perfusion produced maximal vasodilation that was unaffected by intravital differences in vascular tone.

After one and three weeks of 3-VO we further examined the diameter of the anterior and middle cerebral arteries, the internal carotid artery and Heubner's dorsal leptomeningeal anastomoses. We expected that arteriogenic growth would also take place in regions of smaller arteriolar connections, as described by Wei and coworkers in rats after stroke[10]. However, after one week the only significant difference in vessel diameter

3-VO

immediate   1 week

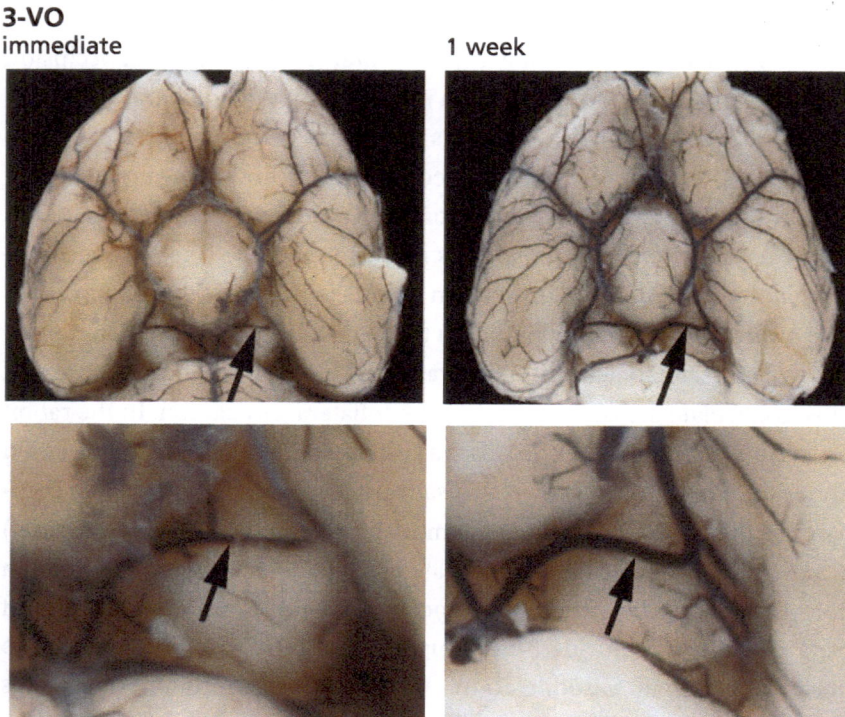

Fig. 2

Visualization of cerebral angioarchitecture by intravascular latex perfusion. Basal view of control brain. Brains inspected immediately or 1 week after 3-vessel-occlusion. The arrows point to the ipsilateral posterior cerebral artery.

was observed in the ipsilateral posterior cerebral artery (PCA). After three weeks a significant increase in vessel size was also detected in the ipsilateral anterior cerebral artery (ACA) and the contralateral PCA. At this time the diameter of the ipsilateral PCA had increased significantly from 187±27 to 322±50 µm (plus 72%), that of the contralateral PCA from 196±29 to 261±38 µm (plus 33%) and that of the ipsilateral ACA from 251±37 to 322±42 µm (plus 28%). Other supplying arteries did not change in diameter during the observation period. Heubner's leptomeningeal anastomoses did not change either: in control animals the mean diameter was 37±4µm ipsi- and contralateral; after 3-VO it was 38±2µm on the ipsilateral and 37±3µm on the contralateral side, and after GM-CSF treatment it insignificantly changed on the ipsilateral side to 39±6µm and on the contralateral side to 36±4µm. Any other supplying arteries did not change.

Functional parameters of collateral growth in the brain

The hemodynamic consequences of 3-VO were tested by measuring the alterations of blood flow during ventilation with 6% CO_2 on the surface of both hemispheres via Laser-Doppler flow transcranial Laser-Doppler flowmetry (LDF). The skull above the fronto-parietal cortex was bilaterally exposed, and laser probes were placed directly on the bone. Changes in blood flow were expressed in percent of pre-ischemic baseline value.

The hemodynamic reserve describes the amount of flow impairment brain vessels may compensate by reducing the vascular resistance. At decreasing brain perfusion pressure – induced either by cardiovascular reduction of systemic blood pressure or occlusion of the main supplying arteries – brain arterioles dilate to maintain blood flow at a constant level (cerebrovascular autoregulation). A reduced hemodynamic reserve is equivalent to an increased risk of suffering ischemic injury under such conditions[11-13]. In fact, this has been confirmed by measurements of hemodynamic reserve for predicting the clinical outcome of patients with internal carotid artery occlusions[14-16].

Here we observed a similar increase of arterial pCO_2 in all four groups: by 21±7mmHg in the control animals, and by 21±9mmHg, 24±4mmHg and 20.5±6mmHg in the animals examined immediately or one and three weeks after 3-VO, respectively (NS).

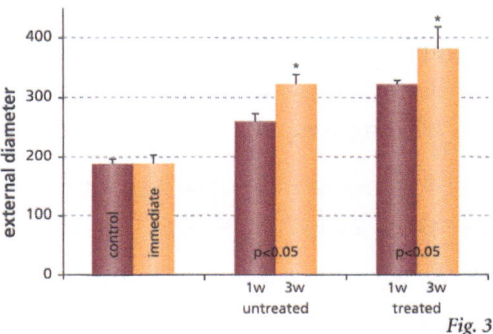

Fig. 3

External diameter of posterior cerebral artery (PCA) in control rats and in rats studied immediately, 1 week or 3 weeks after 3-VO with or without GM-CSF treatment. Note gradual extension of vessel diameter in ipsilateral-hemisphere. * p<0.05 as compared to control.

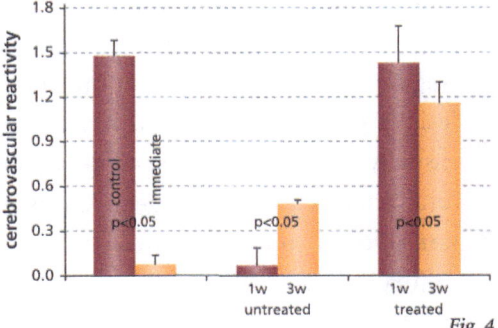

Fig. 4

CO_2 reactivity of cerebral blood flow in normal rat (control) and after different times (immediately, 1 and 3 weeks) after 3-vessel-occlusion with or without GM-CSF treatment. Blood flow was measured during ventilation with 6% CO_2 by Laser-Doppler flowmetry (LDF) in the parietal cortex of the ipsilateral hemisphere. CO_2 reactivity is expressed as percent change of LDF per mmHg increase of arterial pCO_2.

In the non-ischemic controls, LDF (Laser-Doppler flow reflecting changes in cerebrovascular reactivity) increased during CO_2 ventilation by 1.48±0.3 % /mmHg apCO_2 in the right and by 1.1±0.2 %/mmHg in the left hemisphere (no significant difference). Immediately after 3-VO, the cerebrovascular response was reduced to 0.07±0.16 %/mmHg in the ipsilateral and to 0.17±0.3 %/mmHg in the contralateral hemisphere (Fig. 4). After one week survival, this reduction only slightly improved (ipsilateral 0.06±0.35/mmHg, contralateral 0.18±0.6 %/mmHg) but after three weeks CO_2 reactivity returned to 0.48±0.08 %/mmHg in the ipsilateral and to 0.3±0.39 %/mmHg in the contralateral hemisphere. These values amount to about 32 % of the control response. Arteriogenesis thus markedly improves the hemodynamic capacity of the hypoperfused brain.

Regional differences between angiogenesis and arteriogenesis in the brain

In patients with peripheral vascular disease the spatial dissociation between capillary sprouting (angiogenesis) and collateral artery growth (arteriogenesis) is obvious: collateral growth may be found in the thigh, whereas clinical signs of ischemia are located in the foot. In the brain however such dissociations have not been explicitly described, but may be concluded from published data. During focal brain ischemia, the angiogenic factor VEGF is upregulated within the ischemic territory, whereas proliferation of collateral pathways occurs outside the ischemic region in the posterior part of the circle of Willis[4,17-19]. Whereas angiogenesis is observed mainly within the ischemic territory, arteriogenesis is usually temporally and spatially dissociated from this region[20,21]. Collateral arteries grow in oxygen rich tissue and, in contrast to angiogenesis, are able to supply blood from outside the risk region to prevent ischemic injury[22]. Indeed these data support our theory about the regional differences between angiogenesis and arteriogenesis. In the coronary situation it was believed for a long time that collateral growth is closely linked to ischemia. Due to the complex coronary architecture of the coronary arteries, collaterals were often found in regions with low oxygen tension. However, in the last years we have learned that ischemia and collateral growth are two independent variables which may occur at the same time ("three dimensional myocardium") but are not directly linked to each other (in arterio-venous shunt situation for instance collateral growth is induced, whereas ischemia or low oxygen tension are absent).

Monocyte invasion and proliferation of brain collateral anastomoses

In our previous investigations one important key feature of arteriogenesis was the active proliferation of collateral arteries detected either with Brd-U or with Ki-67 and the invasion of circulating mononuclear cells. When we analyzed histological sections of the posterior cerebral artery monocytes (detected via the ED-1 antibody in paraffin sections) as well as the proliferation marker Ki-67 were not detectable in quiescent non-

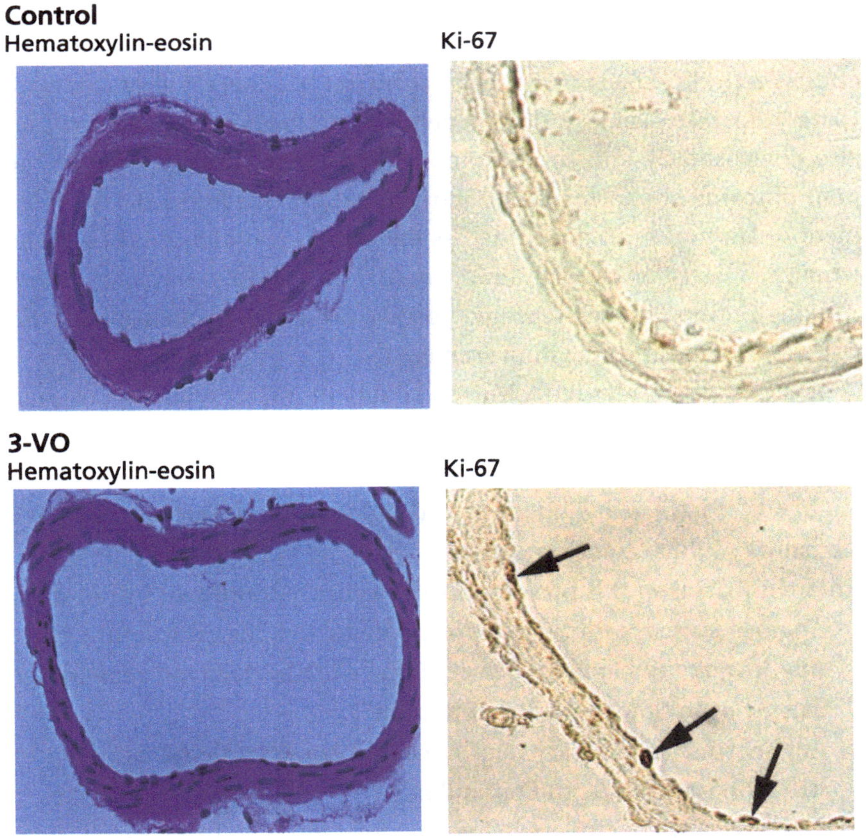

Control
Hematoxylin-eosin   Ki-67

3-VO
Hematoxylin-eosin   Ki-67

Fig. 5

Cross-section of ipsilateral posterior cerebral artery of intact rat (control) and 1 weeks after 3-VO. Note 3-VO-induced enlargement of vessel lumen, positive staining of endothelial cells with the proliferation marker Ki-67 (arrows).

ischemic controls, but could be detected in the enlarged PCA at three days after 3-VO (Fig. 5). Proliferation was mainly located in endothelial cells, whereas the vast majority of macrophages was found in the adventitia of the PCA. Interestingly, hypoxia-dependent angiogenesis markers such as VEGF could neither be detected in controls nor 3-VO animals.

Therapeutic induction of arteriogenesis

In the past, attempts have repeatedly been made to improve blood flow to the brain upon vascular stenosis. One approach was the pharmacological dilation of vessels with vasoactive compounds to improve collateral flow (e.g. prostacyclin, nimodipin). However, blood flow to the ischemic territory did not change or only marginally improved, since the concomitant drop in systemic blood pressure counteracted any positive effects on the decline of the vascular collateral resistance. Other strategies (parasympathetic denervation, hyperglycemia, hemoconcentration) did also not positively influence the reduction in infarct size. Moreover the poor outcome of pharmacological treatment options led to the development of surgical procedures such as the end-to-end anastomoses of the temporal artery with pial branches of the middle cerebral artery. Although several groups reported positive results, controlled studies did not confirm a substantial improvement.

A second point referred to the possibility of infarct reduction or even prevention by therapeutical induction of neo-angiogenesis. Since the focus was primarily set on angiogenesis, it was believed that the brain might suffer irreversible injury before any ischemia-induced angiogenic mediators could become operative.

Now, ten years later this presumption is explicitly confirmed by our data:
1. Angiogenesis is too slow to compensate for arterial occlusion
2. Any increase in capillary density (area of risk) does not remedy the deficiency in flow to the ischemic zone
3. Any increase in capillary density cannot compensate for arterial obstruction (law of Hagen Poiseuille)
4. Arteriogenesis takes place before any ischemia is to be expected (prophylactic approach).

Since several experimental studies in the periphery and the myocardium had meanwhile shown that the speed of arteriogenesis is not limited to its natural time course (infusion of fibroblast growth factors (FGF), CC-chemokines (MCP-1), Placenta like growth factor (PlGF), or the granulocyte-macrophage colony-stimulating factor (GM-CSF) into the peripheral or coronary collateral circulation led to a significant increase in collateral conductance as compared to untreated animals) we decided to transfer these data to the cerebral situation. In the experimental model of the rabbit hind limb, we tested whether the application of pro-arteriogenic cytokines could enhance the speed of collateral growth.

In our 3-VO rat model of hypoperfusion we choose GM-CSF (Granulocyte-Macrophage Colony-Stimulating-Factor) due to the availability of this factor via the subcutaneous route. We hypothesized according to our peripheral studies, that one important mode of action of GM-CSF was the adhesion and transmigration of mononuclear stem cells/monocytes to arteriolar collateral pathways. Interestingly, recent clinical trials demonstrated a positive effect of GM-CSF on therapeutically enhanced arteriogenesis in patients with coronary artery disease.

GM-CSF in hypoperfused rat brain

Sprague-Dawley rats were submitted to 3-VO occlusion. After 7 days of continuous s.c. treatment with either GM-CSF (treated) or Ringer's infusion (untreated) cerebral angiographies confirmed the PCA as the main collateral pathway to the left hemisphere: the untreated 3-VO led to a significant increase in the diameter of the left PCA, measured after maximal vasodilation by latex infusion. Upon GM-CSF treatment every second day the increase in diameter during natural arteriogenesis could be therapeutically enhanced by 24 % after 1 week and 18 % after 3 weeks (Fig. 6, left side). On the functional level blood flow measured in both hemispheres via Laser-Doppler flowmetry under normal air ventilation as well as during ventilation with additional 6 % CO_2. The increase in arterial pCO_2 under CO_2 ventilation reached comparable levels in all three groups. In non-ischemic control animals Laser-Doppler flow increased during 6 % CO_2 ventilation by 1.48 ± 0.3 % per mmHg $apCO_2$ change in the left hemisphere and by 1.1 ± 0.2 % per mmHg $apCO_2$ in the right hemisphere. One week after 3-VO, untreated animals showed a severe reduction of CO_2 reactivity. In the left hemisphere (i.e., ipsilaterally to the occluded common carotid artery) CO_2 reactivity declined to 0.006 ± 0.35 %

and in the right hemisphere to $0.18 \pm 0.6\%$ per mmHg. These values represent 4% and 16% of the control response, respectively. At 3 weeks after 3-VO CO_2 reactivity of untreated animals slightly improved on the left side to $0.48 \pm 0.08\%$ and on the right side to $0.30 \pm 0.39\%$ per mmHg apCO$_2$, representing 32% and 27% of the control response, respectively. Following GM-CSF treatment the hemodynamic reserve of the brain almost completely recovered (Fig. 6, right side). On the left (ipsilateral) hemisphere CO_2 reactivity returned to $1.43 \pm 0.68\%$ per mmHg apCO$_2$ after 1 week, and to $1.16 \pm 0.44\%$ per mmHg after 3 weeks, i.e., 97% and 78% of the control response, respectively. In the right (contralateral) hemisphere the corresponding values were $1.12 \pm 1.1\%$ and $0.7\pm 0.16\%$ per mmHg apCO$_2$ after 1 and 3 weeks. These values represent 101% and 64% of control and reflect the substantial therapeutic improvement by the arteriogenesis-promoting drug.

To test the effect of GM-CSF-induced arteriogenesis for the prevention of ischemic injury, we developed a hemodynamic stroke model of rat brain by combining 3-VO with hemorrhagic hypotension (Schneeloch et. al. submitted). One week after 3-VO arterial blood pressure was lowered to 20 mmHg to reduce blood flow in the hemisphere ipsilateral to the carotid artery occlusion below the threshold of energy metabolism. The volume of energy-depleted tissue was determined by bioluminescence imaging of tissue ATP content. Treatment with subcutaneous injections of GM-CSF every other day for 1 week significantly decreazed the volume of ischemic energy failure from $48.4 \pm 44.2\%$ to $15.8 \pm 17.4\%$ of the ipsilateral hemisphere ($p<0.05\%$ of total hemisphere volume).

Immunohistochemistry with an antibody recognizing the ED-1 antigen from rats revealed significant differences among the numbers of macrophages accumulating in the adventitia of proliferating collateral pathways. In the non-ischemic control group mononuclear cells were rarely detectable. 3-VO without treatment resulted in the appearance of a small number of macrophages in the adventitia of the posterior cerebral artery. Upon GM-CSF treatment the number of these mononuclear cells markedly increased.

In summary, this study provided the following data: Cytokines influencing monocyte survival and adhesion (e.g. GM-CSF) enhance the

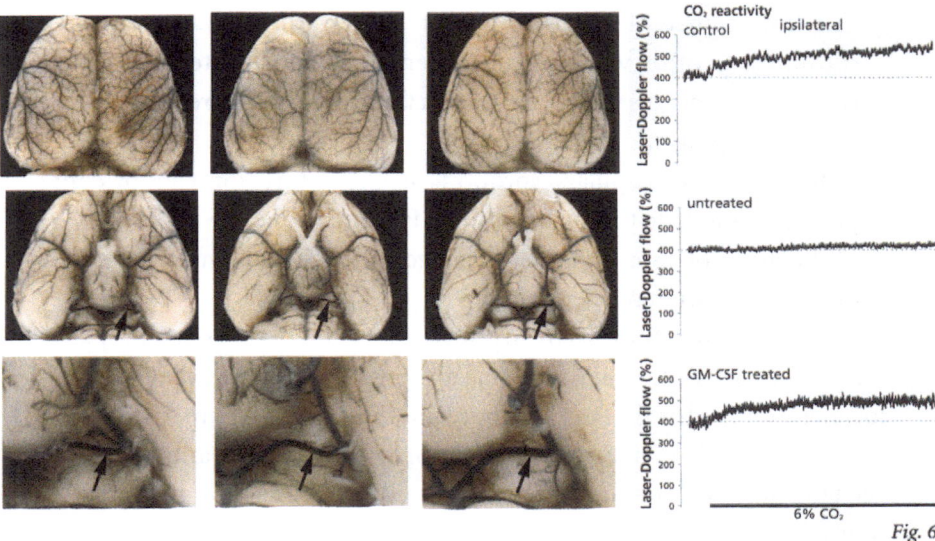

Fig. 6

Visualization of cerebral angioarchitecture and corresponding CO-2 reactivity in control rats and rats after 3-VO, untreated and treated with GM-CSF. Note marked enlargement of ipsilateral PCA (arrows) in GM-CSF-treated animals compared with control and untreated animals.

adaptive proliferation of collateral pathways in the brain; GM-CSF in particular may be given subcutaneously; GM-CSF acts by promoting invasion of mononuclear cells (macrophages) at the site of vascular collateral proliferation.[23]

The terminology of "arteriogenesis" has been controversially discussed over the last year[24]. One major criticism of our opponents was that it is not legitimate to create a supplemental terminology for collateral growth, since angiogenesis covers basically all issues related to neovascularization. Although we agree that all forms of vascular growth show a certain overlap, we could not follow these arguments, since the growth of collateral arteries obeys mechanisms very different from angiogenesis. Moreover the transfer of our concept of arteriogenesis to the cerebral circulation clearly confirmed this point of view. Nearly all observation from the heart and the periphery could be confirmed in the brain:

1. An increase in perfusion in hypoperfused brain regions can be clearly linked to collateral enlargement
2. These collateral pathways provide the ischemic zone from outside the risk region with blood.

3. The time-course of collateral growth exceeds the speed of capillary sprouting, in other words small caliber changes in collateral pathways (law of Hagen-Poiseuille) are more efficient than the relatively slow speed of angiogenic sprouting.

4. Enhancement of capillary sprouting in the risk region cannot compensate for a deficit in in-flow to the ischemic zone.

5. Modulation of monocyte/macrophage function influences the speed of monocyte driven arteriogenesis

In fact, in our model of brain hypoperfusion, the main collateral pathways are not arterioles but functional arteries. We feel, however, that arteriogenesis defined as the "positive outward remodeling of preexistent collateral pathways" is a proper descriptor of this important biological mechanism. Current and future studies will further explore the molecular and cellular basis of this adaptive rescue mechanism.

From the therapeutic point of view our data are (to the best of our knowledge) the first *in vivo* studies providing evidence that a single pro-arteriogenic growth factor may significantly improve collateral growth in the brain. This observation is supported by our infarction studies (Schneeloch et al. unpublished) revealing that the growth of collaterals is directly linked with an increase in perfusion and thus a reduction in ischemic energy failure.

References

1. HOSSMANN K-A. *Collateral Circulation of the Brain.* Kluwer Academic Publishers;1993.
2. KLUYTMANS M, VAN DER GROND J, VIERGEVER MA. Gray matter and white matter perfusion imaging in patients with severe carotid artery lesions. *Radiology.* 1998;209:675-82.
3. COYLE P, JOKELAINEN PT. Differential outcome to middle cerebral artery occlusion in spontaneously hypertensive stroke-prone rats (SHRSP) and Wistar Kyoto (WKY) rats. *Stroke.* 1983;14:605-611.
4. HENDRIKSE J, HARTKAMP MJ, HILLEN B, MALI WP, VAN DER GROND J. Collateral ability of the circle of Willis in patients with unilateral internal carotid artery occlusion: border zone infarcts and clinical symptoms. *Stroke.* 2001;32:2768-73.
5. RINGELSTEIN EB, WEILLER C, WECKESSER M, WECKESSER S. Cerebral vasomotor reactivity is significantly reduced in low-flow as compared to thromboembolic infarctions: the key role of the circle of Willis. *J Neurol Sci.* 1994;121:103-9.

6. BUSCH HJ, BUSCHMANN IR, MIES G, BODE C, HOSSMANN KA. Arteriogenesis in hypoperfused rat brain. *J Cereb Blood Flow Metab.* 2003;May;23(5):621-8.

7. PULSINELLI WA, BRIERLEY JB. A new model of bilateral hemispheric ischemia in the unanesthetized rat. *Stroke.* 1979;10:267-72.

8. PULSINELLI WA, LEVY DE, DUFFY TE. Cerebral blood flow in the four-vessel occlusion rat model. *Stroke.* 1983;14:832-4.

9. KAWATA Y, SAKO K, YONEMASU Y. Sequential changes in cerebrovascular reserve capacity in three-vessel occlusion rats. *Brain Res.* 1996;739:330-4.

10. WEI L, ERINJERI JP, ROVAINEN CM, WOOLSEY TA. Collateral growth and angiogenesis around cortical stroke. *Stroke.* 2001;32:2179-84.

11. CLIFTON GL, HADEN HT, TAYLOR JR, SOBEL M. Cerebrovascular CO_2 reactivity after carotid artery occlusion. *J Neurosurg.* 1988;69:24-28.

12. KLEISER B, WIDDER B. Course of carotid artery occlusions with impaired cerebrovascular reactivity. *Stroke.* 1992;23:171-4.

13. MILLER JD, SMITH RR, HOLADAY HR. Carbon dioxide reactivity in the evaluation of cerebral ischemia. *Neurosurgery.* 1992;30:518-521.

14. MARKUS H, CULLINANE M. Severely impaired cerebrovascular reactivity predicts stroke and TIA risk in patients with carotid artery stenosis and occlusion. *Brain.* 2001;124:457-67.

15. WHITE RP, MARKUS HS. Impaired dynamic cerebral autoregulation in carotid artery stenosis. *Stroke.* 1997;28:1340-4.

16. WIDDER B, KLEISER B, KRAPF H. Course of cerebrovascular reactivity in patients with carotid artery occlusions. *Stroke.* 1994;25:1963-7.

17. HILLEN B, HOOGSTRATEN HW, VAN OVERBEEKE JJ, VAN DER ZWAN A. Functional anatomy of the circulus arteriosus cerebri (WillisII). *Bull Assoc Anat (Nancy).* 1991;75:123-6.

18. COYLE P, PANZENBECK MJ. Collateral development after carotid artery occlusion in Fischer 344 rats. *Stroke.* 1990;21:316-321.

19. COYLE P, HEISTAD DD. Development of collaterals in the cerebral circulation. *Blood Vessels.* 1991;28:183-189.

20. BUSCHMANN I, SCHAPER W. Arteriogenesis versus angiogenesis: Two mechanisms of vessel growth. *News Physiol Sci.* 1999;14:121-125.

21. CARMELIET P, DOR Y, HERBERT JM, FUKUMURA D, BRUSSELMANS K, DEWERCHIN M, NEEMAN M, BONO F, ABRAMOVITCH R, MAXWELL P, KOCH CJ, RATCLIFFE P, MOONS L, JAIN RK, COLLEN D, KESHERT E, KESHET E. Role of HIF-1alpha in hypoxia-mediated apoptosis, cell proliferation and tumour angiogenesis. *Nature.* 1998;394:485-90.

22. STEPP DW, MERKUS D, NISHIKAWA Y, CHILIAN WM. Nitric oxide limits coronary vasoconstriction by a shear stress- dependent mechanism. *Am J Physiol Heart Circ Physiol.* 2001; 281:H796-803.

23. BUSCHMANN I, BUSCH H, MIES G, HOSSMANN K. Therapeutic induction of arteriogenesis in hypoperfused rat brain via Granulocyte-Macrophage Colony-Stimulating Factor. *Circulation.* 2003;108:610-615.

24. CHILIAN WM. Editorial Comment on Arteriogenesis - is this terminolgy necessary? *Basic Res Cardiol.* 2003;98:6-7.

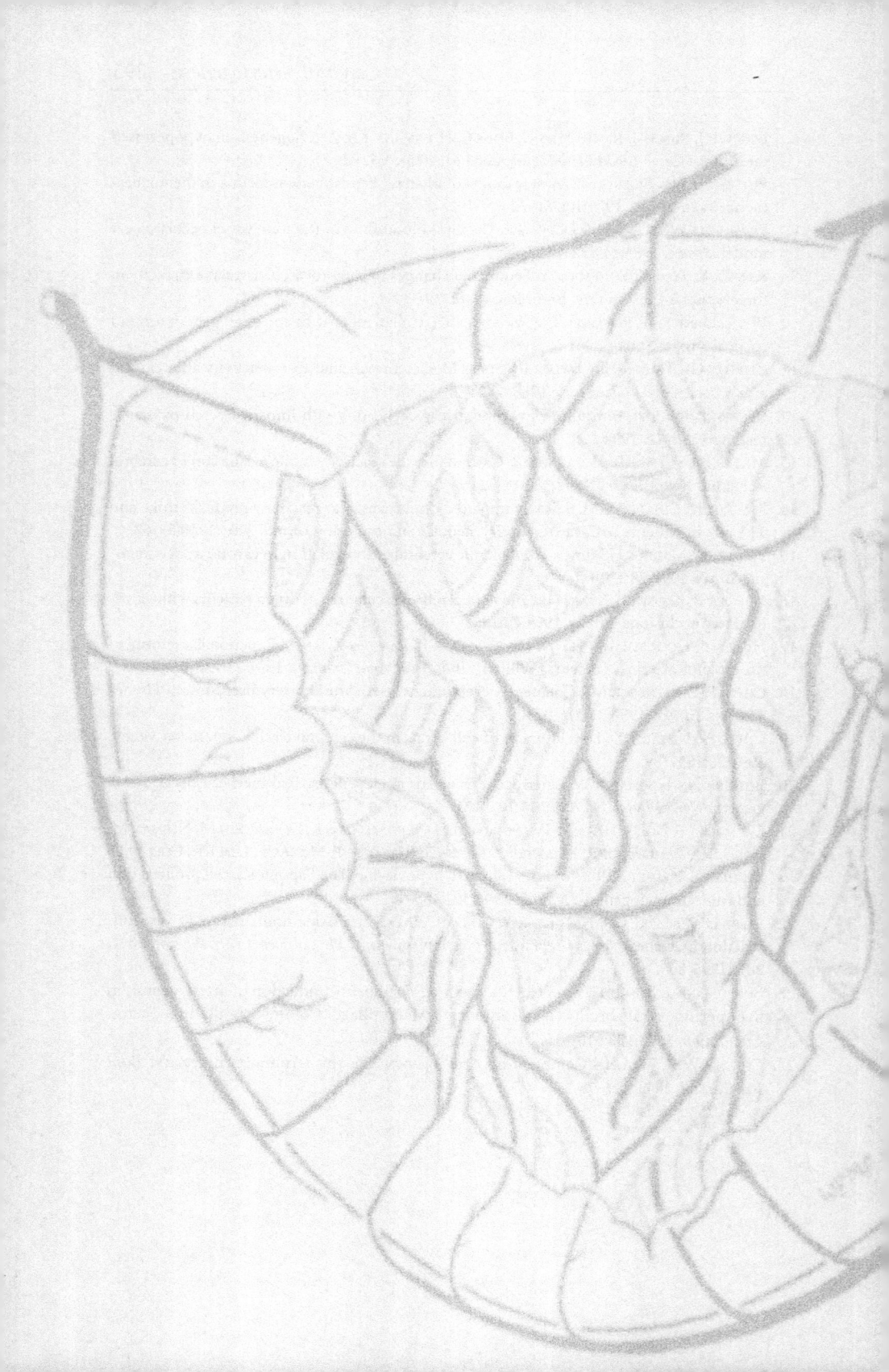

Chapter 16

The Coronary Collateral Circulation in Man

William F.M. Fulton and Niels van Royen

Introduction

Intercommunication in the coronary arterial circulation has been a focus of interest for over 3 centuries. The evidence on the collateral circulation depended for a long time on anatomical and pathological studies. But in the latter third of the twentieth century and continuing, evidence has been explored in clinical studies. There is an important difference to be recognized between these two disciplines. Carefully conducted pathological studies can provide evidence that is more detailed and precise than can be determined *in vivo* but for the most part pathology examines the situation at the time of death and the full picture as it evolved must remain conjectural; whereas clinical investigation assesses the situation in non-fatal lesions, although they may be life-threatening; and the contribution made by the collateral circulation is becoming increasingly accessible to modern methods. The first part of this chapter is devoted to the morphology as studied post mortem. The second part deals with the methods of measurement of the function of the collateral circulation in life, enabling the determination of the protective role of the collateral circulation as witnessed clinically. Much insight into enlargement of anastomoses and their protective effect after coronary occlusion has been derived from experimental studies which are described in detail in this volume.

A: Morphology of the collateral circulation in the human heart

William F.M. Fulton

When I entered this field in 1952, there was general agreement that comparatively large communicating arterial vessels could be found in severe ischaemic heart disease; but the existence of such anastomoses in the normal heart was surprisingly still controversial. Failure by some workers to demonstrate arterial collaterals in the normal heart led to speculation on the origin of the enlarged vessels in disease. That they arose from the capillary bed or *de novo* was widely entertained: and possibly still is. There was evident need for better definition. The development of a technique which included a more penetrating injection medium and stereo-arteriography allowed the demonstration of numerous arterial anastomoses in the normal human heart post mortem. All stages from them to the enlarged communicating vessels in disease could be traced. Based on detailed structural evidence, the conclusion was reached that the prime stimulus for vessel enlargement was the effect on the vessel wall of augmented blood flow; and this in turn was governed by differential pressures consequent on coronary artery obstruction.

Exploration of factors which might translate the effect of blood-flow into vessel growth was beyond the scope of my investigation but the need for such enquiry cried out. At a conference organised in 1967 by Wolfgang Schaper, I commented that "..if some means could emerge.. of encouraging the rate at which normal coronary arterial anastomoses enlarge to form the wide channels of collateral blood flow in disease then a considerable potential advantage would be gained in the management of ischaemic heart disease [1].

This challenge was already being taken up by Schaper and his colleagues; and has been addressed more recently by many others. This aspect of the subject features in other chapters of this volume.

Some historical comments

This is but a synoptic account up to the 1960's. Further reference can be made to Gross[2], Spalteholz[3], Gould[4] and Fulton[5]. The existence of normal coronary arterial communication has been demonstrated in several ways:

a. By introducing fluid into one coronary artery post mortem and observing its arrival in the other. Remarkably this was undertaken in 1669 by Lower[6]. Others included Crainicianu[7], Dock[8], Barmeyer[9], and it formed a small part in the technique of Fulton[5].

b. By section of a coronary artery in the experimental animal beyond a ligature and observing retrograde arterial blood flow from the distal vessel[10].

c. By the observation that the extent of ischaemic myocardial damage is often less than the entire territory of an acutely occluded coronary artery[11]. Non of these methods of course revealed the pathways that were followed.

The anatomy of coronary arterial anastomoses requires some form of injection technique, especially in normal hearts. Many have been the methods used and the list of over 70 presented in Fulton[5] is undoubtedly far from complete. Extensive review of methods and observations is to be found in Gross[2], Spalteholz[3] and Schoenmackers[12]. Several methods of visualisation of the injected vessels have been employed:

a. **Corrosion,** leaving only the cast of the arterial lumen. By this method Hyrtl[13] and Henle[14] failed to demonstrate communications in normal hearts; but convincing demonstration was obtained by Baroldi et al.[15] and by James and Burch[16]. A major disadvantage is that all evidence other than the arterial lumen is destroyed.

b. **Clearing** in organic solvents after injection with an opaque medium was developed by Spalteholz[17]. This achieved the demonstration of even the smallest calibre anastomoses in normal hearts. Disadvantages were visualisation of vessels for only a few mm below the surface and the removal of all lipids from the vessel wall. Gross[2] also resorted to clearing for the demonstration of small vessels, finding radiological demonstration less adequate at that time.

c. **Arteriography,** injection of radio-opaque medium followed by X-ray exposure on film is the most widely used method. Not surprisingly the quality of evidence varies greatly between different studies. Notwithstanding the shortcomings of 2-dimensioal radiography for the demonstration of small-calibre anastomoses, it has been widely adopted. Stereoarteriography was used by the author for all stages in the investigation. Only in 3-dimensions can distinction be made with confidence between continuity of lumen and mere overlap, especially with finer vessels and in the thickness of the left ventricular wall where anastomoses are most abundant. Stereoarteriography has been used by Jamin and Merkel[18], Gross[2], Crainicianu[7] Vastesaeger et al[19] and a number of others, including Schaper[20].

Controversy about collateral vessels in normal hearts

The issue of whether arterial anastomoses exist in normal hearts is fundamental to our understanding of the collateral circulation in disease. The pendulum of opinion has swung several times. The authoritative statement in 1881 by Cohnheim and von Schulthess-Rechberg[21] that the coronary arteries (in the dog) were "end arteries" probably stultified progress for many years.

However Spalteholz[3,17], Gross[2], Crainicianu[7] and Campbell[22], found that coronary arterial anastomoses were abundant in normal human hearts and were able to give a detailed description of them. Unfortunately this knowledge was eclipsed by the advent of a simplified technique of 2-dimensional arteriography[23].

A single radiograph was made of the "unrolled" heart, after the interventricular septum, (perhaps the most important site of anastomoses!) had been excised. Schlesinger concluded that the coronary arteries of man were end-arteries in the sense used by Cohnheim. This was later modified, (after an astonishingly large series of over 1000 hearts), to anastomoses being present in less then a quarter of 244 normal hearts examined[24].

Notwithstanding the most valuable contribution made in coronary artery disease by this group, these numerically over-whelming negative findings left the origin of the larger calibre anastomoses in diseases open to speculation- which still persists in some quarters. It is well to bear in mind that absence of demonstration is not proof of absence.

The findings derived from the Schlesinger method, which has been employed by many others, were in stark contrast to those of earlier workers (Spalteholz, Gross, Crainicianu and Campbell)[2,3,7,22] and with my own findings[5,25]. The discrepancy depends on differences in technique.

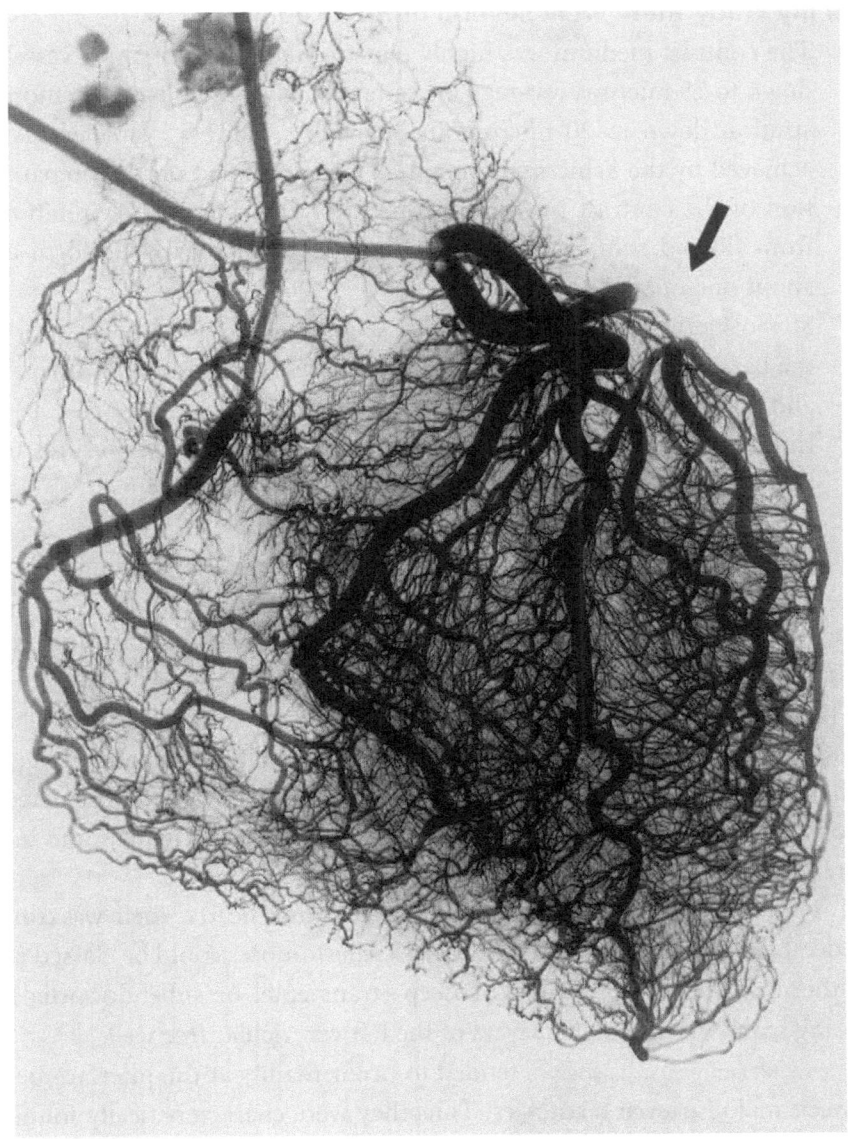

Fig. 1

Arteriogram of a normal heart. Radiological exposure by the immersion method, which almost entirely eliminated tissue shadow and gave the same exposure to all vessels.
Ligation of a branch of the left circumflex artery was performed before injection. The existence of anastomotic communication was demonstrated by retrograde filling of the distal artery in less than 20 seconds. x 1.

In my study there were several differences

a. The contrast medium was highly penetrating. Filling of small vessels down to 15 microns was regularly attained, with radiological demonstration down to 20 microns in diameter – some x 5 smaller than achieved by the Schlesinger method. This depended on the preparation of the contrast medium, Bismuth oxychloride, by precipitation from filtered solutions; so that particle size was nearly uniform at about one micron.

b. Stereoarteriography was used at all stages including the intact heart, the basal portion after opening out, transventricular section(s), apex and atrial "cap".

c. Immersion radiography allowed the same radiological exposures to all vessels, independent of the thickness of the myocardium[26] as can be seen in figure 1.

d. Fine-grain X-ray film and viewing in the stereoscope at x 5 magnification.

Description of the collateral circulation in normal human hearts based on the author's study.

The description which follows is but a summary. Greater detail can be found in Fulton[5,25]. The findings in nearly normal hearts (slightly larger than accepted normal) and in valvular heart disease with unobstructed coronary arteries were essentially similar to normal but with some increase in calibre.

Numerous anastomoses were found in all normal hearts. There was considerable difference between individuals. Anastomoses could be classed as either superficial (epicardial) or deep (transseptal or subendocardial), being scanty in the middle layers of the left ventricular free wall.

Superficial anastomoses tended to occur mainly at the interface between major arterial territories. Thus they were characteristically found on the anterior wall of the right ventricle between the anterior descending artery and the right coronary artery, or conus artery where present; at or on either side of the posterior interventricular groove, between the territories of the right and left circumflex arteries; and near the apex where anterior descending, artery and marginal branches of right and/or left circumflex arteries may converge (Fig. 2). A readily demonstrable network was usually found in the atrial wall especially of the left (and in interatrial septum) (Fig. 3).

Deep anastomoses: These were more numerous than superficial and often of larger calibre (100-200 µm). They comprised the trans-interventricular septal, subendocardial plexus of the left ventricle and the subendocardial plexus of the right ventricle.

a. Interventricular septum. Numerous communicating arterial vessels traversed the interventricular septum connecting the anterior descending artery (LAD) with the posterior interventricular branch of the right coronary artery or, less commonly the circumflex artery, rarely both. They coursed nearly parallel to the atrio-ventricular groove (Fig. 4).

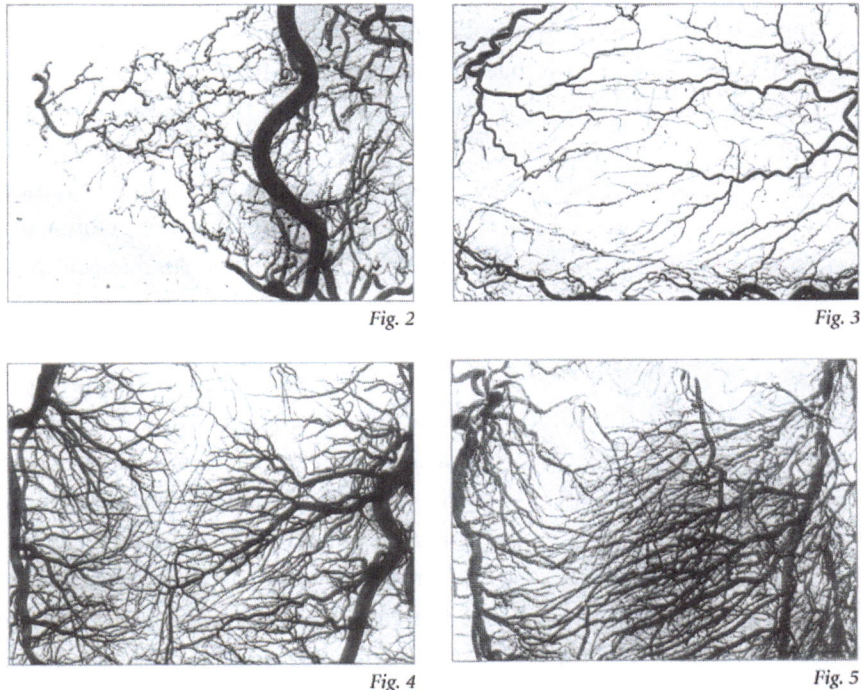

Fig. 2   *Fig. 3*

Fig. 4   *Fig. 5*

2) Apex of a normal heart. Communications can be traced between the anterior descending artery (LAD) and a marginal branch of the right coronary artery. x 0.7.

3) Enlarged arteriogram of left atrial wall in a normal heart. Small caliber anastomoses can be traced. x 2.

4) Interventricular septum, upper part, of a normal heart. Some communications can be traced, even in 2D, linking the anterior descending (LAD) and posterior descending arteries. A few running nearly at right angles to the general course are part of the subendocardial plexus. x 0.5.

5) Interventricular septum, upper part, in coronary artery disease. Enlarged anastomoses carry blood flow from the posterior descending artery on the left to the anterior descending artery, which was obstructed. x 0.5.

(When enlarged in disease they are much more readily demonstrable post mortem (Fig. 5) and may often be identified in clinical coronary angiography.)

b. The subendocardial plexus of the left ventricle (Figs. 6 and 7) is a network of intercommunicating arterial vessels in the inner 1/3 of the free wall, largely in relation to the columnae carneae. It continues onto the innermost layers of the interventricular septum, where the vessels tend to run nearly at right angles to the transseptal vessels.

The subendocardial plexus of the left ventricle was well described in normal hearts by Spalteholz[17] and confirmed by Gross[2] and thereafter appears to have been overlooked until "rediscovered" by me in the early 1950's; and its role in ischaemic heart disease had received no mention. Because that role has great importance, I shall give it special attention.

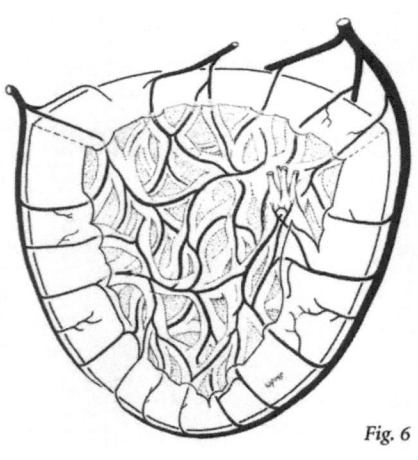

Fig. 6

The subendocardial plexus of the left ventricle: schematic drawing. Note the deep network is supplied by vessels with few branches, directly from epicardial arteries.

Also not only in disease the deep network may perhaps serve a circulatory function in normal hearts, which is improbable for other normal anastomoses.

The inner third or thereby of the left ventricle is particularly vulnerable in respect of its blood supply. This is not only due to its distance from the epicardial arteries but because on systole its blood vessels are emptied by compression, with reversal of blood flow in the arteries[10,27]. The inner zone of the ventricular wall therefore depends entirely on return of blood flow in diastole. (Fig. 8). To meet this problem the deep network has been advantaged by special supply vessels which pass directly from the epicardial arteries through the heart wall with few side branches and little or no reduction in calibre. This feature has been confirmed by Farrer-Brown[28] and by Estes et al.[29]. It is tempting to speculate that this adaptation may have a survival role, allowing return of blood flow to the inner zone with the minimum of delay in the short diastolic intervals in tachycardia as from exertion. There is no doubt about its importance in disease.

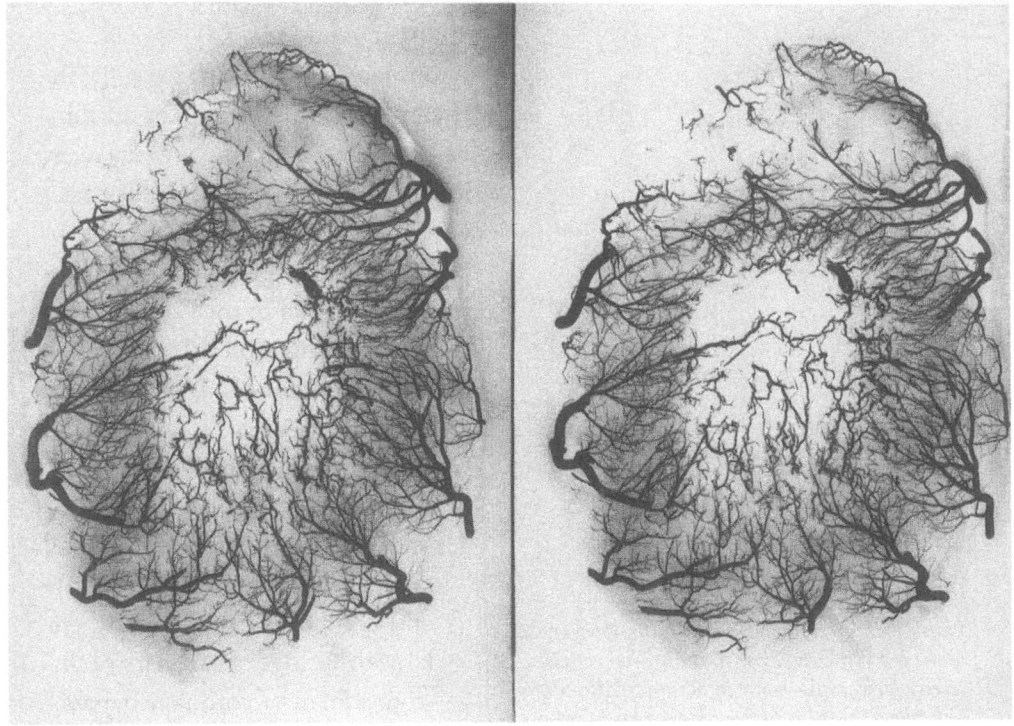

Fig. 7

Subendocardial plexus of the left ventricle in a slightly enlarged heart with a healthy coronary circulation. In the preparation of this transventricular section the floor of the left ventricle just above the apex remained in contact with the free wall. This has given a display fo of the deep network and its vessels of supply. Stereoscopic image. x 1.0.

The deep network interconnects all the vessels, which supply the left ventricle; they are therefore not only intercoronary as with most other anastomoses but also intracoronary. In obstructive coronary artery disease the subendocardial network can undergo very great enlargement. This may be dominantly local in 1- or 2- vessel disease but is characteristically global in multi-vessel obstruction (Fig. 9) and exerts a major influence on the extent and distribution of ischaemic damage. It is surprising that it has received so little attention in the literature. This may be partly due to difficulty in its display in clinical coronary angiography, possibly because of the phasic conditions of blood flow referred to above. In postmortem investigation its recognition is favoured by stereoarteriography and by transventricular sections, procedures that are not often applied.

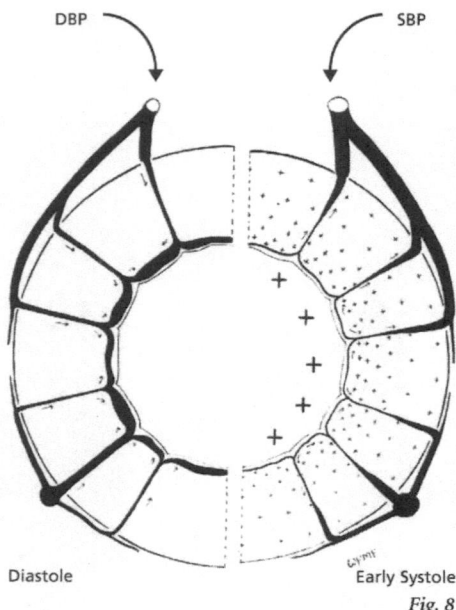

DBP   SBP

Diastole   Early Systole

Fig. 8

Phasic conditions of blood flow in the deep vessels of the left ventricle. Note that the deep vessels receive forward flow only in diastole. DBP - diastolic blood pressure, SBP - systolic blood pressure.

c. Subendocardial plexus of the right ventricle.

A similar deep network exists in the right ventricle but because of the thinness of the wall it is more easily overlooked. Identification is made easier where that chamber is hypertrophied. Interestingly it is partly supplied by a septal branch of the anterior descending artery (LAD) which courses across the moderator band.

Other coronary intercommunications

1. Vasa vasorum: these very small calibre vessels often communicate and sometimes may greatly enlarge to "bridge" a coronary occlusion, a form of coronary bypass.
2. Extracoronary connections.

a. atrial-mediastinal communications were common in my studies. They were usually of small calibre in normal hearts but one of 800 μm diameter was recorded. It is conceivable that a contribution to blood supply to the atria and SA node could occur where atrial arteries have been obstructed at their origins.

Communication with vasa vasorum of aorta and pulmonary arteries was witnessed. Also leakage of injection medium beside pulmonary veins required control, but their destination was not part of my procedure. For more information see, Gross[2] and Schoenmackers[12].

Measurement and enumeration.

Anastomoses were measured and counted in normal hearts and at all sites. Methods, observations and calculations are detailed in Fulton[5,30].

Superficial anastomoses measured 20-200 μm in diameter, being most numerous when less than 100 μm in diameter and only a few were greater than 200 μm in diameter. Deep anastomoses tended to be of larger calibre and more numerous, the greater number being between 100-200 μm in diameter; but many were over 200 μm in diameter.

The same exercise was undertaken in the other groups in the series, and the results from the coronary artery disease group was compared to the normal in figure 10. This shows that large calibre anastomoses are frequent in coronary artery disease, mostly 200-800+ μm in diameter while those less than 100 μm are fewer. There has been, so to speak, a "shift to the right".

The important finding is that sufficient numbers of anastomoses are to be found in normal hearts to account for the numbers of anastomoses of larger calibre found in coronary artery disease. Moreover, there were no patterns of anastomoses found in coronary disease that did not have their counterparts of smaller scale in normal hearts. These observations validate the concept that the large collateral arterial vessels seen in ischaemic heart disease can arise by enlargement of preexisting arterial communications of smaller size.

At the time that I made these observations I found no comparable arteriographic studies with measurement and enumeration of anastomoses. Remarkably, however, Prinzmental et al perfused normal hearts

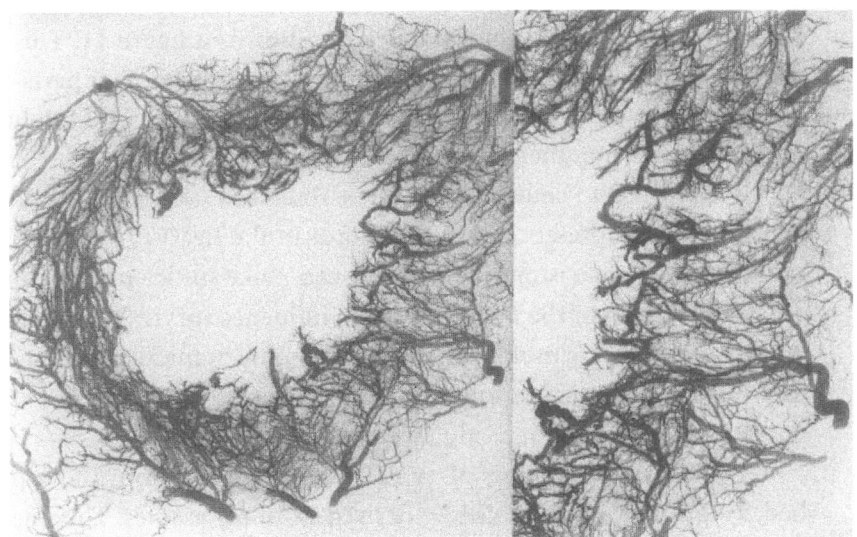

Fig. 9

Generalized enlargement of the subendocardial plexus of the left ventricle in severe long-standing multivessel coronary artery disease. x 1, x 2.4.

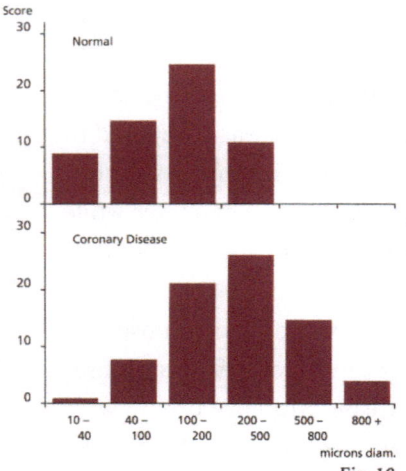

Fig. 10

Comparison of numerical distribution of coronary anastomoses in normal controls and total coronary artery disease group.

with a medium that contained graduated glass spheres and recorded measurements of 70-180 μm lumen diameter for interarterial communications[31]. Also the measurements made by Baroldi et al were in accord with mine[15].

Anatomical origin of coronary anastomoses.

Sufferers from ischaemic heart disease are fortunate that their hearts are endowed with arterial anastomoses with the potential to mitigate the effect of coronary artery obstruction. But it would be teleological and unscientific, and therefore wrong, to suppose that they are there for such a beneficial purpose. In my view, they are remnants of the retiform, early stages of arterial development, of angiogenesis in foetal life; and the advantages they present may be fortunate but are fortuitous. Arterial anastomoses were described in the foetal human heart by Vaestesaeger et al[19] and in neonates by Reiner et al.[32]. The persistence of an obvious network in a normal heart is shown in figure 11. This is an unusually rich network; and the anastomotic pattern in other parts of the same heart was the most abundant that I have witnessed. This might suggest a genetic component or perhaps something else.

I am reluctant to embrace Darwinian/Wallacean "survival-of-the-fittest" grounds for the presence of anastomoses in the heart of man. It seems unlikely that the anastomotic network can make sufficient contribution to the circulation of the normal heart to influence survival of the species. An advantage that is usually manifest today only in middle-aged and elderly men and women is unlikely to have favoured the survival of our ancestors during their reproductive period of life.

On the possible genesis of anastomotic channels from the capillary bed, no positive evidence can be derived from my studies. The injection medium did not enter the capillary bed except in traces. A single rare exception to this is illustrated in figure 6:12 in Fulton[5]. In an area of long-term ischaemia with inner-zonal fibrosis the capillaries themselves were dilated. I have however no evidence in this or any other case of connection being made between two arteries through capillaries. Having already remarked that absence of demonstration is not proof of absence, I prefer to leave the question open. The demonstration of abundant pre-capillary arterial communications however, reduces the need to invoke a capillary origin for collateral vessel development.

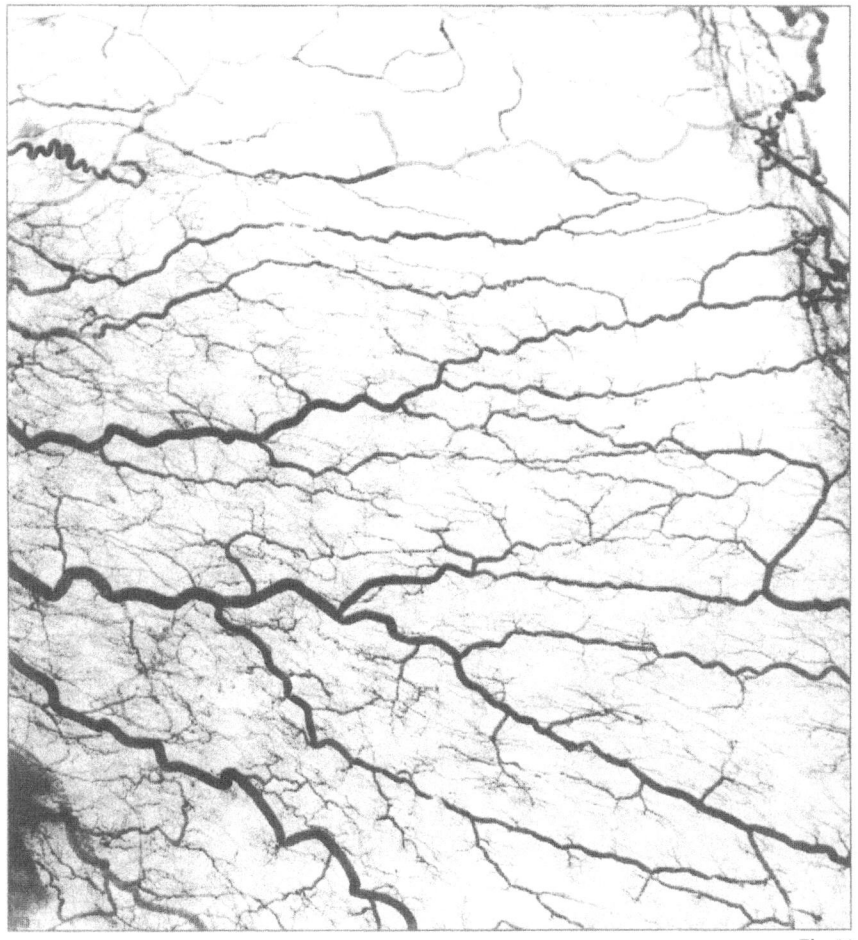

Fig. 11

Radiograph of left atrial wall showing unusually rich network of arterial anastomoses. Vessels could be traced down to 20 microns diameter. x 4.0.

Factors in the enlargement of coronary anastomoses.

It is generally accepted that the main underlying stimulus for anastomotic enlargement is coronary artery occlusion or severe stenosis, that the differential pressure gradient so caused promotes augmented blood flow from the well-provided donor artery into the ischaemic territory, and that increased blood flow provokes vessel enlargement. Although it may exert an influence, simple vasodilatation can account only for a small increase in diameter and blood flow[10]. It is evident that the major increase in diameter which occurs must involve actual growth of the vessel wall, increase for instance from 50 to 500 μm lumen diameter involves increase in circumference of the order of 30 times.

Careful study of the structure involved reveals that the donor, non-ischaemic, portion of the collateral vessels characteristically enlarges to a similar degree as does the recipient portion in the area of ischaemia (Fig. 12).

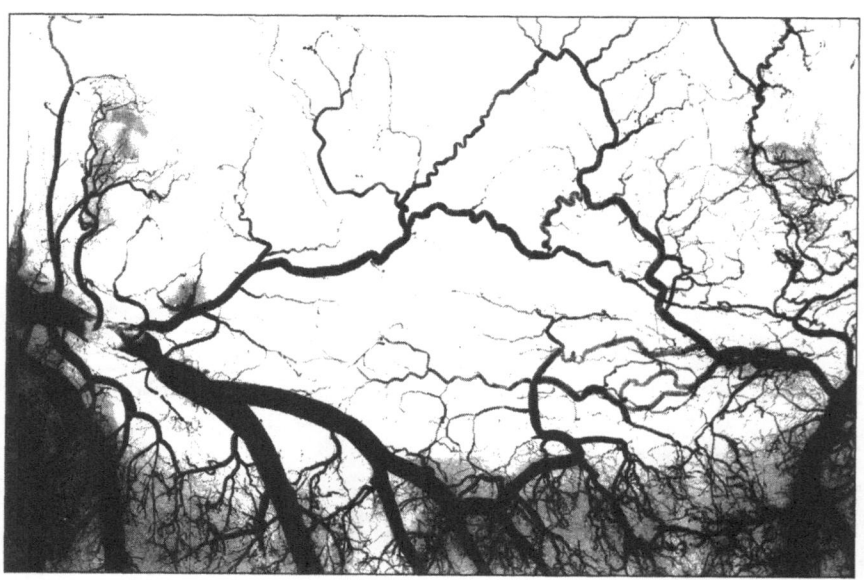

Fig. 12

Enlargement of atrial anastomoses in coronary artery disease. An acute (fatal) occlusion of the left circumflex artery is seen.
Before this event the circumflex artery had been supplying the territory of the right coronary artery, which was completely occluded 1 1/2 years earlier. There is no difference in degree of enlargement of the donor, non-ischemic vessels and the recipient vessels in the ischemic area on the right of the picture. x 1.2.

This reinforces the concept of blood flow as the prime stimulus; and goes against a primary role for ischaemia itself. Indeed it is not only the collateral vessels themselves that respond to the stimulus of blood flow but in course of time some arterial branches feeding them and even the main stems may respond. The complex factors which translate flow stimulus into vessel growth have been addressed by the Schapers and by others and will receive attention elsewhere.

Enlargement of anastomoses depends not only on the intensity of the stimulus but also on its duration. Short of complete occlusion, for strong stimulation to be exerted by stenosis, reduction in the epicardial artery lumen requires to be of the order of 10% of cross sectional area[33]. Yet it is conceivable that lesser degrees of stenosis will also be effective over long periods of time; indeed my studies are in keeping with this being so. Final thrombotic occlusion is nearly always preceded by previous episodes of encroachment on the lumen, not always so severe as suggested above; yet sufficient collateral enlargement has been engendered for the protection of much of the myocardial territory of the freshly occluded artery.

Enlargement of anastomoses does not take place in anticipation of need, as has been suggested. It is a pathological response to, and therefore a sequel to, coronary artery obstruction. Accordingly it is no surprise that the response lags behind the threat and ultimate completion of occlusion usually finds the protection insufficient to prevent some degree of ischaemic damage.

It would appear that in man a much longer period of time is required than has been reported in the dog. Instead of weeks we need to think in terms of months and years. When I divided cases into three categories according to duration of ischaemic histories (0-3 months, 6 months, 2 years and 7-14 years) there was a progressive increase in the number of anastomoses of 500-800 µm; and only in cases with the longer histories were vessels greater than 800 µm diameter found[5,34]. These were largely in the subendocardial plexus of the left ventricle. It is important to recognise that these observations refer only to the state of the collateral circulation at the time of death and give no precise information on the anastomotic status at the time of old occlusions that had been survived. The process initiated by coronary artery occlusion evidently continues for years.

While enlargement of an anastomotic channel may indicate that at one time it had been carrying augmented blood flow, it must not be assumed that it had continued to do so to the end. The situation in coronary artery disease is so often complex that every detail must be taken into account before a valid relationship between structure and function can be reached. Thus a donor vessel that had been contributing substantial relief blood flow will cease to do so when it in turn becomes obstructed - as happens frequently. This may result in infarction not only of its own territory (ipsi-regional infarction) but of much of the territory of its neighbour, which it had till then being supporting (eg case 22,[5] Fig. 11, Fulton 1964[35]). This event gives us convincing retrospective evidence of the extent to which collateral blood flow had indeed supported a neighbouring territory. This phenomenon, which I refer to as pararegional infarction, occurs only where occlusion involves at least a second artery; and in varying degree is common in these circumstances. It can be recognised with certainty only where arterial territories have been identified by arteriography. It has been described by others (e.g. Blumgart et al[36]).

Another circumstance where enlarged vessels cannot carry increased forward flow is found in long-standing multi-vessel disease where, as already described, the subendocardial plexus has become a network of wide-bore interconnecting channels. Yet they are unable to relieve ischaemia because total inflow to the coronary circulation is severely curtailed by obstruction of all epicardial arteries. But they do serve to arrange an equitable distribution of the severely impoverished blood supply. When further adverse events, be they fresh complete arterial occlusion or one of many extra-coronary factors, carry ischaemia beyond a degree critical for myocardial survival, the entire inner zone of the left ventricle suffers, and infarction takes the form of multiple areas of focal necrosis[5,35,37]. The great enlargement of the vessels of the deep plexus is not immediately in accord with concepts of blood flow as the prime stimulus. I believe this paradox can be resolved if we allow that non-laminar ebb- and -flow can exert a stimulus to vessel growth similar to augmented forward flow[38].

Anastomotic enlargement and ischaemic myocardial damage

The most important single factor in determining the extent and distribution of myocardial infarction following coronary artery occlusion is the pattern of anastomotic enlargement present at the time[35]. In individual hearts all gradations and combinations of coronary artery obstruction, ischaemic myocardial damage and patterns of collateral circulation may be found and the situation may be highly complex. Nevertheless some general principles emerge.

Very little protection is afforded by a collateral circulation that has increased only slightly from the normal. This occurs where the evolution of arterial disease to occlusion has been rapid, the history - if present - short; and the myocardial damage is characteristically massive. The other extreme in long-standing multi-vessels disease has already been discussed. Where the evolution of obstructive diseases has taken place over longer periods of time enlargement of anastomoses can mitigate the effects of occlusion to the extent that the resultant damage may be much limited and even, uncommonly, absent.

Credit is commonly given to enlargement of superficial anastomoses and also transinterventricular vessels, but the subendocardial plexus has been overlooked. In my findings, this deep network played a major role in regional infarction as well as in inner-zonal (diffuse subendocardial) infarction.

In my series of fatal myocardial infarction coronary occlusion was always complete or nearly so, so that precise observations could usually be made on the collateral status at the time. But it could have been otherwise in non-fatal infarction, for two reasons. Firstly the anastomotic enlargement at the time must remain speculative because much of the observed enlargement may have resulted from occlusion, the process having continued after the event. Secondly there is often the possibility that the occlusion may not have been complete or had been complete for only a short period of time so that the smaller size of old infarcts may have been related to the incompleteness of the obstructive lesion rather than to the degree of anastomotic enlargement at the time[39,40]. In a later series most infarct-related old coronary occlusions were incomplete at death[41].

There is a further point about the protective effect of coronary anastomoses that has relevance to early interventions in evolving myocardial infarction. It is probable that the time-period occlusion to necrosis may be prolonged. Thus, for instance, thrombolytic therapy may still be appropriate several hours after onset, and not be constrained to the very short interval that acute experimental occlusion in normal subjects might suggest.

In a second series, 48 cases of fatal myocardial infarction were ana-lysed in detail in respect of the final occlusion, old obstructive lesions, distribution of old and new infarction, anastomotic enlargement and the patency or otherwise of donor vessels. The concept that the collateral cir-culation modifies the extent and distribution of ischaemic myocardial damage resulting from coronary occlusion was upheld in 92% of cases. In 4 cases (8%) some of the anastomotic evidence had been obliterated in necrosis. Importantly, no case ran counter to the above concept[42].

Following non-fatal coronary artery occlusion augmentation of the collateral circulation continues, for the stimulus has not only increased but persists: provided of course that the foster artery remains patent. This brings progressive security to the myocardium that has survived and favours restoration of function and reduction in ischaemic symptoms. In this context my studies suggest a major role for collateral blood flow. But amelioration may also result from recanalisation of the occluded artery. Indeed both processes may co-exist and possibly compete.

My studies of obstructive coronary artery disease indicated that it is not, as sometimes supposed, a gradual process but that it evolves by episodes. Each episode may elicit a degree of anastomotic enlargement. Many sub-clinical episodes may occur over a long period before anginal symptoms are manifest. The background to stable (effort) angina is commonly one of multi-vessel obstructive coronary artery disease with considerable en-largement of the collateral circulation. In long-standing angina severe multi-vessel disease with great enlargement of the subendocardial plexus of the left ventricle is characteristic[37]. Ultimately the stage of so called "acute coronary insufficiency"[43] or status anginosus as some prefer, e.g. Papp and Smith[44], is reached on a basis of severe chronic disease; aggravation of symp-toms is commonly due to extracoronary factors or to further obstruction of the coronary arteries. On the other hand the precise pathology underly-ing unstable angina that has been survived is hard to determine. One may expect that survival may well be favoured by the collateral circulation at the time, as with coronary artery occlusion and myocardial infarction. In fatal cases studied by me, pre-infarction unstable angina was related to epi-sodic acute changes in the occlusive lesion with intimal dissection preced-ing thrombotic occlusion[45]. The pathogenesis of unstable angina has been reviewed by Conti[46], without assessing the role of collateral circulation.

Editorial comment by W. Schaper

Dr. Fulton has shown more than 40 years ago that collateral vessel growth during evolving coronary artery disease in man depends on the presence of preexisting arteriolar connections within and between vascular territories. Even today one finds in the literature reports that assume recruitment of smooth muscle cells by newly formed capillaries as a mechanism of arteriogenesis in adult organism[47].

We have often shown that such a "neo-arteriogenesis" is rarely observed and that the old Fulton dogma is much more likely. If no arteriolar interconnecting vessels preexist collateral vessels cannot develop in response to arterial stenosis. A case in point is the heart of the domestic pig that lacks preexistent collaterals. The fact that slowly occurring coronary occlusions in this species is tolerated with only small infarctions or even only minor scarring is an apparent contradiction of the above stated dogma. However, angiographic and his-

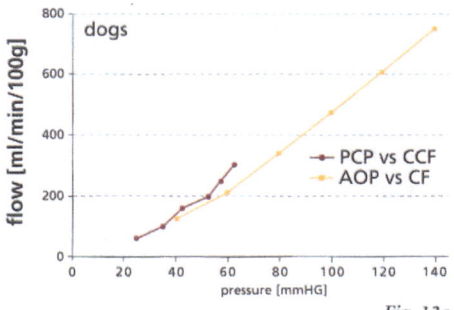

Fig. 13a

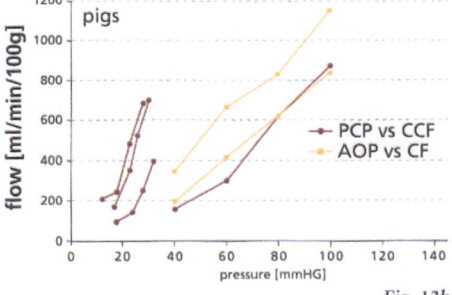

Fig. 13b

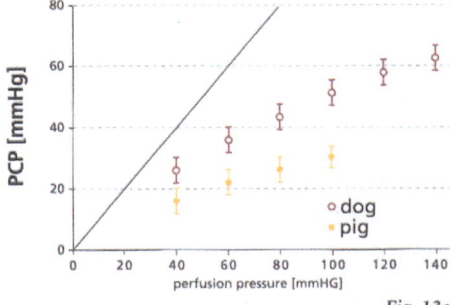

Fig. 13c

Relationship between aortic perfusion pressure (AOP) and blood flow to the normal myocardium of hearts with one constricted coronary artery and between peripheral coronary pressure (PCP) and collateral blood flow (CCF).

Panel a. Pressure flow relationships in dog hearts with chronic coronary occlusion. The relationship PCP vs collateral flow overlaps with AOP vs coronary flow and suggests that minimal vascular resistance in the recipient bed was not changed. Panel b: In the three pig hearts available for detailed pressure-flow studies the relationship PCP vs collateral flow is much steeper than that of AoP vs coronary flow, suggesting a substantially decreased minimal resistance of the recipient bed. Panel c: Relationship between aortic perfusion pressure and peripheral coronary pressure (measured in the distal stump of the occluded artery) determined during maximal coronary vasodilation with adenosine. In canine hearts PCP is much higher than in porcine hearts.

tological studies had shown that in contrast to the dog heart (where large muscular arteries develop subepicardially) many capillaries had enlarged and served as collateral vessels that were located mainly in the subendo- and mid-myocardium, were thin-walled and lacked an arterial coat. The fact that cardiac myocytes are closely apposed to the endothelial/pericyte structure, thereby supporting the fragile vessel wall, and the low intra-vascular pressure prevented their rupture. These vessels are the product of the strong angiogenic response that occurred during the ischemic phase and their genesis lowered the total resistance of the sum of serial resistors, which is composed of the conduit- resistance and micro-vessels (capillaries). Reductions of the minimal resistance of the microcircula-tion can be demonstrated by varying the perfusion pressure of isolated blood-perfused pig hearts with a chronically occluded left circumflex artery: although the peripheral stump/wedge pressure is significantly lower than in the dog under comparable conditions, any increment in pressure moves significantly more blood flow into the collateral supplied myocardial regions compared to flow in normally perfused regions of the same heart (Fig. 13) in the pig compared to the dog where no angiogenic but a strong arteriogenic response occurs[48].

The low intra-vascular pressure of the capillary-derived pig collaterals and their location close to the endocardium makes them vulnerable for rises in the left ventricular enddiastolic pressure which reduces perfusion in that region and may lead to ischemia and infarction. In contrast to the canine heart where the left circumflex plus the right coronary artery can be oc-cluded in a graded manner without ensuing infarction, the pig heart will not survive such an operation because of its inability to generate a second-ary network of collaterals. Thus: pig hearts devoid of preexisting arterio-lar connections between perfusion territories are unable to produce mus-cular collateral vessels. Their numerous enlarged interconnecting capillar-ies are unable to recruit smooth muscle. The low wedge pressures may be the result of the low pressure that normally exists in the capillary system from which the capillary collaterals emerge but also because collateral flow is transported by many small tubes that lead to cumulative energy losses.

B: Clinical measurements, tools and demonstration of its protective role during the course of coronary artery disease

Niels van Royen

Before the 1960's, research on the collateral circulation was focused on the central issue whether arterial anastomoses are present in normal human hearts and whether they enlarge in the course of coronary artery disease. This debate was emphatically settled by Fulton around 1965 [5,25,30] by showing unequivocally that preexistent anastomoses are abundant in human hearts and that their caliber, and not their number, increases in the course of coronary artery disease. *In vivo* studies on the human coronary collateral circulation that were performed thereafter, in the last third of the 20th century, can be roughly divided into three categories: methodology of measurements at the collateral circulation in the clinical setting, protective role of the collateral circulation in coronary artery disease and pharmacological modulation of the collateral circulation (the latter is beyond the focus of this chapter).

Measurements of the collateral circulation in patients

Balloon inflation for accurate measurement of the collateral circulation

To make exact measurements of the collateral circulation, antegrade inflow in the recipient artery needs to be interrupted in order to determine the contribution of the collateral circulation to the perfusion of a jeopardized vascular territory. The introduction of balloon angioplasty has made such observations possible in the clinical setting and it was Feldman who first did so by applying brief balloon occlusions and measuring simultaneously the pressure deficit over the occlusion to detect the development of the collateral circulation [49]. Since we believe such coronary total occlusions are of paramount importance for the reliable measurement of the functionality of the collateral circulation, the methodology section of this chapter will be dedicated mainly to techniques in which such short-term balloon occlusions are implemented.

Angiography

Using brief coronary occlusions, recruitment of the collateral circulation can be visualized by angiography. This is the basis of the Rentrop classification [50] requiring repeated contrast injections, which is rarely used today in its original form. Other methods are based on angiographically measured diameter of the recipient artery [51] or washout of contrast agent during balloon occlusion [52].

ST-segment changes

Brief coronary occlusions also provoke ST-segment changes and the magnitude of these changes can be used as a measure of collateral flow [53-55], whereas in cases of significant collateral artery development ST-changes can be completely absent. ST-segment changes thus provide an indication of the extent of the collateral circulation in individual patients. However, ischemic preconditioning can obscure the relationship.

Intracoronary derived pressure measurements

Probably the most valuable parameters during brief coronary occlusion are the pressure deficit over the occluded arterial segment and the residual flow in the recipient coronary artery. Feldman performed a balloon inflation in the proximal LAD in a group of 19 patients [49]. Based on the pressure deficit over the occlusion and venous flow from the great cardiac vein, he found that collateral resistance was about 45% lower in patients with retrograde angiographic filling of the occluded LAD, as compared to patients without such retrograde filling [49]. Probst then showed in a larger group of 63 patients with single-vessel disease that the distal pressure during balloon inflation correlated with the extent of the non-provoked spontaneously visible collateral circulation [56]. Meier showed that distal coronary pressure is higher in patients with either spontaneously visible or recruitable collateral arteries than in patients without visible collateral arteries. He also showed that values for distal pressure of 30 mmHg or more were only found in patients with spontaneously visible or recruitable collateral arteries [57]. In order to obtain a more precise calculation of the pressure index, Pijls subtracted venous pressure from both aortic and coronary wedge pressure [59], a calculation that is nowadays referred to as pressure derived collateral flow index (CFI) [60].

Flow velocity measurements and resistance index calculation

As mentioned above, Feldman used venous flow return in combination with pressure deficit to determine collateral resistance during balloon inflation[49]. The venous circulation of the heart is characterized by several anastomotic connections, so that venous flow return does not necessarily represent collateral flow. Later studies therefore attempted to measure collateral flow directly in the recipient artery. Ofili was the first to report data on residual flow in the recipient artery as obtained with a Doppler-tipped angioplasty guidewire[61]. Seiler's group was the first to compare velocity data with pressure-derived indices and with the intracoronary ECG[60]. Subsequently, Kern reported that collateral flow, in a group of patients that received angioplasty, was approximately 30% of post-procedural antegrade flow[62]. During balloon occlusion of the LAD, Kyriakidis measured flow increase in the right coronary artery that served as donor artery for the collateral circulation to the diseased LAD. He found that in patients with spontaneously visible collateral arteries flow in the RCA increased during LAD occlusion with a mean of 66% in patients with spontaneously visible collateral arteries as compared to no significant change of flow in patients without visible collateral arteries[63]. These studies also paved the way for the calculation of resistance from the combined measurement of collateral flow and pressure in the donor and/or the recipient coronary artery[64,65], which can be used to document for example the pharmacological responsiveness of the collateral vascular bed to vasodilators[66]. Three main pitfalls in collateral flow measurements from the recipient artery are to be noted. First of all, flow measurements with Doppler guidewires are actually flow velocity measurements. To calculate true flow, also the diameter of the vessel needs to be known, for example with the use of quantitative angiography (QCA) or intravascular ultrasound (IVUS). Secondly, flow measured in the recipient artery will vary with the position of the Doppler sensor in the recipient artery. When the sensor is proximal to a major re-entry of the collateral circulation in the recipient artery, a very different signal will be found as compared to a position directly distal from such a re-entry. Finally, flow (but also pressure) measurements are not feasible in case of a non-revascularizable total occlusion. Nevertheless, resistance measurements directly reflect the capacity of the collateral circulation. It is to be expected that

future methodological studies will be focused on techniques which measure this parameter reliably since it would serve best as an endpoint for
studies on pharmacological modulation of the collateral circulation.

The protective role of the coronary collateral circulation in man

Acute myocardial infarction

The protective potential of collateral arteries in the human heart was
already recognized at their first discovery in 1669 by Richard Lower. He
described the following: "Coronary vessels describe a circular course to
ensure a better general distribution, and encircle and surround the base
of the heart. From such an origin they are able to go off respectively to
opposite regions of the heart, yet around the extremities they come together again and here and there communicate by anastomoses. As a result
fluid injected into one of them spreads at one and the same time through
both. There is everywhere an equally great need of vital heat and nour-
ishment, so deficiency of these is very fully guarded against by such anastomoses"[67]. As described in the first part of this chapter, research in subsequent centuries was dedicated to the very existence of collateral anastomoses in the heart and the preexisting nature of these vessels. After the
publication of highly detailed post-mortem studies by Fulton finally settled this debate by around 1963, attention was now fully focused on the
functionality and the protective role of the collateral circulation.

The introduction of coronary angiography made it possible to determine the extent of the collateral circulation in living patients[68]. Consequently, the extent of the collateral circulation could also be linked to
outcome after myocardial infarction. In 1976 Williams showed in a group
of 20 patients with acute myocardial infarction, that "adequate" collateral vessels, as observed with angiography, were associated with a lower LV
end-diastolic pressure, a better cardiac index and ejection fraction as well
as a smaller area of dyskinesia as compared to patients with an "inadequate" collateral vasculature. It was also found that patients with "adequate" collateral vessels more frequently reported preceding angina pectoris. Finally, Williams observed that all patients with "adequate" collateral vessels survived myocardial infarction whereas in the group with

inadequate collateral vessels 10 patients had cardiogenic shock and 8 patients died[69]. Schwartz et al showed that residual flow in the infarct related artery, either due to subtotal occlusion or due to a well developed collateral circulation, preserves left ventricular function after myocardial infarction[70]. It was also shown that in the scenario of an acute myocardial function, myocardial damage as measured by creatin kinase level can be limited by the presence of a well developed collateral circulation[71]. Not only outcome directly upon AMI but also long-term (10 year) survival depends on the extent of the collateral circulation. Probably, one of the reasons for this long-term benefit is the prevention by collateral arteries of LV aneurysm formation as a result of extensive transmural infarction as shown by Hirai in patients with unsuccessful thrombolytic reperfusion therapy[73]. In another study from this group it was shown that preinfarction angina is linked to a better functional preservation of the left ventricle and they claim that this is caused by stimulation of the development of the collateral circulation by repetitive brief ischemic periods[74]. In our opinion, this merely reflects the differences between slow and rapid progression of arterial obstruction, whereby in the case of slow progression the collateral circulation can adapt better to the increased demand of blood flow. The collateral circulation can also serve as a bridge between the acute event and a late-stage revascularization procedure. Sabia et al showed that success of late-revascularization of an occluded infarct-related artery strongly depends on the percentage of the infarcted area that is supplied by collateral flow. Patients in which 50 % or more of the infarct bed is supplied by collateral flow, show better improvement of wall motion score after revascularization[75].

In contrast to the above mentioned studies on the protective role of the collateral circulation during AMI, Boehrer et al. found no relation between angiographic evidence of collateral filling and long-term survival or cardiac function after AMI[76].

It should be noted though that in this study, no Rentrop score was performed and patients were simply divided in a group with and without collateral filling of the infarct related artery, resulting in a large number of patients (120 out of 146) assigned to the group with angiographic evidence of collateral filling. It can be postulated that a more refined system of collateral circulation grading would have resulted in a different outcome.

Taken together, we feel that it can be safely concluded that a well developed collateral circulation preserves left ventricular function and results in a better outcome after AMI.

Chronic coronary artery disease

The protective role of the collateral circulation in situations of chronic coronary artery disease is most dramatically shown in a small subgroup of patients that present with total occlusion of the stem region of the left main coronary artery and well preserved left ventricular function. Several of such observations in small series of patients have been published [77-82]. In most of these cases, a dominant right coronary is described from which collateral arteries towards the left coronary artery originate. Hamby performed a retrospective study on 465 patients with complete obstruction of either the LAD or the RCA. In his studies he found that the collateral circulation towards a chronically obstructed LAD is of great functional significance with regard to preservation of ventricular function [83]. Cohen and Rentrop showed in patients with chronic coronary artery disease that poor filling of the collateral circulation upon balloon occlusion was associated with anginal pain, ST-segment changes and ventricular asynergy during the procedure [53]. These results were confirmed in a later study by Norell et al [55]. Using thallium scintigraphy, Nakatsuka et al found that post-infarction patients with fixed defects that were associated with akinesia had a relative underdevelopment of the collateral circulation as compared to patients with still viable myocardium [84]. In a population that was referred to the catheterization lab for elective coronary angioplasty it was observed that patients with a well developed collateral circulation (based on intracoronary pressure measurements) are at lower risk for future ischemic events [59]. These results were confirmed in a study with 403 patients undergoing PTCA for stable angina pectoris. It was shown that patients with a well developed collateral circulation were at a significantly lower risk for major cardiac ischemic events [85]. The protective role of collaterals was also shown in patients that received an LAD bypass graft in a beating heart procedure. During coronary occlusion, patients with a well developed collateral circulation had a superior preservation of left ventricular function as measured with transoesophageal echocardiography and thermodilution [86]. Van Liebergen showed that patients with good collateralization, based on either intracoronary derived pressure or flow measurements during balloon occlusion, were best protected against ischaemic episodes resulting from occlusion[87].

Thus, also in patients with chronic stable coronary artery disease, a well developed collateral circulation salvages myocardial function and in addition reduces the risk for future ischemic events.

Morphologic preservation

In a very elegant study by Schwarz, the protective role of collateral vessels was shown on a morphological level rather than a functional level. During open heart surgery, transmural myocardial biopsies were taken from patients with severe stenosis of the LAD. Patients with a poorly developed collateral circulation showed increased myocardial fibrosis as compared to patients with a well developed collateral circulation[88]. Vanoverschelde et al showed profound morphological changes like cellular swelling, loss of myofibrillar content, and accumulation of glycogen in patients with a total coronary obstruction and a poorly developed collateral circulation[89].

Protective role during exercise

Whether development of the collateral circulation is stimulated by exercise remains controversial although most studies did not find a significant effect of exercise on collateral artery growth[90-95]. What has been shown though is that coronary collateral arteries are of importance in maintaining left ventricular function during exercise. Goldberg et al showed that in a group of patients with at least one severe stenosis and a mean left ventricular ejection fraction at rest of about 50 %, the decrease in ejection fraction was significantly more pronounced in patients with a poorly developed collateral circulation[96]. Bonetti et al observed that after termination of exercise, ECG returned to baseline more rapidly in patients with a well developed collateral circulation, indicating a faster recovery from exercise-induced ischemia[97]. This was confirmed in a study showing that the recovery of left ventricular dysfunction after dobutamine stress echocardiography is also related to the extent of the collateral circulation[98]. Using exercise thallium-scintigraphy, Wainwright et al found that especially the right coronary bed benefits from collateral flow during exercise[99].

With the same technique, Iskandrian showed that the protective value of collateral vessels largely depends on patency of feeder vessels[100]. This dependency of the collateral circulation on feeder vessels was also found in a study by Dilsizian et al[101]. They showed in patients with multi-vessel disease and a non-revascularizable or re-obstructed stenosis of the LCX that collateral flow and function of the jeopardized territory is improved after bypass surgery to an obstructed feeder vessel (either LAD or RCA).

Summary

The first part of this chapter starts with a brief historical account. The description of coronary arterial anastomoses in normal and diseased human hearts is based mainly on the author's study (Fulton), using a technique, which included stereoarteriography. From these studies the following can be concluded:

- Anastomotic vessels were found in all normal hearts. The coronary arteries of man are not end-arteries. Their distribution, enumeration and measurement are described, in normal hearts and in the presence of coronary artery disease.

- The enlarged collateral vessels present in ischaemic heart disease are derived from preexisting arterial anastomoses. These are present in normal hearts in sufficient numbers to account for the numbers found in disease. The difference is of calibre, not of number.

- The main stimulus to collateral vessel growth is coronary artery occlusion or severe obstruction. The resultant pressure gradients promote increased blood flow from neighbouring donor arteries to the arteries in the ischaemic area distal to the obstruction. Morphological evidence is in keeping with blood flow as the prime stimulus for vessel enlargement.

  Attention is directed to the importance of the deeply placed anastomoses which in the human heart are often more numerous and of larger calibre than the superficial. Emphasis is given to the subendocardial plexus of the left ventricle, which has been largely overlooked.

- The role of collateral blood flow in determining the extent and distribution of ischaemic myocardial damage resulting from coronary artery occlusion is described and discussed.

The second part of this chapter (van Royen) is dedicated to a review of methods that enable functional measurement of the collateral circulation during life. It is emphasized that total occlusion of the recipient artery, either due to underlying occlusive disease or by means of artificial coronary balloon occlusion, is a prerequisite for exact measurements of the functionality of the collateral circulation. Sensitive measurements of the collateral circulation will gain further importance in the nowadays-evolving field of clinical studies on the stimulation of collateral artery development. It is our belief that intracoronary derived pressure and flow measurements will be of great value in determining efficacy of such therapeutic approaches. Finally, a brief summary is given of clinical studies that have been performed in the last third of the 20th century that unequivocally show the protective role of collateral arteries during exercise, in chronic coronary artery disease as well as during acute coronary occlusion. The human collateral circulation is capable of salvaging myocardial tissue, preventing it from undergoing necrosis, fibrotic degradation and aneurysm formation, preserving left ventricular function and limiting the extent of myocardial ischaemia. A well-developed collateral circulation constitutes a natural escape from the devastating consequences of coronary artery disease.

References

1. FULTON WFM. The morphology of coronary arterial anastomoses in health and disease and their influence on ischaemic myocardial damage. *Acta Cardiol.* 1969;Suppl XII:38-67.
2. GROSS L. *The Blood Supply to the Heart:* Oxford University Press; 1921.
3. SPALTEHOLZ W. *Die Arterien der Herzwand. Anatomische Untersuchungen an Menschen- und Tierherzen.* Leipzig: Hirzel; 1924.
4. GOULD SE. *The Pathology of the Heart.* Springfield: Charles C. Thomas; 1953.
5. FULTON WFM. *The Coronary Arteries-Arteriography, microanatomy and pathogenesis of obliterative coronary artery disease.* Springfield: Charles C. Thomas; 1965.
6. LOWER R. *Tractatus de corde, item de motu et colore sanguinis, et chyle in cum transito.* Amsteldami; 1669.
7. CRAINICIANU A. Anatomische Studien über die Koronararterien und experimentelle Untersuchungen über ihre Durchgängigkeit. *Virchows Arch Path Anat.* 1922;238:1.
8. DOCK W. The capacity of the coronary bed in cardiac hypertrophy. *J Exp Med.* 1941;74:177.
9. BARMEYER J. Postmortem measurement of intercoronary anastomotic flow in normal and diseased hearts: a quantitative study. *Vascular Surgery.* 1971;5:239-248.
10. GREGG DE. *Coronary Circulation in Health and Disease.* London: Kimpton; 1950.
11. HIRSCH C, SPALTEHOLZ W. Koronararterien und Herzmuskel. Anatomische und experimentelle Untersuchungen. *Deut Med Wochenschr.* 1907;i:790.
12. SCHOENMACKERS. Die Blutversorgung des Herzmuskels und ihre Störungen. In: *Lehrbuch der speziellen pathologischen Anatomie.* Berlin: Walter de Gruyter & Co; 1967.
13. HYRTL. *Wiener Sitz-Ber.* 1885;XIV:73.
14. HENLE. *Handbuch der systematischen Anatomie des Menschen.* Braunschweig; 1866.
15. BAROLDI G, MANTERO O, SCOMAZZONI G. The collaterals of the coronary arteries in normal and pathologic hearts. *Circ Res.* 1956;4:223-229.
16. JAMES TN, BURCH GE. Blood supply of the human interventricular septum. *Circulation.* 1958;17:391.
17. SPALTEHOLZ W. Die Koronararterien des Herzens. In: *Verhandl Anat Gesell.* 30 ed; 1907:141.
18. JAMIN F, MERKEL H. *Die Koronararterien des menschlichen Herzens in stereoskopischen Röntgenbildern.* Jena: Gustav Fischer; 1907.
19. VASTESAEGER MM, VAN DER STRAETEN PP, FRIART J, CANDAELE G, GHYS A, BERNARD RM. Les anastomoses intercoronariennes telles qu'elles apparaissent à la coronarographie postmortem. *Acta Cardiol.* 1957;12:365.
20. SCHAPER W. *The Collateral Circulation of the Heart.* Amsterdam London: Elsevier North Holland Publishing Company; 1971.
21. COHNHEIM J, VON SCHULTHESS-RECHBERG A. Über die Folgen der Kranzarterienverschliessung für das Herz. *Virchows Arch Path Anat.* 1881;85:503.
22. CAMPBELL JS. Stereoscopic radiography of the coronary system. Quart *J Med.* 1929;22:247.
23. Schlesinger MJ. An injection plus dissection study of coronary artery occlusions and anastomoses. *Am Heart J.* 1938;15:528.
24. ZOLL PM, WESSLER S, BLUMGART HL. Angina Pectoris: a clinical and pathological correlation. *Am J Med.* 1951;11:331.
25. FULTON WFM. Arterial anastomoses in the coronary circulation. I. Anatomical features in normal and diseased hearts demonstrated by stereoarteriography. *Scot Med J.* 1963;8:420.
26. FULTON WFM. Immersion radiography of injected specimens. *Brit J Radiol.* 1963;36:685.

27. HOFFMAN JIE, BUCKBERG GD. Pathophysiology of subendocardial ischaemia. *Br Med J.* 1975;1:76-9.
28. FARRER-BROWN G. Nornal and diseased vascular pattern of myocardium of human heart. I. Normal pattern in the left ventricular free wall. *Br Heart J.* 1968;30:527-36.
29. ESTES EH, JR., ENTMAN ML, DIXON HB, 2ND, HACKEL DB. The vascular supply of the left ventricular wall. Anatomic observations, plus a hypothesis regarding acute events in coronary artery disease. *Am Heart J.* 1966;71:58-67.
30. FULTON WFM. Arterial anastomoses in the coronary circulation. II. Distribution, enumeration and measurement of coronary arterial anastomoses in health and disease. *Scot Med J.* 1963;8:466.
31. PRINZMETAL M, SIMKIN B, BERGMAN HC, KRUGER HE. II. The collateral circulation of the normal human heart by coronary perfusion with radioactive erythrocytes and glass spheres. *Am Heart J.* 1947;33:420.
32. REINER L, MOLNAR J, JIMENEZ AF, FREUDENTHAL RR. Interarterial coronary anastomoses in neonates. *Arch Path.* 1961;71:103-112.
33. SEWELL WH. Physiologic and technical requirements for experimental strong stimulation of coronary collateral arteries. *Circulation.* 1961;24:1036.
34. FULTON WFM. The time factor in the enlargement of anastomoses in coronary artery disease. *Scot Med J.* 1964;9:18.
35. FULTON WFM. Anastomotic enlargement and ischaemic myocardial damage. *Br Heart J.* 1964;26:1.
36. BLUMGART HL, SCHLESINGER MJ, ZOLL PM. Angina pectoris, coronary failure and acute myocardial infarction. *JAMA.* 1941;116:91.
37. FULTON WFM. Chronic generalised myocardial ischaemia with advanced coronary artery disease. *Br Heart J.* 1956;18:341.
38. FULTON WFM. The dynamic factor in enlargement of coronary arterial anastomoses and paradoxical changes in the subendocardial plexus. *Br Heart J.* 1964;26:39.
39. DEWOOD MA, SPORES J, NOTSKE R, MOUSER LT, BURROUGHS R, GOLDEN MS, LANG HT. Prevalence of total coronary occlusion during the early hours of transmural myocardial infarction. *N Engl J Med.* 1980;303:897-902.
40. DAVIES MJ, THOMAS AC. Plaque fissuring—the cause of acute myocardial infarction, sudden ischaemic death, and crescendo angina. *Br Heart J.* 1985;53:363-73.
41. FULTON WFM. Koronaratherosklerose, Fissurbildung der Plaque und Thrombose. In: de Bono DP, Brochier ML, Hugenholtz PG, Kuebler W, Verstraete M, eds. *Thrombolytische Therapie des akuten Herzinfarkts.* Berlin, Heidelberg, New York, London, Paris, Tokyo: Springer Verlag; 1987.
42. FULTON WFM. Intercoronary anastomoses studied by post-mortem stereoarteriography: relationship to coronary occlusion and myocardial damage. In: KALTENBACH M, LICHTLEN P, BALCON R, BUSSMANN WD, EDS. *Coronary Heart Disease.* Stuttgart: Georg Thieme Verlag; 1978.
43. MASTER AM, GUBNER R, DACK S, JAFFE HL. Differentation of acute coronary insufficiency with myocardial infarction from coronary occlusion. *Arch Int Med.* 1941;67:646.
44. PAPP C, SHIRLEY SMITH K. Status Anginosus. *Br Heart J.* 1960;22:259.
45. FULTON WFM. Pathogenesis of unstable angina preceding acute myocardial infarction. In: RAFFLENBEUL W, LICHTLEN P, BALCON R, EDS. *Unstable Angina Pectoris.* Stuttgart, New York: Georg Thieme Verlag; 1981.

46. CONTI CR. Unstable angina: thoughts on pathogenesis. In: Hugenholtz PG, Goldman BS, eds. *Unstable angina*. Stuttgart: Schattauer; 1985:55-64.

47. CARMELIET P. Mechanisms of angiogenesis and arteriogenesis. *Nature Med* 2000;6:389-395.

48 GOERGE G, SCHMIDT T, ITO BR, PANTELY GA, SCHAPER W. Microvascular and collateral adaptation in swine hearts following progressive coronary artery stenosis. *Basic Res Cardiol.* 1989;84:524-535.

49. FELDMAN RL, PEPINE CJ. Evaluation of coronary collateral circulation in conscious humans. *Am J Cardiol.* 1984;53:1233-8.

50. RENTROP KP, COHEN M, BLANKE H, PHILLIPS RA. Changes in collateral channel filling immediately after controlled coronary artery occlusion by an angioplasty balloon in human subjects. *J Am Coll Cardiol.* 1985;5:587-92.

51. FUJITA M, OHNO A, MIWA K, MORIUCHI I, MIFUNE J, SASAYAMA S. A new method for assessment of collateral development after acute myocardial infarction. *J Am Coll Cardiol.* 1993;21:68-72.

52. SEILER C, BILLINGER M, FLEISCH M, MEIER B. Washout collaterometry: a new method of assessing collaterals using angiographic contrast clearance during coronary occlusion. *Heart.* 2001;86:540-6.

53. COHEN M, RENTROP KP. Limitation of myocardial ischemia by collateral circulation during sudden controlled coronary artery occlusion in human subjects: a prospective study. *Circulation.* 1986;74:469-76.

54. MACDONALD RG, HILL JA, FELDMAN RL. ST segment response to acute coronary occlusion: coronary hemodynamic and angiographic determinants of direction of ST segment shift. *Circulation.* 1986;74:973-9.

55. NORELL MS, LYONS JP, GARDENER JE, LAYTON CA, BALCON R. Protective effect of collateral vessels during coronary angioplasty. *Br Heart J.* 1989;62:241-5.

56. MIWA K, FUJITA M, KAMEYAMA T, NAKAGAWA K, HIRAI T, INOUE H. Absence of myocardial ischemia during sudden controlled occlusion of coronary arteries in patients with well-developed collateral vessels. *Coron Artery Dis.* 1999;10:459-63.

57. PROBST P, ZANGL W, PACHINGER O. Relation of coronary arterial occlusion pressure during percutaneous transluminal coronary angioplasty to presence of collaterals. *Am J Cardiol.* 1985;55:1264-9.

58. MEIER B, LUETHY P, FINCI L, STEFFENINO GD, RUTISHAUSER W. Coronary wedge pressure in relation to spontaneously visible and recruitable collaterals. *Circulation.* 1987;75:906-13.

59. PIJLS NH, BECH GJ, EL GAMAL MI, BONNIER HJ, DE BRUYNE B, VAN GELDER B, MICHELS HR, KOOLEN JJ. Quantification of recruitable coronary collateral blood flow in conscious humans and its potential to predict future ischemic events. *J Am Coll Cardiol.* 1995;25:1522-8.

60. SEILER C, FLEISCH M, GARACHEMANI A, MEIER B. Coronary collateral quantitation in patients with coronary artery disease using intravascular flow velocity or pressure measurements. *J Am Coll Cardiol.* 1998;32:1272-9.

61. OFILI E, KERN MJ, TATINENI S, DELIGONUL U, AGUIRRE F, SEROTA H, LABOVITZ AJ. Detection of coronary collateral flow by a Doppler-tipped guide wire during coronary angioplasty. *Am Heart J.* 1991;122:221-5.

62. KERN MJ, DONOHUE TJ, BACH RG, AGUIRRE FV, CARACCIOLO EA, OFILI EO. Quantitating coronary collateral flow velocity in patients during coronary angioplasty using a Doppler guidewire. *Am J Cardiol.* 1993;71:34D-40D.

63. KYRIAKIDIS MK, PETROPOULAKIS PN, TENTOLOURIS CA, MARAKAS SA, ANTONOPOULOS AG, KOUROUCLIS CV, TOUTOUZAS PK. Relation between changes in blood flow of the contralateral coronary artery and the angiographic extent and function of recruitable collateral vessels arising from this artery during balloon coronary occlusion. *J Am Coll Cardiol.* 1994; 23:869-78.

64. PIEK JJ, VAN LIEBERGEN RA, KOCH KT, PETERS RJ, DAVID GK. Comparison of collateral vascular responses in the donor and recipient coronary artery during transient coronary occlusion assessed by intracoronary blood flow velocity analysis in patients. *Journal of the American College of Cardiology.* 1997;29:1528-35.

65. PIEK JJ, VAN LIEBERGEN RA, KOCH KT, PETERS RJ, DAVID GK. Clinical, angiographic and hemodynamic predictors of recruitable collateral flow assessed during balloon angioplasty coronary occlusion. *Journal of the American College of Cardiology.* 1997;29:275-82.

66. PIEK JJ, VAN LIEBERGEN RA, KOCH KT, DE WINTER RJ, PETERS RJ, DAVID GK. Pharmacological modulation of the human collateral vascular resistance in acute and chronic coronary occlusion assessed by intracoronary blood flow velocity analysis in an angioplasty model [see comments]. *Circulation.* 1997;96:106-15.

67. LOWER R. *Early Science in Oxford.* Oxford: Oxford University Press; 1932.

68. GENSINI GG, BRUTO DA COSTA BC. The coronary collateral circulation in living man. *Am J Cardiol.* 1969;24:393-400.

69. WILLIAMS DO, AMSTERDAM EA, MILLER RR, MASON DT. Functional significance of coronary collateral vessels in patients with acute myocardial infarction: relation to pump performance, cardiogenic shock and survival. *Am J Cardiol.* 1976;37:345-51.

70. SCHWARTZ H, LEIBOFF RL, KATZ RJ, WASSERMAN AG, BREN GB, VARGHESE PJ, ROSS AM. Arteriographic predictors of spontaneous improvement in left ventricular function after myocardial infarction. *Circulation.* 1985;71:466-72.

71. NOHARA R, KAMBARA H, MURAKAMI T, KADOTA K, TAMAKI S, KAWAI C. Collateral function in early acute myocardial infarction. *Am J Cardiol.* 1983;52:955-9.

72. HANSEN JF. Coronary collateral circulation: clinical significance and influence on survival in patients with coronary artery occlusion. *Am Heart J.* 1989;117:290-5.

73. HIRAI T, FUJITA M, NAKAJIMA H, ASANOI H, YAMANISHI K, OHNO A, SASAYAMA S. Importance of collateral circulation for prevention of left ventricular aneurysm formation in acute myocardial infarction. *Circulation.* 1989;79:791-6.

74. HIRAI T, FUJITA M, YAMANISHI K, OHNO A, MIWA K, SASAYAMA S. Significance of preinfarction angina for preservation of left ventricular function in acute myocardial infarction. *Am Heart J.* 1992;124:19-24.

75. SABIA PJ, POWERS ER, JAYAWEERA AR, RAGOSTA M, KAUL S. Functional significance of collateral blood flow in patients with recent acute myocardial infarction. A study using myocardial contrast echocardiography. *Circulation.* 1992;85:2080-9.

76. BOEHRER JD, LANGE RA, WILLARD JE, HILLIS LD. Influence of collateral filling of the occluded infarct-related coronary artery on prognosis after acute myocardial infarction. *Am J Cardiol.* 1992;69:10-2.

77. FRYE RL, GURA GM, CHESEBRO JH, RITMAN EL. Complete occlusion of the left main coronary artery and the importance of coronary collateral circulation. *Mayo Clin Proc.* 1977;52:742-5.

78. TRNKA KE, FEBRES-ROMAN PR, CADIGAN RA, CRONE RA, WILLIAMS TH. Total occlusion of the left main coronary artery: clinical and catheterization findings. *Clin Cardiol.* 1980;3:352-5.

79. WARD DE, VALANTINE H, HUI W. Occluded left main stem coronary artery. Report of five patients and review of published reports. *Br Heart J.* 1983;49:276-9.

80. WATT AH, PENNY WJ, RUTTLEY MS. Left main coronary artery occlusion with preserved left ventricular function: a report of three cases. *Br Heart J.* 1987;57:344-7.

81. SLUNGA L, ERIKSSON P, OSTERMAN G. Complete occlusion of the left main coronary artery: clinical and angiographic observations in five cases. *J Intern Med.* 1989;225:123-7.

82. TOPAZ O, DISCIASCIO G, COWLEY MJ, LANTER P, SOFFER A, WARNER M, NATH A, GOUDREAU E, HALLE AA, 3RD, VETROVEC GW. Complete left main coronary artery occlusion: angiographic evaluation of collateral vessel patterns and assessment of hemodynamic correlates. *Am Heart J.* 1991;121:450-6.

83. HAMBY RI, AINTABLIAN A, SCHWARTZ A. Reappraisal of the functional significance of the coronary collateral circulation. *Am J Cardiol.* 1976;38:304-9.

84. NAKATSUKA M, MATSUDA Y, OZAKI M, OGAWA H, MORITANI K, KHONO M, MIURA T, SHIMIZU T, FURUTANI Y, KUSUKAWA R. Coronary collateral vessels in patients with previous myocardial infarction. *Clin Cardiol.* 1987;10:791-5.

85. BILLINGER M, KLOOS P, EBERLI FR, WINDECKER S, MEIER B, SEILER C. Physiologically assessed coronary collateral flow and adverse cardiac ischemic events: a follow-up study in 403 patients with coronary artery disease. *J Am Coll Cardiol.* 2002;40:1545-50.

86. KOH TW, CARR-WHITE GS, DESOUZA AC, FERDINAND FD, PEPPER JR, GIBSON DG. Effect of coronary occlusion on left ventricular function with and without collateral supply during beating heart coronary artery surgery. *Heart.* 1999;81:285-91.

87. VAN LIEBERGEN RA, PIEK JJ, KOCH KT, DE WINTER RJ, SCHOTBORGH CE, LIE KI. Quantification of collateral flow in humans: a comparison of angiographic, electrocardiographic and hemodynamic variables. *J Am Coll Cardiol.* 1999;33:670-7.

88. SCHWARZ F, SCHAPER J, BECKER V, KUBLER W, FLAMENG W. Coronary collateral vessels: their significance for left ventricular histologic structure. *Am J Cardiol.* 1982;49:291-5.

89. VANOVERSCHELDE JL, WIJNS W, DEPRE C, ESSAMRI B, HEYNDRICKX GR, BORGERS M, BOL A, MELIN JA. Mechanisms of chronic regional postischemic dysfunction in humans. New insights from the study of noninfarcted collateral-dependent myocardium. *Circulation.* 1993;87:1513-23.

90. SIM DN, NEILL WA. Investigation of the physiological basis for increased exercise threshold for angina pectoris after physical conditioning. *Journal of Clinical Investigation.* 1974;54:763-70.

91. FERGUSON RJ, PETITCLERC R, CHOQUETTE G, CHANIOTIS L, GAUTHIER P, HUOT R, ALLARD C, JANKOWSKI L, CAMPEAU L. Effect of physical training on treadmill exercise capacity, collateral circulation and progression of coronary disease. *American Journal of Cardiology.* 1974; 34:764-9.

92. KENNEDY CC, SPIEKERMAN RE, LINDSAY MI, JR., MANKIN HT, FRYE RL, MCCALLISTER BD. One-year graduated exercise program for men with angina pectoris. Evaluation by physiologic studies and coronary arteriography. *Mayo Clinic Proceedings.* 1976;51:231-6.

93. NOLEWAJKA AJ, KOSTUK WJ, RECHNITZER PA, CUNNINGHAM DA. Exercise and human collateralization: an angiographic and scintigraphic assessment. *Circulation.* 1979;60:114-21.

94. FROELICHER V, JENSEN D, ATWOOD JE, MCKIRNAN MD, GERBER K, SLUTSKY R, BATTLER A, ASHBURN W, ROSS J, JR. Cardiac rehabilitation: evidence for improvement in myocardial perfusion and function. *Archives of Physical Medicine & Rehabilitation.* 1980;61:517-22.

95. BELARDINELLI R, GEORGIOU D, GINZTON L, CIANCI G, PURCARO A. Effects of moderate exercise training on thallium uptake and contractile response to low-dose dobutamine of dysfunctional myocardium in patients with ischemic cardiomyopathy. *Circulation.* 1998;97:553-61.

96. GOLDBERG HL, GOLDSTEIN J, BORER JS, MOSES JW, COLLINS MB. Functional importance of coronary collateral vessels. *Am J Cardiol.* 1984;53:694-9.

97. BONETTI F, MARGONATO A, MAILHAC A, CARANDENTE O, CAPPELLETTI A, BALLAROTTO C, CHIERCHIA SL. Coronary collaterals reduce the duration of exercise-induced ischemia by allowing a faster recovery. *Am Heart J.* 1992;124:48-55.

98. TSOUKAS A, IKONOMIDIS I, COKKINOS P, NIHOYANNOPOULOS P. Significance of persistent left ventricular dysfunction during recovery after dobutamine stress echocardiography. *J Am Coll Cardiol.* 1997;30:621-6.

99. WAINWRIGHT RJ, MAISEY MN, EDWARDS AC, SOWTON E. Functional significance of coronary collateral circulation during dynamic exercise evaluated by thallium-201 myocardial scintigraphy. *Br Heart J.* 1980;43:47-55.

100. ISKANDRIAN AS, HAKKI AH, SEGAL BL, KANE SA, AMENTA A. Assessment of the myocardial perfusion pattern in patients with multivessel coronary artery disease. *Am Heart J.* 1983; 106:1089-96.

101. DILSIZIAN V, CANNON RO, 3RD, TRACY CM, MCINTOSH CL, CLARK RE, BONOW RO. Enhanced regional left ventricular function after distant coronary bypass by means of improved collateral blood flow. *J Am Coll Cardiol.* 1989;14:312-8.

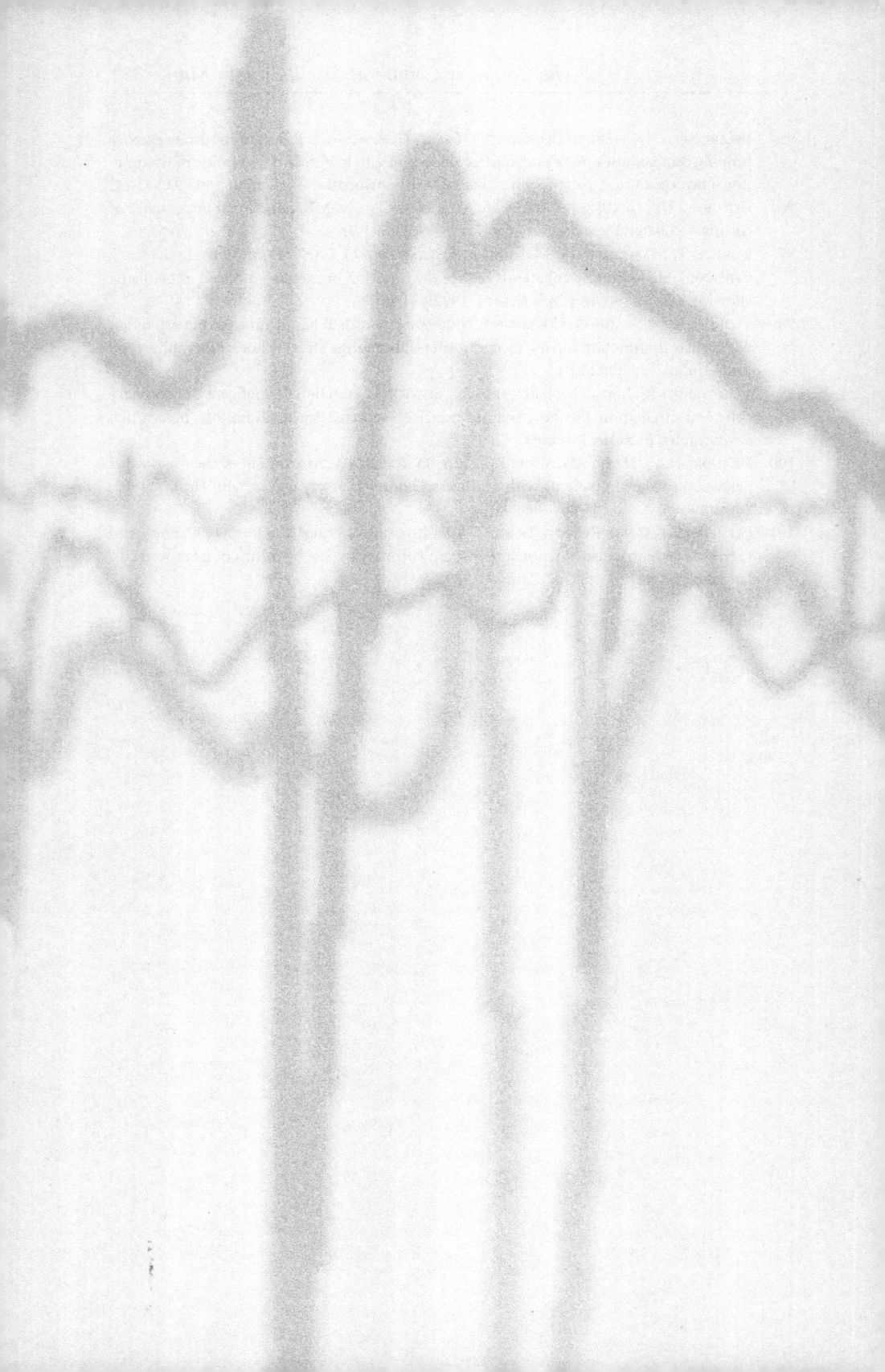

Chapter 17

Function of the Coronary Collateral Circulation in Man

Christian Seiler

Abstract

Well developed coronary collateral arteries in patients with coronary artery disease (CAD) mitigate myocardial infarcts with less ventricular aneurysm formation and improved ventricular function, they reduce future cardiovascular events, and improve survival. Myocardial infarct size is a product of coronary artery occlusion time, area at risk for infarction and the inverse of collateral supply. Collateral arteries preventing myocardial ischemia during brief vascular occlusion are present in 1/3 of patients with CAD. Collateral flow sufficient to prevent myocardial ischemia during coronary occlusion amounts to ≥25% of the normal flow through the open vessel. Among individuals without relevant coronary stenoses, there are preformed collateral arteries preventing myocardial ischemia in 20-25%.

Coronary collateral flow can be assessed only during vascular occlusion of the collateral-receiving artery. Presently, the gold standard for clinical coronary collateral assessment is the measurement of intracoronary occlusive pressure- or velocity-derived collateral flow index which expresses collateral function as a fraction of flow during vessel patency.

Clinical variables predicting the development of collateral arteries are the hemodynamic severity of coronary stenoses and the duration of myocardial ischemic symptoms.

One fifth to one third of patients with CAD cannot be revascularized by percutaneous coronary intervention or coronary artery bypass grafting; therapeutic promotion of collateral growth appears to be a valuable treatment strategy in those patients. Promotion of collateral growth should aim at inducing the development of large conductive collateral arteries (i.e. arteriogenesis) and not so much at the sprouting of capillary like vessels (i.e. angiogenesis). So far, the largest controlled clinical angiogenesis trials on the efficacy of VEGF and basic FGF have been negative with regard to treadmill exercise time and myocardial scintigraphic data. Large conductive collateral arteries (i.e. arteriogenesis) appear to be effectively promoted via the activation of monocytes/macrophages.

List of abbreviations

AR	area at risk for myocardial infarction
bFGF	basic fibroblast growth factor
CAD	coronary artery disease
CFI	collateral flow index (no unit)
CVP	central venous pressure (mmHg)
GM-CSF	granulocyte-macrophage colony-stimulating factor
IS	infarct size
P_{ao}	mean aortic pressure (mmHg)
P_{occl}	mean coronary occlusive or wedge pressure (mmHg)
VEGF	vascular endothelial growth factor
V_{occl}	intracoronary occlusive blood flow velocity (cm/s)
$V_{\varnothing\text{-}occl}$	intracoronary non-occlusive blood flow velocity (cm/s)

Introduction

Cardiovascular diseases, in particular coronary artery disease (CAD), are the leading cause of death in industrialized countries. Established options for revascularization include angioplasty and surgical bypass, both of which are not or only partly suitable in 1/5 to 1/3 of patients in whom the extent of coronary atherosclerosis is especially severe[1]. An alternative treatment strategy for revascularization is therefore warranted, both to control symptoms as well as to alter the course of advanced CAD. An ideal candidate to fill in this gap is therapeutic promotion of coronary collateral growth, i.e., the induction of natural bypasses. In order to reach this goal, a comprehensive understanding of the function of the coronary collateral circulation in man regarding its relevance, accurate assessment, pathogenetic and pathophysiological aspects as well as therapeutic promotion is mandatory.

Relevance of the coronary collateral circulation

The coronary collateral circulation has been recognized for a long time as an alternative source of blood supply to a myocardial area jeopardized by ischemia. More than 200 years ago, Heberden described a patient who had been nearly cured of his angina pectoris by sawing wood each day[2], a phenomenon called warm-up or first effort angina which was traditionally ascribed to coronary vasodilation with opening of collateral vessels to support the ischemic myocardium. Alternatively and more recently,

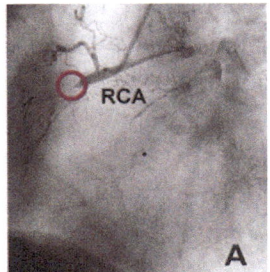
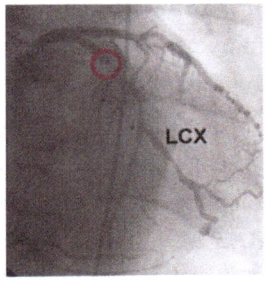
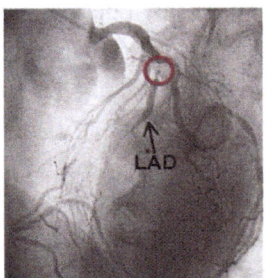

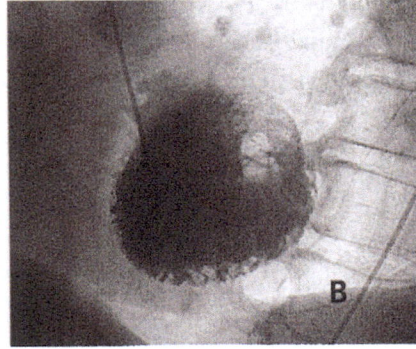
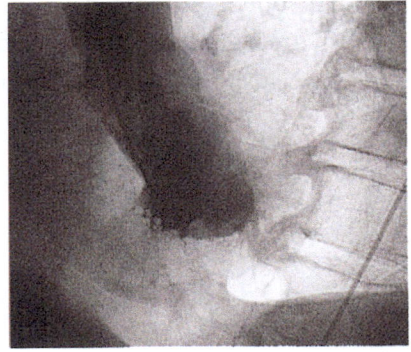

Fig. 1

Coronary angiogram in a patient with triple arterial occlusion (red circles; upper panels) and normal left ventricular angiogram (lower panels). Contrast injection into the right coronary artery (RCA; upper left panel) reveals proximal vascular occlusion with faint appearance of the RCA distal to the occlusion and of the left anterior descending coronary artery (LAD). Proximal occlusion of the left circumflex coronary artery (LCX; upper middle panel) is shown using an right anterior oblique caudal projection. The LCX distal of the blockage is entirely filled via collateral arteries from the LAD (angiographic collateral degree of 3). The LAD is entirely obstructed distal to its first diagonal branch (left anterior oblique cranial projection; right upper panel). There is also 3rd degree angiographic retrograde filling of the LAD. Furthermore, retrograde filling of the RCA can be seen during left coronary injection (at least 2nd degree angiographic collaterals). All of the three major coronary artery supply areas (imaged in left anterior oblique view at end-diastole and during systole, respectively; left and right lower panels, respectively) reveal normal systolic wall motion.

"walk-through angina" has been interpreted as a biochemical (i.e. ischemic preconditioning) rather than biophysical (i.e. collateral recruitment) event leading to the heightened tolerance against myocardial ischemia. Even more likely, both mechanisms contribute to the described phenomenon which is easily obtainable by careful history taking of the patient[3,4]. Aside from controversies just alluded to, there have been numerous investigations demonstrating a protective role of well versus poorly grown collateral arteries in man (Fig. 1) showing smaller infarcts[5], less ventricular aneurysm formation[6], improved ventricular function[5], fewer future cardiovascular events[7], and improved survival[8]. However, the functional relevance of coronary collateral vessels in humans had also been a matter of debate for many years[9]. Much of this controversy was likely due to inadequate means for gauging human coronary collaterals and to the investigation of populations too small to be representative for all the patients with CAD. The latter is well illustrated by the fact that among patients with hemodynamically significant atherosclerotic lesions, only about 1/3 have functionally sufficient coronary collaterals which are able to prevent signs of myocardial ischemia during brief vascular occlusions (Fig. 2;[10]). In the absence of stenoses, it has been tradi-

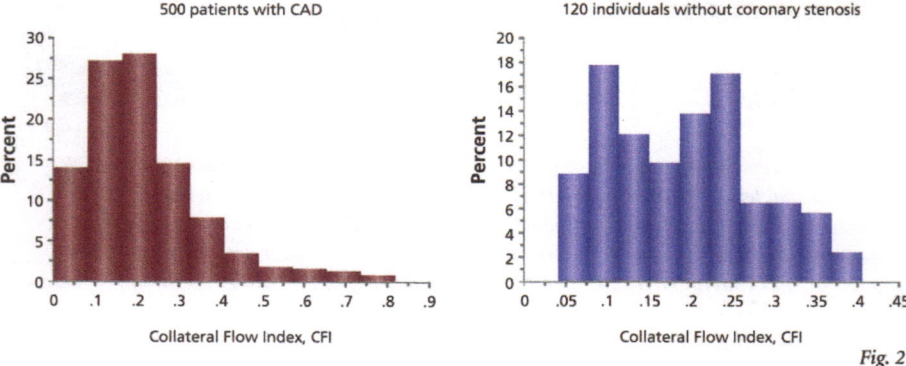

Fig. 2

Frequency distribution (in percent of the entire population, vertical axis) of collateral flow obtained during coronary artery balloon occlusion relative to normal flow during vessel patency (collateral flow index, horizontal axis). The left side shows the distribution in 500 patients with hemodynamically relevant coronary artery stenoses. On the right side, the distribution in 120 individuals without coronary stenoses is depicted.

tionally assumed that coronary arteries are functional end-arteries[11]. Using direct and quantitative intracoronary collateral measurements (see below), it has, however, been documented very recently that the notion of the human coronary circulation being built without preformed functioning anastomoses between vascular territories is a myth rather than reality; in the absence of obstructive CAD or even in entirely normal hearts, there has been collateral flow to a briefly occluded coronary artery sufficient to prevent ECG signs of myocardial ischemia in one fifth to one fourth of the population studied (Fig. 2;[12]).

Assessment

Natural coronary occlusion model (chronic total occlusion model)

In the situation of a spontaneously occurring coronary artery occlusion without myocardial infarction, a well developed collateral circulation must be the reason for the salvaged cardiac muscle (Fig. 1). A pathophysiological alternative to this scenario is indicated by the following equation describing infarct size (IS), and it consists of an exceedingly small ischemic myocardial area at risk (AR)[13]:

$$IS = \text{coronary occlusion time} \times AR \times \text{collateral supply}^{-1}$$

The entire filling of a chronically occluded, collateral-receiving (i.e. ipsilateral) coronary artery from a collateral-supplying (i.e. contralateral) vessel (Fig. 1) illustrates that AR is closely and inversely dependent on collateral flow, to the extent that the AR of a certain vessel may disappear in the presence of well grown collaterals. The validity of the concept described in equation 1 has been recently confirmed in the clinical setting by documenting that coronary occlusion time no longer plays a role as a predictor for IS in the presence of a collateral relative to normal flow (collateral flow index; see below) $\geq 25\%$[14]. Thus, to detect normal ventricular wall motion (Fig. 1) in the presence of a proximal or mid chronic occlusion represents a way of qualifying "good" collateral flow. The major disadvantage of this qualitative method for collateral assessment is that it requires coronary angiography to detect vascular occlusion. Having established the diagnosis of an entirely blocked coronary artery, various myocardial perfusion tracers (different radioactive tracers, echocontrast media) are in principle appropriate to measure the gold standard of collateral function (i.e. absolute perfusion in ml/min/g of tissue) non-invasively by positron emission tomography or Doppler echocardiography[15-18].

Artificial coronary occlusion model (angioplasty model)

At present, invasive cardiac examination is a prerequisite for reliable qualitative or quantitative assessment of coronary collaterals. In the natural occlusion model, it is necessary to confirm total vascular obstruction, in the artificial occlusion model, it is essential to briefly block the vessel using an angioplasty balloon catheter. In addition, systematically consistent and *exclusive* collateral characterization in man (Fig. 3) requires the permanent or temporary occlusion of the epicardial collateral-receiving artery yielding the so called recruitable as opposed to spontaneously visible collateral flow. Employing the angioplasty model, there are several qualitative and quantitative methods subsequently described which can be used to characterize the collateral circulation.

Angina pectoris and intracoronary ECG during vessel occlusion: The simplest but rather imprecise way to qualify collateral vessels is to ask the patient about the presence of angina pectoris shortly before the end of the one- to two-minute arterial balloon occlusion. The predictive value of absent or present chest pain for collaterals sufficient or insufficient, respectively, to prevent ischemia as detected by intracoronary ECG (Fig. 4)

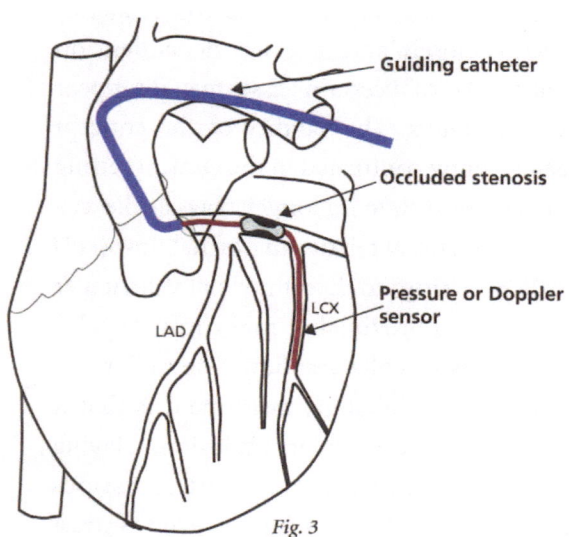

Guiding catheter

Occluded stenosis

Pressure or Doppler sensor

LCX

LAD

Fig. 3

Schematic drawing illustrating the principle of collateral assessment during coronary artery balloon occlusion using an angioplasty sensor guidewire (red line). This pressure or Doppler guidewire is positioned distal to the occluded site. Pressure signals (except for venous back pressure) or flow velocity signals detected during vascular occlusion originate from collateral vessels supplying the blocked vascular region.

is rather low[19,20]. The use of an intracoronary ECG lead obtained via the angioplasty guidewire for collateral assessment provides a good representation of the pertinent myocardial area. Intracoronary ECG ST-segment changes of >0.1mV constitute the definition of collaterals insufficient to prevent ischemia in the respective myocardial territory[19]. A current analysis of our data base including 564 patients with one or more coronary stenotic lesions undergoing invasive ECG- and sensor-derived

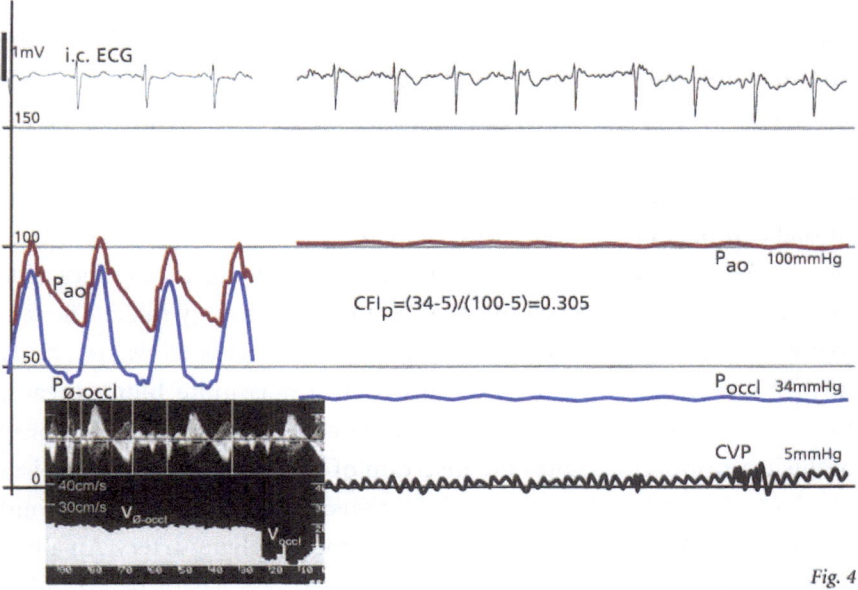

Fig. 4

Sufficient coronary collaterals. Simultaneous recordings of an intracoronary (i.c.) ECG lead (top), phasic (left side) and mean (right side) aortic (P_{ao}, mmHg), coronary occlusive (P_{occl}, mmHg) and central venous pressures (CVP, mmHg). Pao is gauged via a 6 French coronary artery guiding catheter, P_{occl} via a pressure guidewire positioned distal of a stenosis to be dilated and CVP via a right atrial catheter. To the right of the phasic pressure tracings obtained during coronary artery patency, mean pressures are recorded during and after angioplasty balloon deflation. During inflation, there are no relevant ECG ST-segment changes indicating collateral vessels sufficient to prevent myocardial ischemia. Collateral flow index (CFI) is calculated as follows: $CFI_p = (P_{occl}-CVP)/(P_{ao}-CVP)$.

The insert shows intracoronary Doppler flow velocity signals obtained simultaneously as the pressure recordings using a 0.014 inch, 20MHz Doppler angioplasty guidewire. Upper panel: Instantaneous occlusive flow velocity profile recorded over time (horizontal axis). Bi-directional velocity signals indicate collateral flow towards and away from the Doppler sensor which is located at the tip of the guidewire. Lower panel: Flow velocity trend obtained over 90s. Doppler-derived collateral flow index roughly corresponds to the ratio of flow velocity during occlusion (V_{occl}, cm/s) divided by flow velocity at the same site during vessel patency ($V_{\emptyset-occl}$, cm/s).

collateral assessment during balloon occlusion provides the following results: Individuals with ECG signs of ischemia in the collateralized region had a sensor-derived flow to this area amounting to $16.7\pm8.8\%$ of normal antegrade flow through the patent vessel, those without ischemia showed a corresponding value of $35.5\pm17.8\%$ ($p<0.0001$). The best cut-off to distinguish between present and absent ischemia was equal to a collateral relative to normal flow of 25%.

Angiographic methods: The coronary angiographic method for collateral qualification most widely used is similar but not identical to the one first described by Rentrop and coworkers[21]. The latter provides a score from 0-3 for recruitable collateral vessels upon occlusion of the ipsilateral artery, the former an identical score for spontaneously visible collaterals without artificial vascular occlusion. The score describes epicardial coronary artery filling with radiographic contrast dye via collaterals as follows: 0=no filling, 1=small side branches filled, 2=major side branches of the main vessel filled, 3=main vessel entirely filled. The fact that in clinical routine, only spontaneously visible collaterals are scored further impairs the method's sensitivity, which is quite blunt already. Recruitable collateral vessel grading in the absence of chronic coronary occlusion, however, requires the insertion of two coronary catheters, i.e., one for balloon occlusion of the collateral-receiving vessel and the second for injection of contrast dye into the collateral-supplying artery. An alternative, semi-quantitative angiographic method consists of determining the number of heart beats during coronary occlusion needed to wash out the angiographic medium injected into the ipsilateral artery immediately before balloon occlusion (i.e. washout collaterometry,[22]). The contrast dye caught distal to the occlusive balloon can only be washed out by collateral flow. A washout time of ≤11 heart beats accurately predicts collaterals sufficient to prevent ischemia during a brief coronary occlusion.

Intracoronary pressure or Doppler sensor measurements: Today, pressure- or Doppler-sensor-tipped angioplasty guidewires are available which are almost equivalent to regular guidewires in their handling properties. The theoretical basis for the use of intracoronary pressure or blood flow velocity measurements to determine collateral flow relates to the fact that perfusion pressure (> central venous "back" pressure) or flow velocity signals obtained distal to an occluded stenosis originate from collateral vessels (Fig. 3). The measurement of aortic and intracoronary pressure or velocity provides the basic variables for the calculation of a pressure-derived or velocity-derived collateral flow index (CFI) [19], both of which express the amount of flow via collaterals to the vascular region of interest as a fraction of the flow via the normally patent vessel. Pressure-derived CFI is determined by simultaneous measurement of mean aortic (P_{ao}), mean distal coronary occlusive (P_{occl}) and central venous pressure (CVP) (Figs. 4 and 5):

$$CFI = (P_{occl} - CVP)/(P_{ao} - CVP)$$

Velocity-derived CFI is measured by obtaining distal occlusive coronary flow velocity (V_{occl}) and coronary flow velocity during vessel patency ($V_{\emptyset occl}$) taken at the same location and following occlusion-induced reactive hyperemia: $CFI = V_{occl}/V_{\emptyset occl}$ (Fig. 4). CFI measurements have been documented to be very accurate with regard to ECG-derived dichotomous collateral assessment, with regard to each other, but also with regard to quantitative ^{99m}Tc-sestamibi imaging during balloon occlusion [19,20,23]. Pressure- and Doppler-derived intracoronary collateral measurements are regarded as the reference method for clinical assessment of coronary collateral flow. Preliminary data from our laboratory have shown that real-time myocardial contrast echocardiography can be reliably employed to measure absolute myocardial perfusion in ml/min/g [17]. This for the first time provides the opportunity to directly obtain coronary collateral perfusion not only in patients with chronic coronary occlusions but in all individuals undergoing a brief coronary balloon occlusion. Among 24 patients undergoing simultaneous invasive pressure-derived CFI measurement and quantitative contrast echocardiography of the collateralized myocardial territory, absolute collateral perfusion ranged from 0.06 ml/min/g to 0.88 ml/min/g corresponding to a collateral perfusion index (CPI, no unit; i.e. absolute perfusion in the myocardial region of interest during to that at identical location after coronary angioplasty and after cessation of reactive hyperemia) between 0.045 and 0.671. The agreement between pressure-derived CFI and contrast-echoderived CPI was good: CPI = 1.05CFI + 0.01, $r^2 = 0.96$, $p < 0.0001$ [18].

Pathogenesis

Clinical or "environmental" factors consistently described to influence the development of coronary collaterals in humans are the severity of coronary artery stenoses [10,21,24], and the duration of myocardial ischemic symptoms [24]. Conversely, there has been discordant information about the influence of metabolic disorders on collateral development such as diabetes mellitus [25-27]. In our experience encompassing 437 non-diabetic and 89 diabetic patients who underwent intracoronary collateral flow measurements, collateral flow index (see above) is practically identical: 0.215±0.146 and 0.209±0.128, respectively (p=0.71). A possible relevance of the cholesterol metabolism on the expansion of the collateral circulation has been indicated only experimentally [28]. The presence of systemic hypertension has also been suggested to promote well grown collaterals. Previous studies on the pathogenesis of collateral vessels in humans have often lacked sufficient patient numbers and/or quantitative means for collateral assessment. Although coronary stenosis severity is the independent predictor for collateral development in humans, CFI may vary for a given stenosis of, e.g., 95% diameter narrowing between 0.0 and 0.70 [10]. Conversely, in the absence of a coronary artery stenotic lesion CFI ranges between 0.05 and 0.4 [12]. Therefore, aside from "environmental" factors just described the influence of a certain genetic background or the temporarily varying up- / down-regulation of genes on the formation of well conductive collateral arteries even before the start of CAD must be very relevant but, so far, only rarely investigated [29].

Functional aspects

Functional, hemodynamic or biophysical aspects of well grown collateral arteries relate to the fact that they constitute a network within the coronary circulation (Fig. 6). Such connections between adjacent vascular territories together with spatially varying vascular resistances to blood flow [30] are the basis for pathophysiological aspects of collaterals rarely considered, such as the redistribution of blood during vasodilation away from a region in need (i.e. coronary steal, Fig. 6; [31,32]), the decrease in collateral flow to a certain vascular region following recanalization of a chronically occluded coronary artery [33,34], and the enhanced risk of coronary restenosis following percutaneous coronary intervention in the presence of high and competitive collateral flow to this area[35]. The latter situation is similar to that of competitive flow between a barely stenotic coronary artery and a bypass graft to this vessel which was unnecessarily implanted; usually, the lifespan of such a bypass is very much abridged.

Regarding the vasomotor response of collateral arteries, experimental studies have illustrated that physical exercise induces a more than two fold perfusion increase in collateral dependent myocardium via beta adrenergic and nitric oxide mechanisms[36]. For comparison, the capacity to increase flow during hyperemia in the normal human coronary circulation amounts to a factor of 3 to 4 (i.e. coronary flow reserve). In 50 patients with chronic CAD undergoing coronary angioplasty and CFI measurements, dynamic handgrip exercise during 3 minutes induced an increase in CFI by a factor of 1.8 among those without β-blocker treatment (Fig. 7)[37]; there was no exercise-induced CFI change in patients under β-blockers.

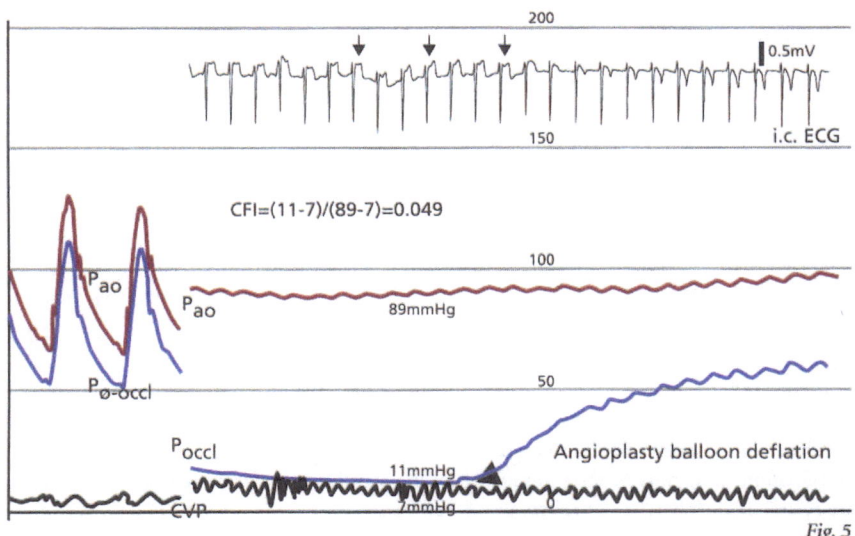

Fig. 5

Insufficient coronary collaterals. Simultaneous recordings of an intracoronary (i.c.) ECG lead (top), phasic (left side) and mean (right side) aortic (P_{ao}, mmHg), coronary occlusive (P_{occl}, mmHg) and central venous pressures (CVP, mmHg). Pao is gauged via a 6 French coronary artery guiding catheter, P_{occl} via a pressure guidewire positioned distal of a stenosis to be dilated and CVP via a right atrial catheter. To the right of the phasic pressure tracings obtained during coronary artery patency, mean pressures are recorded during and after angioplasty balloon deflation. During inflation, there are marked ECG ST-segment elevations (arrows) indicating collateral vessels insufficient to prevent myocardial ischemia. Collateral flow index (CFI) is calculated as follows: CFI=(P_{occl}-CVP)/(P_{ao}-CVP). Abbreviations see Fig. 4.

In up to 50% of patients with chronic total coronary artery occlusions, there may be no infarcted myocardium within the vascular territory supplied by the blocked vessel. It is unknown how many such patients
remain completely asymptomatic, and therefore, must even have a normal collateral coronary flow reserve, i.e., the capacity to augment flow in
response to increased myocardial demand. However, some of the patients
with chronic total occlusions without myocardial infarction suffer from
chest pain on exertion, and they have been found, using positron emission tomography, to exert a reduced collateral dependent flow reserve in
response to dipyridamole[38]; interestingly, the same patients also revealed
impaired systolic function in the collateral supplied left ventricular
region as opposed to individuals with maintained collateral coronary
flow reserve featuring normal regional wall motion.

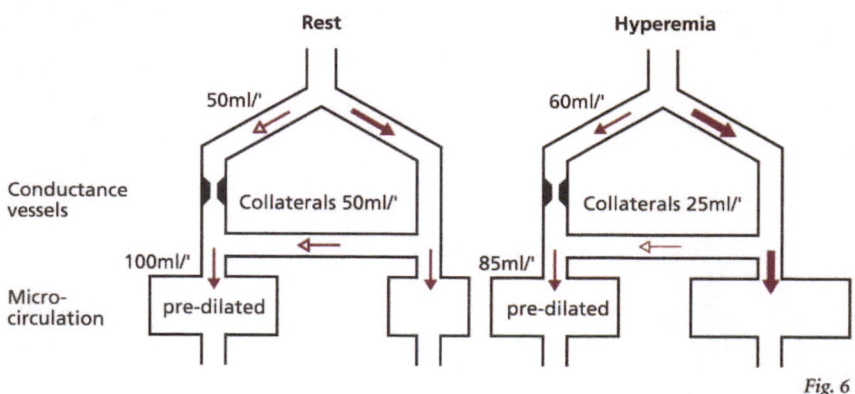

Fig. 6

*Coronary collateral steal. Schematic drawing illustrating the coronary circulation at rest
and during hyperemia as a network of two major epicardial and microcirculatory regions
which are interconnected by a collateral vessel. The thickness of the red arrows indicates the
blood volume flow rate. In the situation of coronary collateral steal, the changing balance of
the microcirculatory vascular resistances at rest versus hyperemia (specified by the size of
the rectangles) leads to an enhanced hyperemic perfusion in the collateral-supplying territory at the expense of a diminished blood flow rate in the vascular area downstream of the
stenotic, collateral-receiving artery. ml/'= ml/min*

Therapeutic promotion

In 1/5 to 1/3 of patients with CAD in whom the extent of coronary atherosclerosis is too severe to allow conventional revascularization, an alternative treatment strategy is needed. Therapeutic angiogenesis/arterio-
genesis are new strategies for revascularizing ischemic myocardial tissue

by formation of "natural bypasses", i.e., collateral vessels. Understanding the many steps and regulatory mechanisms of angio- and arteriogenesis as opposed to vasculogenesis is important for designing such strategies.

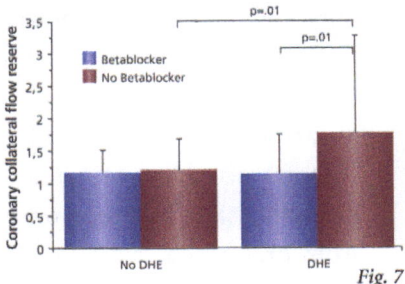

Vasculogenesis: The initial steps for the formation of the vascular system during embryonic life involve the differentiation of mesodermal cells into angioblasts that give rise to endothelial cells forming the first primitive blood vessels[39].

Angiogenesis: New vessels can subsequently develop from the preexisting plexus by sprouting and intussusception. This formation of new vessels from preexisting ones has been called angiogenesis[40]. In addition to endothelial cells, pericytes (for capillaries) and smooth muscle cells (for larger vessels) are necessary for the

Fig. 7

Exercise induced coronary collateral flow reserve. Coronary collateral flow reserve values (vertical axis) obtained during vessel occlusions without and with dynamic handgrip exercise (DHE) in patients with and without betablocker treatment (horizontal axis). Coronary collateral flow reserve without DHE was calculated as collateral flow index (CFI) at the end of 1st or 2nd 1-minute coronary occlusions without DHE divided by CFI at the start of the respective occlusions; coronary collateral flow reserve with DHE was computed as CFI at the start of 1st or 2nd 1-minute coronary occlusions with DHE divided by CFI at the start of occlusions without DHE.

maturation of these newly growing vessels[40]. Angiogenesis and arteriogenesis are not restricted to the growing organism. Tissue repair and regeneration are manifestations of angiogenesis. New capillaries form around zones of tissue ischemia, as it occurs in myocardial infarction and stroke. However, vessel formation and growth is also a part of pathogenic processes like proliferative retinopathies, psoriasis, hemangiomas, tumors and atherosclerotic plaques[41]. Upon angiogenic stimulation, e.g. after tissue injury or ischemia, with hypoxia or hypoglycemia, growth factors and inflammatory mediators are released locally leading to vasodilation, enhanced vascular permeability and accumulation of monocytes and macrophages which in turn secrete more growth factors and inflammatory mediators[42]. These inflammatory cells release metalloproteinases that dissolve the surrounding matrix and the basal membrane of the preformed vessel. Hypoxia sensitizes the local endothelial cells to the chemotactic and proliferative effects of various growth factors by upregulating their receptors. Endothelial cells detach from their neighbors, migrate, proliferate and subsequently form a new vessel with a lumen. Pericytes and smooth muscle cells are also involved in this process.

Arteriogenesis: Invasive cardiologists have long been aware of the occurrence of large and often epicardial collateral vessels after total or subtotal occlusion of a major coronary artery (Fig. 1). These usually become visible within two weeks following an occlusion, and they arise from preformed arterioles. The remodeling process involved in this re-cruitment of already existing collateral vessels has been termed arterio-genesis[43]. Large bridging collaterals are likely much more effective in sal-vaging ischemic myocardium at risk for necrosis than small peri-ischemia capillaries. The complete obstruction of a coronary artery leads to a fall in poststenotic pressure and to a redistribution of blood to pre-existing arterioles. The resulting stretch and shear forces may lead to an increased expression of certain endothelial chemokines, adhesion mole-cules and growth factors. Within days, circulating monocytes attach to the endothelium of the bridging collateral vessels causing a local inflam-matory reaction[42]. Matrix dissolution occurs and the vessels undergo a growth process with active proliferation of their endothelial and smooth muscle cells.

Growth factor candidates: A variety of physiological molecules have been identified that appear to promote angio- and arteriogenesis. Most of them act by stimulating migration and proliferation of endothelial cells and/or smooth muscle cells, like the family of FGFs and VEGFs. Both cause vasodilation by stimulating the release of nitric oxide. It is therefore important in animal as well as clinical studies to differentiate between improved perfusion due to mere vasodilation and true collateral growth. Other growth factor candidates include placental growth factor, angio-poietin 1, transforming growth factor β, platelet derived growth factor, and about half a dozen other cytokines, proteases and proteins[41]. Arteri-ogenesis has been shown to be induced by activated macrophages[44], by lipopolysaccharide[42], monocyte chemotactic protein-1[43], tumor necrosis factor-alpha, FGF, and also via granulocyte-macrophage colony-stimu-lating factor (recombinant human GM-CSF; Molgramostim®)[39,45].

Clinical studies: Angiogenesis may be induced by surgical or catheter-based delivery of various promotors, such as VEGF and FGF, angiogenic agents most often used in current clinical studies[46,47]. Although animal studies have established the principle that collateral function improves after delivering angiogenic growth factors[48], and although first uncontrolled clinical studies have demonstrated safety and feasibility of VEGF and basic FGF[49], efficacy data of angiogenic therapy have been scarce and controversial. The most recent and largest controlled clinical trials using VEGF165 (VIVA, VEGF in Ischemia for Vascular Angiogenesis[50]) and FGF2 (FIRST, FGF Initiating Revascularization Trial[51]) in 178 and in 337 patients with CAD, respectively, have not shown an effect on the study endpoints, i.e., treadmill exercise time, angina pectoris at 60 and 120 days (VIVA), and respectively, exercise tolerance test duration at 90-day-follow-up and changes in the magnitude of myocardial ischemia by Tc99m SPECT. Controversy on the ability of angiogenic growth factors to promote coronary collaterals is likely due to the use of endpoints for their assessment which are too blunt to discern subtle changes in collateral flow. At this early phase of clinical angio-/arteriogenic therapy during which screening for the most effective growth factor among more than a dozen candidates has not even started properly, selection of the best agents ought to be based on accurate and direct invasive measurements of coronary collateral flow (Figs. 3 and 4), i.e., the variable hypothesized to be positively influenced by the growth factors. Equally important, angiogenic factors may have been employed, which induce the formation of small, high resistance capillaries (angiogenesis) rather than large interconnecting arterioles (arteriogenesis), which are required for the salvage of myocardium in the presence of occlusive CAD. In a first randomised placebo-controlled clinical trial, granulocyte-macrophage colony-stimulating factor (GM-CSF) has been shown to be effective with regard to sequentially and invasively obtained collateral flow among 21 patients with CAD[52].

There has been evidence presented in previous studies that adaptive regulation of wall shear stress to flow changes is operative through remodeling of the vessel; its purpose is to maintain wall shear stress at a constant level[53,54]. Arteriogenesis is related to enhanced flow-related shear forces at the vessel wall of preexisting collaterals along a pressure gradient between a normally and abnormally perfused (i.e. stenotic) vascular territory[55]. Correspondingly, physical exercise would be an ideal therapeutic option for inducing arteriogenesis, because cardiac output and thus coronary flow is elevated along the arterial branches of the coronary circulation during exercise. In the absence of CAD, the effect of physical endurance exercise among healthy volunteers appears to correspond well with the mentioned investigations, since an augmented caliber with increased functional capacity of the coronary (non-collateral) circulation can be observed[56]. So far, the only prospective investigation in humans on the effect of exercise regarding collateral growth has employed an insensitive instrument for collateral assessment, i.e., angiographic imaging of spontaneously visible collateral vessels, and has been negative[57]. Preliminary data from our own laboratory suggest that even in the absence of CAD collateral flow as assessed by intracoronary pressure-derived measurements is augmented substantially in response to endurance exercise training[58].

References

1. JONES EL, CRAVER JM, GUYTON RA, BONE DK, HATCHER CRJ, RIECHWALD N. Importance of complete revascularization in performance of the coronary bypass operation. *Am J Cardiol.* 1983;51:7-12.
2. HEBERDEN W. A letter to DR. HEBERDEN, concerning the angina pectoris; and an account of the dissection of one who had been troubled with that disorder. Read at the college November 17, 1772. *Medical Transactions Published by the College of Physicians in London.* 1785;3:1-11.
3. BILLINGER M, FLEISCH M, EBERLI FR, GARACHEMANI AR, MEIER B, SEILER C. Is the development of myocardial tolerance to repeated ischemia in humans due to preconditioning or to collateral recruitment? *J Am Coll Cardiol.* 1999;33:1027-1035.
4. LAMBIASE PD, EDWARDS RJ, CUSACK MR, BUCKNALL CA, REDWOOD SR, MARBER MS. Exercise-induced ischemia initiates the second window of protection in humans independent of collateral recruitment. *J Am Coll Cardiol.* 2003;41:1174-1182.
5. HABIB GB, HEIBIG J, FORMAN SA, BROWN BG, ROBERTS R, TERRIN ML, BOLLI R. Influence of coronary collateral vessels on myocardial infarct size in humans. Results of phase I thrombolysis in myocardial infarction (TIMI) trial. The TIMI Investigators. *Circulation.* 1991;83:739-746.
6. HIRAI T, FUJITA M, NAKAJIMA H, ASANOI H, YAMANISHI K, OHNO A, SASAYAMA S. Importance of collateral circulation for prevention of left ventricular aneurysm formation in acute myocardial infarction. *Circulation.* 1989;79:791-796.
7. BILLINGER M, KLOOS P, EBERLI F, WINDECKER S, MEIER B, SEILER C. Physiologically assessed coronary collateral flow and adverse cardiac ischemic events: a follow-up study in 403 patients with coronary artery disease. *J Am Coll Cardiol.* 2002;40:1545-1550.
8. HANSEN JF. Coronary collateral circulation: clinical significance and influence on survival in patients with coronary artery occlusion. *Am Heart J.* 1989;117:290-295.

9. HELFANT RH, VOKONAS PS, GORLIN R. Functional importance of the human coronary collateral circulation. *N Engl J Med.* 1971;284:1277-1281.

10. POHL T, SEILER C, BILLINGER M, HERREN E, WUSTMANN K, MEHTA H, WINDECKER S, EBEERLI FR, MEIER B. Frequency distribution of collateral flow and factors influencing collateral channel development. Functional collateral channel measurement in 450 patients with coronary artery disease. *J Am Coll Cardiol.* 2001;38:1872-1878.

11. PITT B. Interarterial coronary anastomoses. Occurence in normal hearts and in certain pathologic conditions. *Circulation.* 1959;20:816-822.

12. WUSTMANN K, ZBINDEN S, WINDECKER S, MEIER B, SEILER C. Is there functional collateral flow during vascular occlusion in angiographically normal coronary arteries? *Circulation.* 2003;108:in press.

13. REIMER KA, IDEKER RE, JENNINGS RB. Effect of coronary occlusion site on ischemic bed size and collateral blood flow in dogs. *Cardiovasc Res.* 1981;15:668-674.

14. LEE CW, PARK SW, CHO GY, HONG MK, KIM JJ, KANG DH, SONG JK, LEE HJ, PARK SJ. Pressure-derived fractional collateral blood flow: a primary determinant of left ventricular recovery after reperfused acute myocardial infarction. *J Am Coll Cardiol.* 2000;35:949-955.

15. DEMER LL, GOULD KL, GOLDSTEIN RA, KIRKEEIDE RL. Noninvasive assessment of coronary collaterals in man by PET perfusion imaging. *J Nucl Med.* 1990;31:259-270.

16. DE MARCHI S, SCHWERZMANN M, FLEISCH M, BILLINGER M, MEIER B, SEILER C. Quantitative contrast echocardiographic assessment of collateral derived myocardial perfusion during elective coronary angioplasty. *Heart.* 2001;86:324-329.

17. VOGEL R, NAMDAR M, KAUFMANN P, SEILER C. Absolute quantification of myocardial perfusion using real-time myocardial contrast echocardiography: an *in vitro* study and first *in vivo* results. *Eur Heart J.* 2003;24 (suppl):102 (abstract).

18. VOGEL R, ZBINDEN R, SCHWERZMANN M, WINDECKER S, MEIER B, SEILER C. Quantitative assessment of collateral derived myocardial perfusion using real-time myocardial contrast echocardiography during elective coronary angioplasty. *Eur Heart J.* 2003;24 (suppl):135 (abstract).

19. SEILER C, FLEISCH M, GARACHEMANI A, MEIER B. Coronary collateral quantitation in patients with coronary artery disease using intravascular flow velocity or pressure measurements. *J Am Coll Cardiol.* 1998;32:1272-9.

20. VAN LIEBERGEN RA, PIEK JJ, KOCH KT, DE WINTER RJ, SCHOTBORGH CE, LIE KI. Quantification of collateral flow in humans: a comparison of angiographic, electrocardiographic and hemodynamic variables. *J Am Coll Cardiol.* 1999;33:670-7.

21. RENTROP KP, COHEN M, BLANKE H, PHILLIPS RA. Changes in collateral channel filling immediately after controlled coronary artery occlusion by an angioplasty balloon in human subjects. *J Am Coll Cardiol.* 1985;5:587-92.

22. SEILER C, BILLINGER M, FLEISCH M, MEIER B. Washout collaterometry: a new method of assessing collaterals using angiographic contrast clearance during coronary occlusion. *Heart.* 2001;86:540-546.

23. MATSUO H, WATANABE S, KADOSAKI T, YAMAKI T, TANAKA S, MIYATA S, SEGAWA T, MATSUNO Y, TOMITA M, FUJIWARA H. Validation of collateral fractional flow reserve by myocardial perfusion imaging. *Circulation.* 2002;105:1060-1065.

24. PIEK JJ, KOOLEN JJ, HOEDEMAKER G, DAVID GK, VISSER CA, DUNNING AJ. Severity of single-vessel coronary arterial stenosis and duration of angina as determinants of recruitable collateral vessels during balloon occlusion. *Am J Cardiol.* 1991;67:13-17.

25. MELIDONIS A, TOURNIS S, KOUVARAS G, BALTARETSOU E, HADANIS S, HAJISSAVAS I, TSATSOULIS A, FOUSSAS S. Comparison of coronary collateral circulation in diabetic and nondiabetic patients suffering from coronary artery disease. *Clin Cardiol.* 1999;22:465-71.

26. ABACI A, OGUZHAN A, KAHRAMAN S, ERYOL NK, UENAL S, ARINC H, ERGIN A. Effect of diabetes mellitus on formation of coronary collateral vessels. *Circulation.* 1999;99:2239-2242.

27. WALTENBERGER J, LANGE J, KRANZ A. Vascular endothelial growth factor-A-induced chemotaxis of monocytes is attenuated in patients with diabetes mellitus: A potential predictor for the individual capacity to develop collaterals. *Circulation.* 2000;102:185-90.

28. VAN BELLE E, RIVARD A, CHEN D, SILVER M, BUNTING S, FERRARA N, SYMES JF, BAUTERS C, ISNER JM. Hypercholesterolemia attenuates angiogenesis but does not preclude augmentation by angiogenic cytokines. *Circulation.* 1997;96:2667-74.

29. BOENGLER K, PIPP F, BROICH K, FERNÁNDEZ B, SCHAPER W, DEINDL E. Identification of differentially expressed genes like cofilin2 in growing collateral arteries. *Biochem Biophys Res Commun.* 2003;17:751-756.

30. PIEK JJ, VAN LIEBERGEN AM, KOCH KT, DE WINTER RJ, PETERS RJG, DAVID GK. Pharmacological modulation of the human collateral vascular resistance in acute and chronic coronary occlusion assessed by intracoronary blood flow velocity analysis in an angioplasty model. *Circulation.* 1997;96:106-115.

31. SEILER C, FLEISCH M, MEIER B. Direct intracoronary evidence of collateral steal in humans. *Circulation.* 1997;96:4261-7.

32. BILLINGER M, FLEISCH M, EBERLI FR, MEIER B, SEILER C. Collateral and collateral-adjacent hyperemic vascular resistance changes and the ipsilateral coronary flow reserve. Documentation of a mechanism causing coronary steal in patients with coronary artery disease. *Cardiovasc Res.* 2001;16:600-608.

33. WERNER G, RICHARTZ B, GASTMANN O, AL E. Immediate changes of collateral function after successful recanalization of chronic total coronary occlusions. *Circulation.* 2000;102:2959-2965.

34. POHL T, HOCHSTRASSER P, BILLINGER M, FLEISCH M, MEIER B, SEILER C. Influence on collateral flow of recanalising chronic total coronary occlusions: a case-control study. *Heart.* 2001;86:438-443.

35. WAHL A, BILLINGER M, FLEISCH M, MEIER B, SEILER C. Quantitatively assessed coronary collateral circulation and restenosis following percutaneous revascularization. *Eur Heart J.* 2000;21:1776-1784.

36. KLASSEN CL, TRAVERSE JH, BACHE RJ. Nitroglycerin dilates coronary collateral vessels during exercise after blockade of endogenous NO production. *Am J Physiol.* 1999;277:H918-23.

37. POHL T, WUSTMANN K, ZBINDEN S, WINDECKER S, MEHTA H, MEIER B, SEILER C. Exercise-induced human coronary collateral function: quantitative assessment during acute coronary occlusions. *Cardiology.* 2003;99:in press.

38. VANOVERSCHELDE JLJ, WIJNS W, DEPRÉ C, ESSAMRI B, HEYNDRCKX GR, BORGERS M, BOL A, MELIN JA. Mechansims of chronic regional postischemic dysfunction in humans. New insights from the study of non-infarcted collateral-dependent myocardium. *Circulation.* 1993;87:1513-1523.

39. CARMELIET P. Mechanisms of angiogenesis and arteriogenesis. Nature Med. 2000;6:389-395.

40. RISAU W. Mechanisms of angiogenesis. *Nature.* 1997;386:671-674.

41. FOLKMAN J. Angiogenesis in cancer, vascular, rheumatoid and other disease. *Nature Medicine.* 1995;1:27-31.

42. ARRAS M, WULF DI, SCHOLZ D, WINKLER B, SCHAPER J, SCHAPER W. Monocyte activation in angiogenesis and collateral growth in the rabbit hind limb. *J Clin Invest.* 1998:40-50.

43. ITO WD, ARRAS M, WINKLER B, SCHOLZ D, SCHAPER J, SCHAPER W. Monocyte chemotactic protein-1 increases collateral and peripheral conductance after femoral artery occlusion. *Circ Res.* 1997;80:829-837.

44. POLVERINI PJ, COTRAN RS, GIMBRONE MA, UNANUE ER. Activated macrophages induce vascular proliferation. *Nature.* 1977;269:804-806.

45. BUSCHMANN I, HOEFER I, VAN ROYEN N, KATZER E, BRAUN-DULLEAUS R, HEIL M, KOSTIN S, BODE C, SCHAPER W. GM-CSF: a strong arteriogenic factor acting by amplification of monocyte function. *Atherosclerosis.* 2001;159:343-356.

46. HENDEL RC, HENRY TD, ROCHA-SINGH K, ISNER JM, KEREIAKES DJ, GIORDANO F, SIMONS M, BONOW RO. Effect of intracoronary recombinant human vascular endothelial growth factor on myocardial perfusion. *Circulation.* 2000;101:118-121.

47. LAHAM RJ, CHRONOS NA, PIKE M, LEIMBACH ME, UDELSON JE, PEARLMAN JD, PETTIGREW RI, WHITEHOUSE MJ, YOSHIZAWA C, SIMONS M. Intracoronary basic fibroblast growth factor (FGF-2) in patients with severe ischemic heart disease: results of a phase I open-label dose escalation study. *J Am Coll Cardiol.* 2000;36:2132-2139.

48. SCHAPER W, ITO WD. Molecular Mechanisms of Coronary Collateral Vessel Growth. *Circ Res.* 1996;79:911-919.

49. HELISCH A, SCHAPER W. Angiogenesis and arteriogenesis - not yet for prescription. *Z Kardiol.* 2000;89:239-244.

50. HENRY TD, ANNEX BH, MCKENDALL GR, AZRIN MA, LOPEZ JJ, GIORDANO FJ, SHAH PK, WILLERSON JT, BENZA RL, BERMAN DS, GIBSON CM, BAJAMONDE A, CHEN RUNDLE A, FINE J, MCCLUSKEY ER, INVESTIGATORS FTV. The VIVA Trial. Vascular Endothelial Growth Factor in Ischemia for Vascular Angiogenesis. *Circulation.* 2003;107:1359-1365.

51. SIMONS M, ANNEX BH, LAHAM RJ, KLEIMAN N, HENRY T, DAUERMAN H, UDELSON JE, GERVINO EV, PIKE M, WHITEHOUSE MJ, MOON T, CHRONOS NA. Pharmacological treatment of coronary artery disease with recombinant fibroblast growth factor-2: double-blind, randomized, controlled clinical trial. *Circulation.* 2002;105:788-793.

52. SEILER C, POHL T, WUSTMANN K, HUTTER D, NICOLET PA, WINDECKER S, EBERLI FR, MEIER B. Promotion of collateral growth by granulocyte-macrophage colony-stimulating factor in patients with coronary artery disease: a randomized, double-blind, placebo-controlled study. *Circulation.* 2001;104:2012-7.

53. KAMIYA A, TOGAWA T. Adaptive regulation of wall shear stress to flow change in canine carotid artery. *Am J Physiol.* 1980;239:H14-H21.

54. SEILER C, KIRKEEIDE RL, GOULD KL. Basic structure-function relations of the epicardial coronary vascular tree. Basis of quantitative coronary arteriography for diffuse coronary artery disease. *Circulation.* 1992;85:1987-2003.

55. SCHAPER W, SCHOLZ D. Factors regulating arteriogenesis. *Arterioscler Thromb Vasc Biol.* 2003;23:1143-1151.

56. WINDECKER S, ALLEMANN Y, BILLINGER M, POHL T, HUTTER D, ORSUCCI T, BLAGA L, MEIER B, SEILER C. Effect of endurance training on coronary artery size and function in healthy men: an invasive followup study. *Am J Physiol Heart Circ Physiol.* 2002;282:H2216-H2223.

57. NIEBAUER J, HAMBRECHT R, MARBURGER C, HAUER K, VELICH T, VON HODENBERG E, SCHLIERF G, KUBLER W, SCHULER G. Impact of intensive physical exercise and low-fat diet on collateral vessel formation in stable angina pectoris and angiographically confirmed coronary artery disease. *Am J Cardiol.* 1995;76:771-775.

58. ZBINDEN R, ZBINDEN S, WINDECKER S, MEIER B, SEILER C. Direct demonstration of coronary collateral growth by physical endurance exercise in a healthy marathon runner. *Heart.* 2003:submitted.

Chapter 18

Collateral Circulation in Clinical Practice

Own clinical observations
Ralf Ritter

Natural collaterals, consisting of a network of vessels of varying caliber, can circumvent vessel stenosis or vascular occlusion. Depending on the efficiency of the collateral circulation, basal or even functional metabolism can be maintained in organs requiring an arterial blood supply.

In the human body two collateralization pathways may be distinguished. The first pathway utilises preexisting collateral circulation, such as the circulus arteriosus cerebri, the vertebra-vertebral circulation, Riolan's anastomosis or the pancreatic-duodenal vascular system[1,2,3,4]. The second pathway includes the terminal arterioles in the arterial bloodstream. Here, terminal arterioles undergo transformation into small arteries, which can then bridge a vascular occlusion in a vessel such as the superficial femoral artery.

The capacity of collateral vascularization to overcome vascular occlusion in the human is not the same for all vessels. The efficiency of collateralization is limited by the number and caliber of preexistent arterioles. Another decisive factor is the period of time preceding final vessel occlusion, which means differentiating between acute and chronic, progressive arterial stenosis. Acute occlusion often exceeds the ischemic tolerance of the dependent organ, causing irreparable damage, whereas chronic, gradual arterial occluding processes not only allow basal but also functional metabolism to be maintained. An example is acute versus chronic renal artery occlusion[5] (Fig. 1).

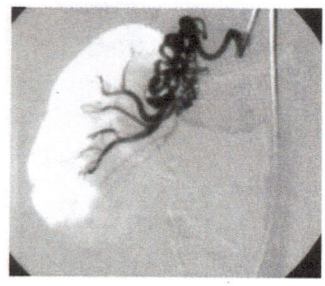

Fig. 1

Occlusion of the right renal artery with blood supply to the kidney via the medial suprarenal artery with flow reversal in the inferior suprarenal artery. Cathetertip in A. suprarenalis media.

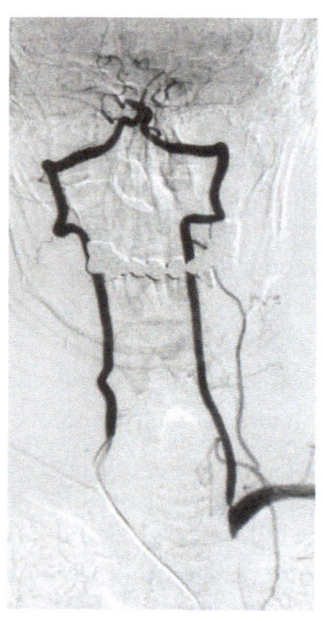

Fig. 2

Occlusion of the left subclavian artery. Flow reversal in the left vertebral artery and blood supply to the left arm via the posterior cerebral circulation. Cathetertip in A. vertebralis dextra.

Tissue served by endarteries cannot be collateralized, since these arteries have no preexisting connection to other arterioles. This is the case in the parenchymal organs: kidney, liver and spleen, and also the brain and the retina. Occlusion of small terminal arteries results in typical, wedge-shaped infarcted areas.

From a clinical point of view, collateral vascularization can be divided into three categories:

Category 1

An occlusion in a conduit vessel can be bypassed by retrograde flow in another conduit vessel, when both arteries are naturally joined. This leads to complete clinical compensation and the occluded transport artery remains asymptomatic. A typical clinical example is occlusion of the proximal subclavian artery[5], which results in retrograde flow in the ipsilateral vertebral artery (subclavian steal phenomenon) (Fig. 2). Another clinical example is occlusion of the celiac trunk, which in the case of a sufficiently extensive pancreatic-duodenal arcade also remains asymptomatic (Fig. 3) [3,6]. The same can be said for occlusion of the superior mesenteric artery, which can be compensated for by Riolan's anastomosis[3] (connection between the inferior and superior mesenteric arteries) (Fig. 4).

Category 2

An occluded conduit vessel can be bypassed by a naturally existing parallel arteriolar network, which previously took part in perfusing the area. During this compensating process, arterioles are transformed into small arteries, which connect

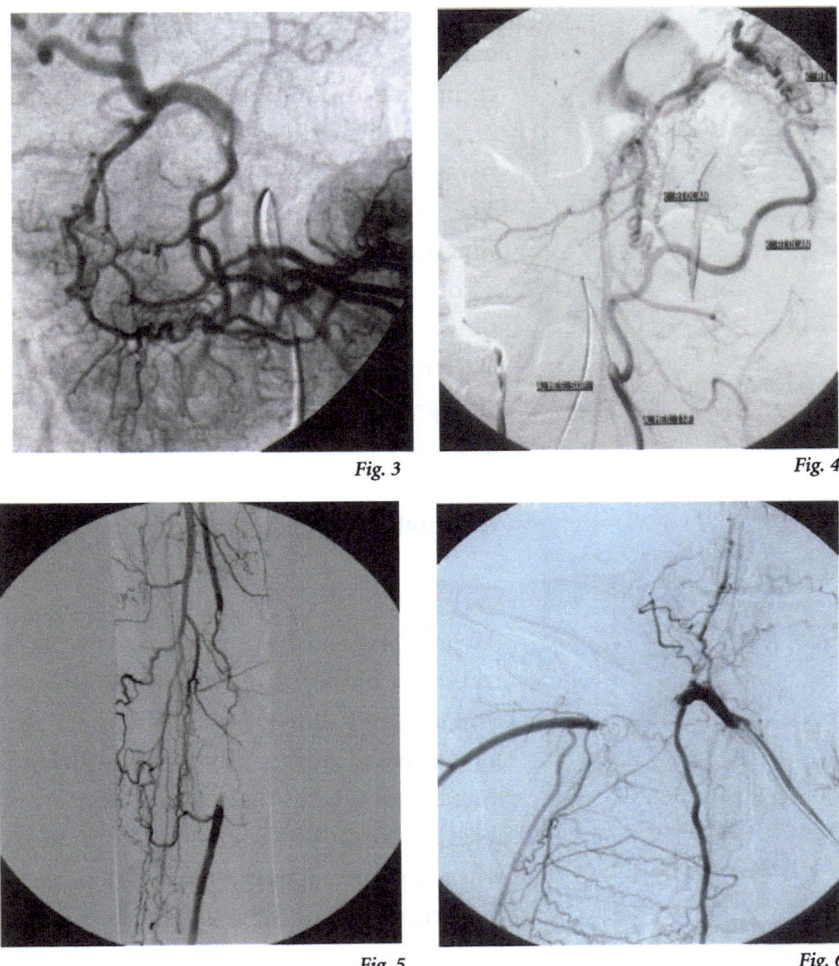

Fig. 3

Fig. 4

Fig. 5

Fig. 6

3) *Occlusion of the truncus coeliacus and blood supply to the liver, stomach, spleen via pancreatic-duodenal arcades supplied from a sidebranch of the upper mesenteric artery with flow reversal in the gastro-duodenal artery. Cathetertip in A. mesenterica superior.*

4) *Occlusion of the upper mesenteric artery and blood supply to the small intestine via the inferior mesenteric artery and Riolan's anastomosis. Cathetertip in the inferior mesenteric artery.*

5) *Occlusion of the superficial femoral artery with blood supply to the leg via collaterals originating from the deep femoral artery and connecting with the supragenuidal part of the popliteal artery, the intact reentry segment.*

6) *Occlusion of the right subclavian artery and blood supply to the right arm via the internal mammary artery and pectoral sidebranches connecting with the thoraco-acromialis artery and to the lateral thoracic artery. Cathertip in A. subclavia dextra.*

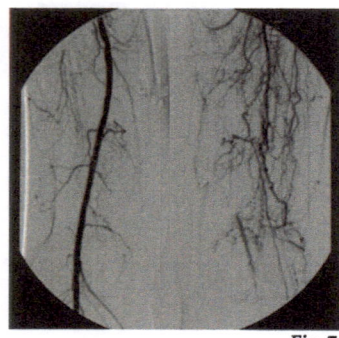

Fig. 7

Occlusion of the left superficial femoral artery together with a significant stenosis in the deep femoral artery at the reentry part in the upper popliteal artery.

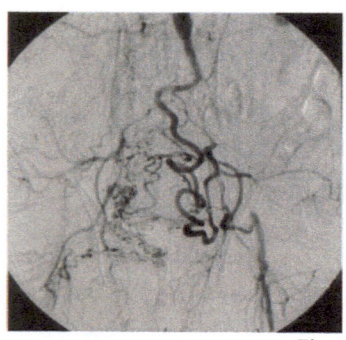

Fig. 8

Infrarenal occlusion of the aorta with blood supply to the legs via the inferior mesenteric artery connecting with the iliacal artery and finally to the common femoral artery (ileomesenteric collaterals) On the right side: collaterals also via ureteral collaterals. Cathetertip in the aorta.

distally to the occluded artery. This type of collateral circulation does not lead to complete compensation and, depending on the degree of physical exertion, there will be discomfort rising from the inadequately perfused area[7]. The classic clinical example is occlusion of the superficial femoral artery with development of a collateral profunda artery circulation[8]. Residual functional limitation in the form of intermittent claudication (Fig. 5) persists. Similarly, brachial claudication can manifest itself, especially when occlusion of the subclavian artery incorporates the entrance to the vertebral artery (Fig. 6).

Category 3

After occlusion of a conduit artery collateralization is hindered or the anatomic localization does not allow collateralization as characterized in categories 1 and 2. Insufficient collateralization takes place by connection of arterioles from different perfusion areas or where the preexisting arteriolar density is not high enough to allow adequate compensation. Such collateralization provides for basal metabolism in the perfusion area but leads to substantial functional impairment[9]. The clinical picture stems from stenosis or occlusion in the feeder artery of the dependent collateral network or in the re-entry segments of the receiving artery. Examples are stenosis in the supragenicular popliteal artery, which serves as the receiving segment of the profunda collateral circulation (Fig. 7), the collateralization of the pelvic blood stream through the inferior mesenteric artery (Fig. 8) or the rete articulare genus to bypass an occlusion of the popliteal artery (Fig. 9).

The severity of peripheral arterial occlusive disease (PAOD) is primarily determined by the quality of collateral vascularization. Making full use of the natural potential for collateralization, i.e., by encouraging exercise, which will increase flow and shear stress, is the mainstay of conservative therapy.

Knowledge of the natural collateral pathways is important for two reasons:

1. Angiographic data show that these pathways are rather uniform and practically always employed (depending on lesion location). No unusual patterns are described which makes the assumption redundant of a "neo-arteriogenesis" starting with sprouting capillaries that recruit smooth muscle and thereby create a completely new artery in places where no arteriolar network had previously existed.

2. Lesion site and collateral pathways determine the outcome of non-surgical therapy. Vessels bridging the groin and the knee may be difficult to stimulate because of their scarceness. This should be considered when recruiting patients for growth factor trials.

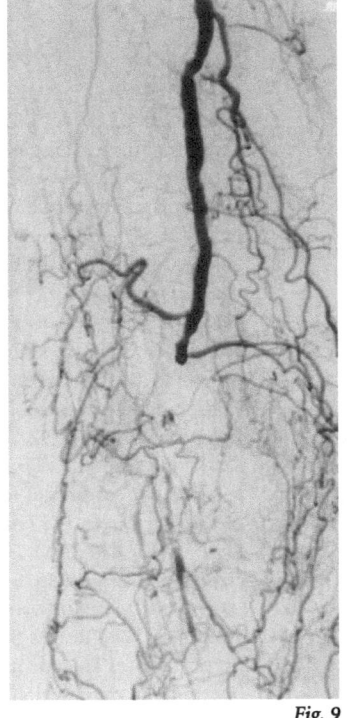

Fig. 9

Occlusion of the popliteal artery. Blood supply to the lower leg via the rete genu.

The success of efforts to stimulate the natural reserves of the body, such as stimulating the growth of the collateral vasculature (arteriogenesis) determines the course PAOD will take. Despite intensive research directed at improving collateralization after arterial occlusion, including the TRAFFIC study published in 2002 (one of the few randomized studies in humans directed towards clinical application of growth factors), the therapeutic implementation of arteriogenesis has fallen short of expectations.[10]

References

1. FISHER DF JR, FRY WJ. Collateral mesenteric circulation. *Surg Gynecol Obstet.* 1987 May; 164(5):487-92
2. GOLABEK R, SZYMCHEL J, RYGLEWICZ D, KRUSZEWSKA J. Collateral circulation via the arterial network of the neck in subclavian artery occlusion. *Neurol Neurochir Pol.* 1980;14(5):485-92.
3. KOSHI T, GOVIL S, KOSHI R. Problem in Diagnostic Imaging: Pancreaticoduodenal Arcade in Splanchnic Arterial Stenosis. *Clinical Anatomy* 11:206–208 (1998)
4. LIEBESKIND DS. Collateral circulation. *Stroke.* 2003 Sep;34(9):2279-84.
5. HIETALA SO, KUNZ R. Collateral circulation in stenosis or occlusion of the renal artery. *Cardiovasc Radiol.* 1979 Nov;2(4):249-55.
6. SPINDLER S, SCHMITT R, HELMBERGER T. Arterial collateral pathways in liver cirrhosis and celiac axis occlusion. *Radiologe.* 1991 Jul;31(7):344-7.
7. BOENDER AC, PERLBERGER RR. An attempt to classify the collateral systems in total occlusions at different levels of the lumbar aorta and pelvic arteries: causes and consequences. *Radiol Clin* (Basel). 1977;46(5):348-63.
8. MACCHI C, GIANNELLI F, CECCHI F, CORCOS L, REPICE F, CANTINI C, BRIZZI E. Collateral circulation in occlusion of lower limbs arteries: an anatomical study and statistical research in 35 old subjects. *Ital J Anat Embryol.* 1996 Apr-Jun;101(2):89-96.
9. BROOKS DH, BRON KM. Postprandial rest pain and claudication of the lower extremity: A case report. *Surgery.* 1975 Nov;78(5):677-81.
10. LEDERMAN RJ, MENDELSOHN FO, ANDERSON RD, SAUCEDO JF, TENAGLIA AN, HERMILLER JB, HILLEGASS WB, ROCHA-SINGH K, MOON TE, WHITEHOUSE MJ, ANNEX BH; TRAFFIC INVESTIGATORS. Therapeutic angiogenesis with recombinant fibroblast growth factor-2 for intermittent claudication (the TRAFFIC study): a randomised trial. *Lancet.* 2002 Jun 15;359(9323):2053-8.

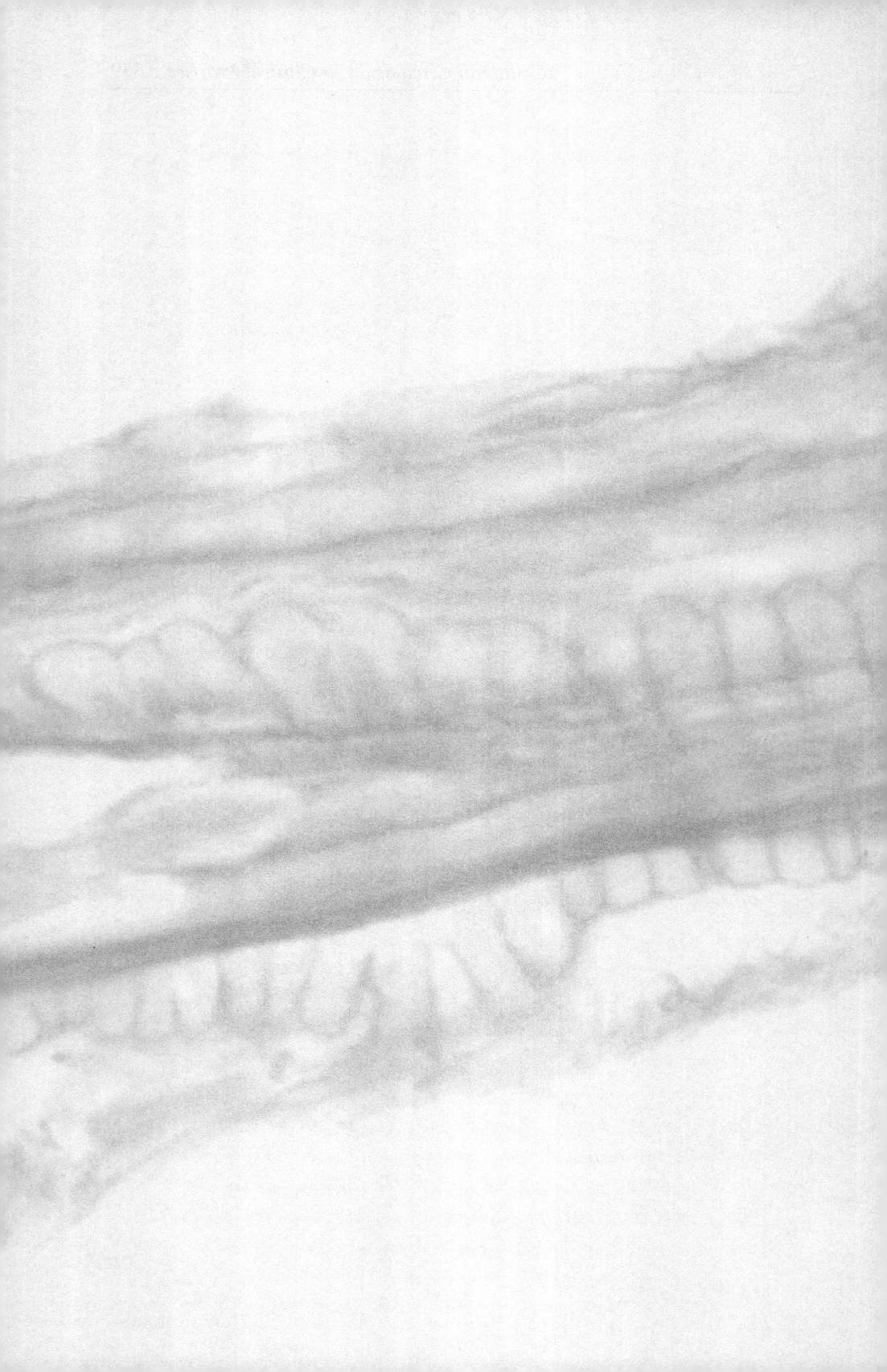

Chapter 19

Arteriogenesis and Atherosclerosis: Strange Bedfellows

Niels van Royen and Wolfgang Schaper

Arteriogenesis, the escape hatch in cases of atherosclerotic occlusions, shares surprisingly many features with the processes leading to occlusion, i.e. atherosclerosis. These are tortuosity, activation of the endothelium, upregulation of adhesion molecules, invasion of monocytes, expression of MCP-1, activation of matrix-metalloproteinases, digestion of elastin, smooth muscle cell (SMC) proliferation, and intima formation. Even outward remodeling, the most striking aspect of collateral artery growth, also occurs in the early stages of atherosclerotic plaque formation. It provides for a constant size of the internal diameter of the artery for a relatively long time. The difference is that the substrate for the atherogenic process is large arteries whereas in arteriogenesis it is small arterioles, which are virtually immune against atherosclerosis except in patients with diabetic microangiopathy. Another common denominator is the damage that is inflicted in both cases: in large arteries this is dysfunctional endothelium and lipid overload and in case of collateral vessels it is endothelium, which is activated by the sudden, marked and long lasting increase in fluid shear stress. In both structures the limited repertoire of arterial defense, which at first consists in monocyte attraction and invasion as a start of the remodeling process, is initiated. Small arterioles, consisting of only one layer of endothelium and one to three layers of smooth muscle, are easily remodeled at first. Later, when the collateral arteriole has attained more SMCs by proliferation, the re-arrangement and migration of the new cells is more difficult, and enlarged collaterals in some aspects resemble atherosclerotic lesions. Large arteries are much too thick to be remodeled by monocytes: After being cut off from their stem cell factor, they will die soon and release their lipid burden, and the damage is increased by the inflammation. Thus, their penetration is limited. In view of the similarities of these processes, difficulties with regard to growth factor therapy for the stimulation of arteriogenesis can be imagined. It can be envisaged that this may constitute a double-edged sword: pro-arteriogenic factors may also be pro-atherogenic. This is particularly significant because most of the classical growth factors are also pro-thrombotic. This aspect will be discussed in detail below.

MCP-1

MCP-1 is a strong and well-documented pro-arteriogenic factor. The efficacy of this compound in stimulating the development of the collateral circulation has been shown in small as well as in large animal species[1-3]. However, MCP-1 has also been associated with atherosclerosis and is expressed in plaque tissue[4]. Moreover, increased levels of circulating MCP-1 are associated with increased rates of myocardial infarction and with acute coronary syndromes[5], suggesting a role of this cytokine in plaque progression and rupture.

More significant evidence for a role of MCP-1 in atherogenesis was provided by two studies showing that a deficiency in either MCP-1 or its receptor CCR2 leads to diminished plaque formation in mice[6,7]. On the other hand, we could show that the receptor knockout almost completely prevents the recovery of blood flow after femoral artery occlusion because collateral artery growth is severely inhibited. Additionally, it was shown that overexpression of MCP-1 next to the vessel wall leads to increased macrophage infiltration and neointima formation[8]. Finally, in irradiated ApoE-deficient mice that were repopulated with bone marrow cells from MCP-1 transgenic mice, the localized overexpression of MCP-1 by macrophages resulted in aggravation of atherosclerosis[9]. These studies show that disruption of the MCP-1/CCR-2 interaction can prevent progression of atherosclerosis and that local MCP-1 expression leads to local aggravation of atherosclerosis. This does not necessarily implicate that pro-arteriogenic therapeutic strategies using local MCP-1 protein infusion bear the risk of invoking atherosclerosis at a coronary or aortic level. To specifically address this question we have conducted a study in both, Watanabe rabbits as well as ApoE [-/-] mice. Two questions were posed for the study: 1st: Is MCP-1 still effective under hyperlipidemic conditions, and 2nd: Does local intra-arterial application of MCP-1 aggravate atherogenesis?

In a first approach, hyperlipidemic Watanabe rabbits were treated with MCP-1 protein[10]. Total treatment period was one week, with a dosage of either 1 or 3.3 µg/kg/week. The protein was infused locally into the proximal stump of the occluded femoral artery. In this manner, substances are delivered directly into the collateral circulation. After 1 week, adenosine-induced hyperemic hind limb flow was measured by means of fluorescent microspheres that were infused into the abdominal aorta. If measured under conditions of maximal vasodilatation, conductance directly reflects the degree of development of the collateral vessels. We could show that 3.3 µg/kg/week of MCP-1 were effective in stimulating the development of the collateral circulation upon femoral artery ligation, whereas 1 µg/kg/week had no effect. The latter dose was used in previous studies in normal New Zealand White (NZW) rabbits of the same age where it produced a pro-arteriogenic effect. It could thus be concluded that MCP-1 efficacy is preserved under conditions of hyperlipidemia, although the dose-response curve is shifted to the right. Furthermore, we aimed at assessing pro-atherogenic effects of local MCP-1 protein infusion. In a follow-up study of 6 months, we did not detect changes of the aortic plaque surface. However, the issue of induction of atherosclerosis was not satisfactorily addressed in this model because the large spread of data on atherosclerotic plaque surface might have caused a type II analytic error.

Therefore, a second study was conducted in ApoE [-/-] mice[11] that were treated with either MCP-1 or PBS after ligation of the femoral artery. Compounds were delivered directly into the collateral circulation of the hind limb via a catheter inserted into the proximal part of the occluded femoral artery. Animals at the age of eight weeks were used to determine the pro-arteriogenic effects as well as the effects on early stages of atherosclerosis, whereas mice aged 6 months served to determine the effects of MCP-1 on terminal stages.

Similar to our results in Watanabe rabbits, we found that collateral conductance was increased in mice treated with MCP-1 (10 µg/kg/week). The finding that the effects of a short-term therapy (one week) were detectable up to two months after initiation of the experiment, was of additional interest. It showed that not only arteriogenesis can be accelerated but that perfusion can be improved by MCP-1 treatment in the long run, as well. The increase in collateral conductance in treated mice was accompanied by increased accumulation of monocytes around proliferating arteries providing further evidence for the mediating role of these cells during arteriogenesis and the feasibility of interfering with this mechanism via MCP-1.

Local MCP-1 treatment also induced activation of circulating monocytes as reflected by increased expression of MAC-1. In young mice, MCP-1 treatment led to an increased intima/media ratio and monocyte adhesion in the aorta. In older mice, an increase in plaque surface was found in a two-month follow up. Furthermore, MCP-1 treatment modulated cellular composition of plaques, resulting in a decrease of smooth muscle cell content. The significance of these experiments for possible treatment of patients is difficult to judge. Our experiments in mammals larger than the mouse have shown that systemic infusion of very high doses of MCP-1 does not stimulate arteriogenesis, most probably because the cytokine is rapidly bound to the membrane of erythrocytes and inactivated via Duffy receptors. For this reason, the acute and subchronic toxicity of MCP-1 is low. Only locally produced MCP-1 or close infusion does produce an effect. Cardiac myocyte-specific overexpression of MCP-1 in transgenic fertile mice leads to chronic low-grade myocarditis but not to atherosclerotic coronary heart disease, as we could show[12]. The increase of lesion size in ApoE mice after continuous infusion of MCP-1 is probably caused by overwhelming Duffy receptor capacity. Furthermore, the ApoE[-/-] model does not reflect all aspects of human thrombogenic atherosclerosis.

GM-CSF

GM-CSF has as well been described to induce arteriogenesis both in experimental[13] as well as clinical settings[14]. The role of GM-CSF during atherogenesis is not yet fully understood. A pro-atherogenic role of GM-CSF has been advocated. GM-CSF was found to be increasingly expressed in human atherosclerotic plaque tissue, located to macrophages, smooth muscle cells and endothelial cells [15]. It has been shown that oxidized low-density lipoproteins strongly induce GM-CSF expression in endothelial cells [16]. GM-CSF is also expressed in plaque-macrophages [17] and monocyte adhesion to endothelial cells results in high levels of GM-CSF mRNA and protein expression [18].

However, in patients treated with GM-CSF for aplastic anemia it has been observed that total cholesterol levels decrease by about one third during the time of therapy [19]. Similar effects were found in hyperlipidemic rabbits [20]. In a group of patients with coronary artery disease, GM-CSF treatment led to a reduction in both total cholesterol as well as HDL-cholesterol, though leaving the ratio of HDL to total cholesterol unchanged [14].

The clearest evidence of interaction between GM-CSF and plaque development was provided in a study showing that long-term treatment with GM-CSF in Watanabe rabbits significantly slowed down plaque progression. It should be noted, however, that plaque progression was accompanied by a decrease in smooth muscle and collagen content and an increase in macrophage content of plaques potentially leading to plaque instability [21]. Such plaque-destabilizing effects were also attributed to GM-CSF in a study showing that myeloperoxidase expression of macrophages is related to GM-CSF expression [22]. These findings on plaque-destabilizing effects of GM-CSF are in strong contrast to conclusions of another study, which suggests that endogenous GM-CSF induces collagen VIII and contributes to plaque stability [23].

Altogether, experimental evidence that exogenously applied GM-CSF partially inhibits plaque progression exists. Exogenously applied GM-CSF additionally modulates serum lipids, although in patients with coronary artery disease both total cholesterol as well as HDL levels decrease without their ratio being affected. The potential plaque-destabilizing role of endogenously produced GM-CSF in atherosclerotic plaques therefore remains uncertain.

TGF-ß$_1$

TGF-ß$_1$ is expressed during natural arteriogenesis and intra-arterial infusion of TGF-ß$_1$ increases the arteriogenic response upon femoral artery ligation in rabbits[24]. The mechanism of induction of collateral artery growth can probably in part be attributed to direct influence of TGF-ß$_1$ on monocytes/macrophages[25]. Interestingly, it has recently been shown that TGF-ß$_1$ also produces a direct effect on the vascular wall of collateral arteries by inducing the expression of cardiac ankyrin repeat protein (carp)[26]. Carp is expressed during natural arteriogenesis and might serve as an upstream regulator of the immediate early gene Egr-1[26]. Egr-1 in turn is a transcriptional regulator of numerous pro-arteriogenic growth factors like PDGF-B, TGF-ß$_1$ and FGF-2[27] but also of ICAM-1, an adhesion molecule that is involved in monocyte adhesion during arteriogenesis[28].

Furthermore, TGF-ß$_1$ is expressed in atherosclerotic plaque tissue in humans, and it has been suggested that it contributes to progression of atherosclerosis via induction of proteoglycan biosynthesis and subsequent lipoprotein retention in the vessel wall[29]. However, other investigators have advocated a plaque-suppressing role of TGF-ß$_1$ by inhibition of inflammation and cell turnover[30]. Grainger et al. showed that serum concentrations of active TGF-ß$_1$ are severely reduced in advanced atherosclerosis. Patients with triple vessel disease showed a marked decrease of the active form of TGF-ß$_1$ to levels less than 25 % compared to patients with chest pain but showing normal coronary angiograms, who showed increased levels of total, active and inactive, TGF-ß$_1$ levels. These data suggest that the active form of TGF-ß$_1$ exerts anti-atherogenic effects, although total concentrations might be increased in atherosclerotic lesions[31].

In addition, experimental evidence is mounting that TGF-ß$_1$ exerts a stabilizing effect on atherosclerotic plaques. Direct gene-transfer of TGF-ß$_1$ to the porcine vessel wall leads to extracellular matrix production[32]. Treatment of ApoE$^{-/-}$ mice with neutralizing antibodies recognizing TGF-ß$_1$, TGF-ß$_2$ and TGF-ß$_3$ interfered with plaque composition, resulting in a more vulnerable phenotype of plaques. These data were confirmed by a later study, in which TGF-ß$_1$ signaling was blocked by the use of soluble TGF-ß$_1$ receptor II, which also resulted in an increase of inflammatory cells and lipids within the plaque, whereas the content of collagens decreased[33].

Conclusion

Progression of atherosclerosis leads to slow or sudden arterial obstruction. Collateral arteries constitute a natural escape mechanism from the devastating effects of progressive atherosclerotic disease. In a large cohort of patients the natural development of the collateral circulation does, however, not preclude the occurrence of clinical symptoms of exercise-induced angina or claudication, and stimulation of arteriogenesis would be of clinical benefit. As every other medical intervention this does bear the potential risk of side-effects and this chapter focused on the interaction of vascular growth and atherosclerosis. Therapies aiming at the induction of vascular growth can be divided into pro-angiogenic and pro-arteriogenic strategies. The induction of angiogenesis might lead to direct induction of atherosclerosis, since angiogenesis is an integral part of atherosclerosis. Indeed, anti-angiogenic compounds inhibit plaque progression, whereas pro-angiogenic compounds like VEGF induce plaque progression. Pro-arteriogenic strategies do not necessarily promote atherosclerosis but it should be noted that depending on the compound chosen, pro-atherogenic effects need to be excluded in pre-clinical studies since the aggravation of atherosclerotic disease would prohibit clinical application of such strategies.

References

1. ITO WD, ARRAS M, WINKLER B, SCHOLZ D, SCHAPER J, SCHAPER W. Monocyte chemotactic protein-1 increases collateral and peripheral conductance after femoral artery occlusion. *Circ Research.* 1997;80:829-37.
2. HOEFER IE, VAN ROYEN N, BUSCHMANN IR, PIEK JJ, SCHAPER W. Time course of arteriogenesis following femoral artery occlusion in the rabbit. *Cardiovasc Res.* 2001;49:609-17.
3. VOSKUIL M, VAN ROYEN N, HOEFER IE, SEIDLER R, GUTH BD, BODE C, SCHAPER W, PIEK JJ, BUSCHMANN IR. Modulation of collateral artery growth in a porcine hind limb ligation model using MCP-1. *Am J Physiol Heart Circ Physiol.* 2003;284:H1422-8.
4. TAKEYA M, YOSHIMURA T, LEONARD EJ, TAKAHASHI K. Detection of monocyte chemoattractant protein-1 in human atherosclerotic lesions by an anti-monocyte chemoattractant protein-1 monoclonal antibody. *Hum Pathol.* 1993;24:534-9.
5. DE LEMOS JA, MORROW DA, SABATINE MS, MURPHY SA, GIBSON CM, ANTMAN EM, MCCABE CH, CANNON CP, BRAUNWALD E. Association between plasma levels of monocyte chemoattractant protein-1 and long-term clinical outcomes in patients with acute coronary syndromes. *Circulation.* 2003;107:690-5.

6. Gu L, Okada Y, Clinton SK, Gerard C, Sukhova GK, Libby P, Rollins BJ. Absence of monocyte chemoattractant protein-1 reduces atherosclerosis in low density lipoprotein receptor-deficient mice. *Mol Cell.* 1998;2:275-81.

7. Boring L, Gosling J, Cleary M, Charo IF. Decreased lesion formation in CCR2$^{-/-}$ mice reveals a role for chemokines in the initiation of atherosclerosis. *Nature.* 1998;394:894-7.

8. Namiki M, Kawashima S, Yamashita T, Ozaki M, Hirase T, Ishida T, Inoue N, Hirata K, Matsukawa A, Morishita R, Kaneda Y, Yokoyama M. Local overexpression of monocyte chemoattractant protein-1 at vessel wall induces infiltration of macrophages and formation of atherosclerotic lesion: synergism with hypercholesterolemia. *Arterioscler Thromb Vasc Biol.* 2002;22:115-20.

9. Aiello RJ, Bourassa PA, Lindsey S, Weng W, Natoli E, Rollins BJ, Milos PM. Monocyte chemoattractant protein-1 accelerates atherosclerosis in apolipoprotein E-deficient mice. *Arterioscler Thromb Vasc Biol.* 1999;19:1518-25.

10. van Royen N, Hoefer I, Buschmann I, Kostin S, Voskuil M, Bode C, Schaper W, Piek JJ. Effects of local MCP-1 protein therapy on the development of the collateral circulation and atherosclerosis in Watanabe hyperlipidemic rabbits. *Cardiovasc Res.* 2003;57:178-85.

11. van Royen N, Hoefer I, Bottinger M, Hua J, Grundmann S, Voskuil M, Bode C, Schaper W, Buschmann I, Piek JJ. Local monocyte chemoattractant protein-1 therapy increases collateral artery formation in apolipoprotein E-deficient mice but induces systemic monocytic CD11b expression, neointimal formation, and plaque progression. *Circ Res.* 2003;92:218-25.

12. Martire A, Fernández B, Buehler A, Strohm C, Schaper J, Zimmermann R, Kolattukudy PE, Schaper W. Cardiac overexpression of monocyte chemoattractant protein-1 in transgenic mice mimics ischemic preconditioning through SAPK/JNK1/2 activation. *Cardiovasc Res.* 2003;57:523-534.

13. Buschmann IR, Hoefer IE, van Royen N, Katzer E, Braun-Dulleaus R, Heil M, Kostin S, Bode C, Schaper W. GM-CSF: a strong arteriogenic factor acting by amplification of monocyte function. *Atherosclerosis.* 2001;159:343-56.

14. Seiler C, Pohl T, Wustmann K, Hutter D, Nicolet P, Windecker S, Eberli FR, Meier B. Promotion of collateral growth by granulocyte-macrophage colony-stimulating factor in patients with coronary artery disease: a randomized, double-blind, placebo-controlled study. *Circulation.* 2001;104:2012-2017.

15. Plenz G, Koenig C, Severs NJ, Robenek H. Smooth muscle cells express granulocyte-macrophage colony-stimulating factor in the undiseased and atherosclerotic human coronary artery. *Arterioscler Thromb Vasc Biol.* 1997;17:2489-99.

16. Rajavashisth TB, Andalibi A, Territo MC, Berliner JA, Navab M, Fogelman AM, Lusis AJ. Induction of endothelial cell expression of granulocyte and macrophage colony-stimulating factors by modified low-density lipoproteins. *Nature.* 1990;344:254-7.

17. Wang J, Wang S, Lu Y, Weng Y, Gown AM. GM-CSF and M-CSF expression is associated with macrophage proliferation in progressing and regressing rabbit atheromatous lesions. *Exp Mol Pathol.* 1994;61:109-18.

18. Takahashi M, Kitagawa S, Masuyama JI, Ikeda U, Kasahara T, Takahashi YI, Furukawa Y, Kano S, Shimada K. Human monocyte-endothelial cell interaction induces synthesis of granulocyte-macrophage colony-stimulating factor. *Circulation.* 1996;93:1185-93.

19. Nimer SD, Champlin RE, Golde DW. Serum cholesterol-lowering activity of granulocyte-macrophage colony-stimulating factor. *JAMA.* 1988;260:3297-3300.

20. Ishibashi T, Yokoyama K, Shindo J, Hamazaki Y, Endo Y, Sato T, Takahashi S, Kawarabayasi Y, Shiomi M, Yamamoto T, et al. Potent cholesterol-lowering effect by human granulocyte-macrophage colony-stimulating factor in rabbits. Possible implications of enhancement of macrophage functions and an increase in mRNA for VLDL receptor. *Arterioscler Thromb.* 1994;14:1534-41.

21. Shindo J, Ishibashi T, Yokoyama K, Nakazato K, Ohwada T, Shiomi M, Maruyama Y. Granulocyte-macrophage colony-stimulating factor prevents the progression of atherosclerosis via changes in the cellular and extracellular composition of atherosclerotic lesions in watanabe heritable hyperlipidemic rabbits. *Circulation.* 1999;99:2150-6.

22. Sugiyama S, Okada Y, Sukhova GK, Virmani R, Heinecke JW, Libby P. Macrophage myeloperoxidase regulation by granulocyte macrophage colony-stimulating factor in human atherosclerosis and implications in acute coronary syndromes. *Am J Pathol.* 2001;158:879-91.

23. Plenz G, Reichenberg S, Koenig C, Rauterberg J, Deng MC, Baba HA, Robenek H. Granulocyte-macrophage colony-stimulating factor (GM-CSF) modulates the expression of type VIII collagen mRNA in vascular smooth muscle cells and both are codistributed during atherogenesis. *Arterioscler Thromb Vasc Biol.* 1999;19:1658-68.

24. van Royen N, Hoefer I, Buschmann I, Heil M, Kostin S, Deindl E, Vogel S, Korff T, Augustin H, Bode C, Piek JJ, Schaper W. Exogenous application of transforming growth factor beta 1 stimulates arteriogenesis in the peripheral circulation. *FASEB J.* 2002;16:432-434.

25. McCartney-Francis N, Mizel D, Wong H, Wahl L, Wahl S. TGF-beta regulates production of growth factors and TGF-beta by human peripheral blood monocytes. *Growth Factors.* 1990;4:27-35.

26. Boengler K, Pipp F, Fernández B, Ziegelhoeffer T, Schaper W, Deindl E. Arteriogenesis is associated with an induction of the cardiac ankyrin repeat protein (carp). *Cardiovasc Res.* 2003;59:573-81.

27. Khachigian LM, Collins T. Inducible expression of Egr-1-dependent genes. A paradigm of transcriptional activation in vascular endothelium. *Circ Res.* 1997;81:457-61.

28. Scholz D, Ito W, Fleming I, Deindl E, Sauer A, Wiesnet M, Busse R, Schaper J, Schaper W. Ultrastructure and molecular histology of rabbit hind limb collateral artery growth (arteriogenesis). *Virch Arch Intern J Pathol.* 2000;436:257-270.

29. Bobik A, Agrotis A, Kanellakis P, Dilley R, Krushinsky A, Smirnov V, Tararak E, Condron M, Kostolias G. Distinct patterns of transforming growth factor-beta isoform and receptor expression in human atherosclerotic lesions. Colocalization implicates TGF-beta in fibrofatty lesion development. *Circulation.* 1999;99:2883-91.

30. Ihling C, Technau K, Gross V, Schulte-Monting J, Zeiher AM, Schaefer HE. Concordant upregulation of type II-TGF-beta-receptor, the cyclin-dependent kinases inhibitor P27Kip1 and cyclin E in human atherosclerotic tissue: implications for lesion cellularity. *Atherosclerosis.* 1999;144:7-14.

31. Grainger DJ, Kemp PR, Metcalfe JC, Liu AC, Lawn RM, Williams NR, Grace AA, Schofield PM, Chauhan A. The serum concentration of active transforming growth factor-beta is severely depressed in advanced atherosclerosis. *Nat Med.* 1995;1:74-9.

32. Nabel EG, Shum L, Pompili VJ, Yang ZY, San H, Shu HB, Liptay S, Gold L, Gordon D, Derynck R. Direct transfer of transforming growth factor beta 1 gene into arteries stimulates fibrocellular hyperplasia. *Proc Natl Acadof Sci USA.* 1993;90:10759-63.

33. Lutgens E, Gijbels M, Smook M, Heeringa P, Gotwals P, Koteliansky VE, Daemen MJ. Transforming growth factor-beta mediates balance between inflammation and fibrosis during plaque progression. *Arterioscler Thromb Vasc Biol.* 2002;22:975-82.

Index

BASIC SCIENCE FOR THE CARDIOLOGIST

1. B. Swynghedauw (ed.): *Molecular Cardiology for the Cardiologist.* Second Edition. 1998   ISBN 0-7923-8323-0
2. B. Levy, A. Tedgui (eds.): *Biology of the Arterial Wall.* 1999
    ISBN 0-7923-8458-X
3. M.R. Sanders, J.B. Kostis (eds.): *Molecular Cardiology in Clinical Practice.* 1999   ISBN 0-7923-8602-7
4. B.Ostadal, F. Kolar (eds.): *Cardiac Ischemia: From Injury to Protection.* 1999
    ISBN 0-7923-8642-6
5. H. Schunkert, G.A.J. Riegger (eds.): *Apoptosis in Cardiac Biology.* 1999
    ISBN 0-7923-8648-5
6. A. Malliani, (ed.): *Principles of Cardiovascular Neural Regulation in Health and Disease.* 2000   ISBN 0-7923-7775-3
7. P. Benlian: *Genetics of Dyslipidemia.* 2001   ISBN 0-7923-7362-6
8. D. Young: *Role of Potassium in Preventive Cardiovascular Medicine.* 2001
    ISBN 0-7923-7376-6
9. E. Carmeliet, J. Vereecke: *Cardiac Cellular Electrophysiology.* 2002
    ISBN 0-7923-7544-0
10. C. Holubarsch: *Mechanics and Energetics of the Myocardium.* 2002
    ISBN 0-7923-7570-X
11. J.S. Ingwall: *ATP and the Heart.* 2002   ISBN 1-4020-7093-4
12. W.C. De Mello, M.J. Janse: *Heart Cell Coupling and Impuse Propagation in Health and Disease.* 2002   ISBN 1-4020-7182-5
13. P.P.-Dimitrow: *Coronary Flow Reserve – Measurement and Application: Focus on transthoracic Doppler echocardiography.* 2002   ISBN 1-4020-7213-9
14. G.A. Danieli: *Genetics and Genomics for the Cardiologist.* 2002
    ISBN 1-4020-7309-7
15. F.A. Schneider, I.R. Siska, J.A. Avram: *Clinical Physiology of the Venous System.* 2003.   ISBN 1-4020-7411-5
16. Can Ince: *Physiological Genomics of the Critically Ill Mouse.* 2004
    ISBN 1-4020-7641-X
17. Wolfgang Schaper, Jutta Schaper: *Arteriogenesis.* 2004
    ISBN 1-4020-8125-1
    eISBN 1-4020-8126-X

KLUWER ACADEMIC PUBLISHERS – DORDRECHT/BOSTON/LONDON